Human Reproductive Biology

Hing-Sing Yu

CRC Press

Boca Raton   Ann Arbor   London   Tokyo

QP251
.Y8
1994

Library of Congress Cataloging-in-Publication Data

Yu, Hing-Sing
   Human reproductive biology / by Hing-Sing Yu.
      p. cm.
   Includes bibliographical references and index.
   ISBN 0-8493-4439-5
   1. Human reproduction. I. Title.
   [DNLM: 1. Reproduction—physiology. 2. Reproduction—genetics.
  3. Sex Hormones. 4. Sex Behavior.   WQ 205 Y94h 1994]
   QP251.Y8   1994
   612.6—dc20
   DNLM/DLC
   for Library of Congress   93-43111
                                                     CIP

International Standard Book Number 0-8493-4439-5
Library of Congress Card Number 93-43111
Printed in the United States of America 1 2 3 4 5 6 7 8 9 0
Printed on acid-free paper

To my wife, Ming-Ying.

AUTHOR

Hing-Sing Yu is Director of the Biorhythm Research Laboratory in the Division of Mathematics, Computer Science, and Statistics at the University of Texas at San Antonio. He graduated from the University of Hong Kong with a B.Sc. (Hon.) in 1979. He received his M.Phil. and Ph.D. degrees in reproductive and developmental biology at the same university. In 1988, Dr. Yu came to the United States as Research Instructor in the Department of Ophthalmology at the University of Texas Health Science Center at San Antonio and later became Assistant Professor. In 1991, he joined the College of Science and Engineering at the University of Texas at San Antonio to teach statistics, applied mathematics, reproductive biology, and cytodifferentiation. Dr. Yu is a member of the American Association for the Advancement of Science, American Society for Cell Biology, Association for Research in Vision and Ophthalmology, International Society for Eye Research, Society for the Study of Endocrinology, Metabolism and Reproduction, Society for the Study of Reproduction and Fertility, and Tissue Culture Association. With Dr. Russel J. Reiter, he has recently edited a book entitled *Melatonin: Biosynthesis, Physiological Effects, and Clinical Applications*. His current research interests include cell culture and computational models in rhythmic biological processes such as melatonin rhythms and cell proliferation.

PREFACE

This book is based on a series of lectures given in a one-semester graduate course. I intended to cover most aspects of reproductive biology and to present current important issues at deeper levels. The only way to achieve both in one volume is to broaden the scope across the chapters and to emphasize selected topics of interests in each chapter. My goal is to arouse the interest of graduate students to pursue research in reproductive biology. At the end of the course, they should have sufficient knowledge to select a favorite project. Interested readers can continue to search for publications cited in each chapter. References are mostly recent reviews, selected original papers and historical publications. The book is also a good reference source for research scientists and medical professionals in areas related to reproductive biology.

Most readers may agree that it is almost impossible to discuss human reproduction without referring to animal models. A comparative approach on mammalian reproduction is sometimes necessary, including cellular mechanisms, hormonal regulation, and the effects of environmental factors. The use of the term "animal model" implies that humans are not animals. We would like to call nonhuman species "animals" and ourselves "humans." I agree. I therefore want to emphasize that if the findings are also valid in humans, I write "... in animals including humans" or "... in primates including humans." Also, the word "humans" refers to all individuals in *Homo sapiens sapiens* with any types of genetics, while "men" are male and "women" female humans.

Sex determination is considered the starting point of the reproductive continuum. The emergence of two morphologically distinct entities, the female and male, is the beginning of sexual reproduction. Reproductive biology is the study of how these two sexes interact to produce offspring successfully. When sex is defined properly, the process leads to sexual union. Fertilization occurs and embryonic development commences. The purpose of reproduction is achieved when the baby is born. I chose not to spend much time on the events after fertilization as these processes are classified under developmental biology. Instead, the behavioral aspect of reproduction is presented in two different chapters (see Chapters 7 and 12). Sexual behavior is an important aspect of the reproductive process during which the organism interacts with others and the environment. Human beings have learned to manipulate the environment and to control reproductive processes in themselves and other species. The pattern of human reproduction and sexuality is attributed to this behavior.

Recent advancement in the understanding of reproductive biology was brought about by experimental research in different related areas including psychological physiology and sociobiology. The first experimental approach to study reproduction was adopted by Berthold in 1849 when a factor from the testis was discovered in the blood. He removed the testis and observed the deficiency caused, followed by transplantation to restore the function. This is still the basic approach to study the role of an endocrine organ. Despite general public opposition to studies of sex organs, the cyclicity of vaginal smears in rats and the estrogenic activity in follicular fluid were reported in the early 1920s. In those years, the National Research Council considered sex research not appropriate for scientific study.

Modern biologists now realize that understanding the reproductive process is crucial not only to human existence but also to other species. Without proper knowledge, it is difficult to cope with problems such as overpopulation, the lack of food, and infertility. We must be grateful to those early, stubborn reproductive biologists who insisted on studying sex and reproduction scientifically. They would be happy to know that human reproductive biology is now a public concern. More people realize that ignorance in this area could ultimately cause the human race's extinction.

Among early reports by German investigators, the findings of Novak and Te Linde[1] on endometrial changes in women during the menstrual cycle were published in the *Journal of the American Medical Association* as early as 1924. All these early findings led to a surge of the interest in reproductive biology. The most important turning point was the publication of *Sex and Internal Secretions,* edited by Edgar Allen in 1932.[2] Its second edition was published in 1939.[3] It was a product of a group of distinguished biologists and biochemists who were willing to devote their time to reproductive biology.

Another milestone in reproductive biology was the isolation and identification of sex steroids. The first sex steroid identified was estrone (3-hydroxy-estra-1,3,5(10)-trien-17-one) which was crystallized from urine of pregnant women by Doisy et al. in 1929.[4] Estradiol-17β, (estra-1,3,5(10)-trien-3,17β-diol), with a chemical structure very similar to estrone, had long been shown to have effects comparable with estrone even *in vitro*.[5] Estrone and estradiol are commonly known as E_1 and E_2, respectively. Estrone is only about 10% of estradiol potency in enhancing the endometrial growth.

Progesterone is another steroid hormone acting on the endometrium in the latter half of the menstrual cycle after ovulation. An early experiment showing progesterone effects was reported by Hisaw et al. on monkeys in 1930.[6] By 1938, it was known that the effect of progesterone in promoting endometrial growth is potentiated by estrogen.[7,8] The understanding of sex steroids and their actions is central to reproductive biology. Recent developments in molecular biology allow the elucidation of steroid receptor mechanisms. With new research tools, our understanding of the reproductive process has increased exponentially.

This brief historical review is an appreciation of these pioneers who performed innovative research and published excellent reviews on reproductive biology. Together with many recent findings, they provide a rich source of information for the present volume. We are therefore indebted to these authors. Many publishers and other organizations have granted us the permission to reproduce or modify the illustrations of their publications. Special thanks should be given to them and specific statements about the sources have been made in the text.

I thank my teachers, Professor B. Lofts, Professor S.T.H. Chan, and Dr. S.F. Pang, who introduced me to the field of reproductive biology. Professors Lofts and Chan provided me a model for teaching reproductive biology in their excellent courses on this subject during my years at the University of Hong Kong. I am also grateful to Dr. R.J. Reiter, Professor of Neuroendocrinology at the University of Texas Health Science Center at San Antonio, for his profound impact on my research and teaching philosophy. I had invited him to give a lecture on "Environment and Reproduction" in my Reproductive Biology course. His lively teaching style, flavored by immense interests and enjoyment in his field made the students excited about pineal gland research.

I wish to acknowledge Dr. Matthew J. Wayner, the former Division Director of Life Sciences, who had recommended me to teach the course. I must also give credit to some of the graduate students, especially Veronica Guel-Gomez, Marilu Vazquez, Phong Nguyen, Darren Levy, and Steven Nowotny. Parts of their excellent reports and projects have been adopted in this book. I am also indebted to Mrs. Alice Adams, who incidentally clarified some misconceptions about Mormonism. Another key person who made this project possible is Mr. Paul Petralia of CRC Press, who enthusiastically guided the book proposal through the difficult review process. Paul and I are also indebted to the secretarial staff of CRC Press.

I would like to express my gratitude to Dr. Shair Ahmad, the Division Director, whose encouragement and support are extremely important throughout the writing process. I greatly appreciate the generous help provided by the administrative and secretarial staff of the division. I should also thank the artists who made the excellent drawings, and the Yates Foundation for using the computer facilities. Some studies in our laboratory were supported in part by grants from the Research to Prevent Blindness, Inc., the Semp Russ Foundation and the Norma Friedrich Ward Trust of the San Antonio Area Foundation.

Finally, the publisher and I welcome criticisms and comments, which will be extremely helpful for our next edition.

H.S. Yu
San Antonio, Texas

REFERENCES

1. **Novak, E. and Te Linde, R.W.,** Endometrium of menstruating uterus, *J. Am. Med. Assoc.,* 83, 900, 1924.
2. **Allen, E., Ed.,** *Sex and Internal Secretions, 1st ed.,* Williams and Wilkins, Baltimore, 1932.
3. **Allen, E., Danforth, C.H., and Doisy, E.A., Eds.,** *Sex and Internal Secretions, 2nd ed.,* Williams and Wilkins, Baltimore, 1939.
4. **Doisy, E.A., Veler, C.D., and Thayer, S.,** Folliculin from urine of pregnant women, *Am. J. Physiol.,* 90, 329, 1929.
5. **Villee, C.A.,** Effects of estrogens and antiestrogens *in vitro, Cancer Res.,* 17, 507, 1957.
6. **Hisaw, F.L., Meyer, R.K., and Fevold, H.L.,** Production of a premenstrual endometrium in castrated monkeys by ovarian hormones, *Proc. Soc. Exp. Biol. Med.,* 27, 400, 1930.
7. **Hisaw, F.L. and Greep, R.O.,** The inhibition of uterine bleeding with estradiol and progesterone and associated endometrial modifications, *Endocrinology,* 23, 1, 1938.
8. **Engle, E. and Smith, P.E.,** The endometrium of the monkey and estrone-progesterone balance, *Am. J. Anat.,* 63, 349, 1938.

TABLE OF CONTENTS

1 Sex and Its Determination

CHAPTER CONTENTS

I. INTRODUCTION

Most species reproduce sexually, including plants, vertebrates, invertebrates, and even protozoa. In its simplest definition, sexual reproduction is the union of genetic materials from two individuals of the same species in producing offspring. For example, two paramecia conjugate, a pair of hermaphroditic snails copulate, frogs perform external fertilization, and cross-pollination occurs in many plant taxa. Almost all vertebrates rely on sexual reproduction. Humans are exclusively sexual.

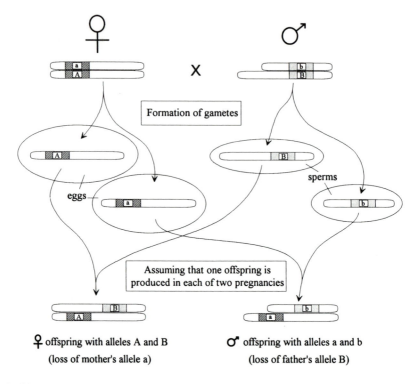

FIGURE 1.1.   Allele loss during sexual reproduction.

The obvious advantage of sexual reproduction is the increased diversity because of genetic exchange. A genetically diverse species has a higher chance of having individuals that can survive through devastating environmental changes. The benefits outweigh the disadvantages of gamete wastage and allele loss.[1] As shown in Figure 1.1, only half a set of the genetic material from each parent is inherited. Despite the allele loss, the offspring is genetically different from the parents. The increased genetic variability provides a greater adaptability of the species against the pressure of natural selection.

A.   DEFINITIONS OF SEX

In the broadest sense, the word "sex" refers to all matters directly or indirectly related to the reproductive process. For a reproductive process to be sexual, it must involve the union of two individuals having appropriate sets of reproductive structures and behavior. Under the pressure of natural selection, abnormal structures and deviant behavior leading to unsuccessful reproduction are unlikely to persist. Although the word "sexuality" is often used to describe human reproductive behavior, "animal sexuality" should be a valid term for all animal behavior associated with sexual reproduction. This is especially true if our experimental inferences are mostly based on animal models.

Psychologists interpret sex in the context of sexual behavior. They may define sex as a motive force bringing two individuals into intimate contact.[2] Geneticists may use the word "sex" to describe chromosomes. Embryologists would like to group neonatal mice according to sex, while sociobiologists refer to sex as gender. Both "sex" and "gender" are adopted to show the existence of females and males in the same species. In humans, these definitions are valid and appropriate. The terms "male" and "female," however, may not be well defined in some lower vertebrates showing sex reversal. In more primitive animals, sex may not be readily distinguishable.

B. SEX DETERMINATION

Sex determination can be interpreted in two different ways. First, by what criteria can we determine the sex of an organism? In normal humans, sex can readily be determined because we have distinct external genitalia. Very often, the outline of the body can lead to an impression about the sex of the individual, though we have no knowledge about the external genitalia. In general, some vertebrates do have intersex or hermaphroditic individuals that possess features of both sexes. This condition is, however, considered abnormal in humans. Under normal conditions, the sex of an organism with well-differentiated sexual apparatus can be determined.

Second, by what mechanisms is an organism determined or destined to develop or differentiate into a female or male? This is a more involved biological question. We are interested in the mechanism involved in storing the information of being a female or male and in passing this information to the next generation. The involvement of genes had long been known, but we are just beginning to understand part of the complex molecular mechanism adopted by this biological information management system for sex.

II. DIFFERENT LEVELS OF SEX DETERMINATION

Sex determination of an organism by an observer based on examination of its external genitalia is only one of the criteria. This method usually correlates with genetic identification of the sex in normal humans. In the human society, we have more complex ways to determine the sex of an individual, though the two main criteria are still genetic constitution and external genitalia. Based on these two basic criteria, there are different levels of determination that can also accommodate variants. All these different levels, however, are interrelated and change dynamically with the development of the organism. As shown in Figure 1.2, there are three basic processes interacting with one another: evolution of sex, genetic expression, and education. The education component is particularly important in humans.

A. LEGAL OR SOCIAL SEX

There is a legal determination of the sex of an individual. Under normal circumstances, this correlates with the genetic sex of the individual. Although it is possible to change the legal sex of an individual, for example, after transsexual operation, the determination is very often controversial. Legal sex determination

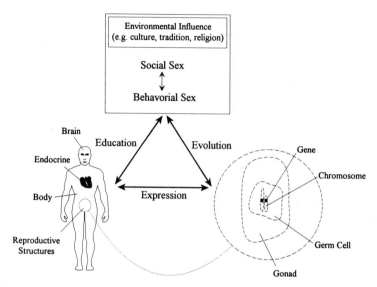

FIGURE 1.2.   Basic processes in the evolution of sex determination.

has become an issue of human rights.[3] Despite one's true biological sex, an individual should have the right to proclaim oneself as the opposite sex. In this case, the issue depends on the consensus among members of a society to establish laws or ethical standards for administrative purposes to maintain harmony. Legal sex is virtually a formalized social sex derived from such a consensus.

Based on the tradition in different cultures, there are defined ways to determine the sex of an individual. Behavior, clothing, and other social roles are criteria adopted by others in the society to determine the sex. This type of social sex determination creates a social pressure for individuals with well-defined biological sex to conform. In a group of male pseudohermaphrodites from the Simbari Anga linguistic group in the Eastern Highlands of Papua New Guinea, their rudimentary external genitalia start to develop at puberty. These infants were originally thought to be females at birth. Now, these individuals are treated socially as boys in infancy, but are still viewed differently from normal males with the understanding that they are destined to assume the male role as adults.[4] In many cultures, parents do impose social sex determination on their children to a certain extent.

B.   BEHAVIORAL SEX

The behavior of an individual is the most important component in social sex determination. Despite clothing and social roles, behavior is the strongest indication of one's sex without physical examination. There are obviously some traditional or cultural criteria for classifying female or male behavior. At best, these are based on the observed behavior of most females and males in the population. No matter how unreliable these criteria are, their use is common practice across different cultures. This is, however, based on the sociological approach of behavioral sex determination of an individual by an observer.

Biologically, behavioral sex can be determined based on the sexual differentiation of the brain, because behavior is governed by the brain. This is known as gender differences in behavior. Maternal behavior is a good example of gender differences. It is a statistical comparison; most females are feminine and most males are masculine. Since behavior can be acquired, behavioral sex should not be considered as a biological constraint that, if it exists, depends on the sexually differentiated brain. A well-defined gender difference in sex behavior is, however, an important factor for reproduction. This subject will be discussed in Chapter 7.

C. BRAIN SEX

If behavioral sex is excluded, brain sex can be defined as sex determination based on gender differences in brain anatomy and activity. Recent studies have shown anatomical differences between female and male brains in humans and laboratory animals.[5] Among these are the hypothalamus, thalamus, corpus callosum, anterior commissure, and Onuf's nucleus.[5,6] It should be noted that anatomical differences in the brain may not be the cause of gender differences in behavior; the latter may instead be the cause of the structural differences. This "cause or effect" problem is still debatable.

In addition, the sex of an unknown brain cannot confidently be identified by locating these anatomical differences. Although examination of the skull or brain may allow gender identification in forensic science, genetic analysis is more reliable. In a recent study on 120 human samples of blood, saliva and semen stains, hair roots, and bone and skin fragments obtained from 30 males and 16 females, Southern blot analysis on the DNA with probe cY97 allowed a more accurate sex determination.[7]

D. BODY SEX

Unlike brain sex, body sex can readily be determined by physical examination of external body structures. The presence of female or male external genitalia is the most convincing indication of body sex. However, secondary sex characteristics (e.g., body figure, developed mammary glands, facial features, and body hairs) contribute to body sex determination. Therefore, body sex determination is only down to the level of external features without considering the internal structures.

E. PHENOTYPIC SEX

According to previous definitions, phenotypic sex is determined on the basis of both external and internal structures discernible by others. A male is characterized by the presence of the testis and the absence of the ovary. A female is characterized by the presence of the ovary but not the testis. A hermaphrodite has both the testis and ovary. These definitions are very restricted to the type of organisms with testis and/or ovary.[8]

Phenotypic sex can be generalized as the sex determined by sex-specific phenotypes that include gross structures discernible by naked eyes or submicroscopic molecules expressed only in one sex. As generally defined, phenotypes are observable features following gene expression. During Mendel's time, phenotypes were almost synonymous to external features, while genotypes were "invisible" genes inside. With advanced technology today, one may describe the phenotype of a mitochondrion that is governed by its genotype. It is also possible to describe the phenotype of a gene segment on a chromosome.

At present, we cannot exclude the possibility of sex-specific phenotypes at submicroscopic levels. It appears necessary to define rigorously what phenotypic sex is in terms of our contemporary knowledge: phenotypic sex is the sex of an individual determined by one's observable characteristics. With this definition, it becomes a collective term for all levels of sex determination except social, behavioral, and genetic sex (see Figure 1.2). For example, brain sex and body sex are subsets of phenotypic sex. Therefore, one must be specific about the phenotype selected when phenotypic sex is discussed.

F.   ENDOCRINE SEX

This is also called hormonal sex. The presence of a testis or ovary implies a subtle difference in internal secretions both during sexual differentiation and in the adult stage. In normal individuals, testosterone level is low in females and high in males. Estrogen and progesterone levels are also characteristic in females. In addition, a sexually differentiated brain also contributes to the endocrine differences. The whole set of unique internal secretions is the basis for defining endocrine sex.

Apparently, discrepancy between endocrine sex and body sex may arise when a hormonal imbalance occurs as a result of disease or drug intake. Gonadal dysfunction and steroid medication can alter plasma steroid levels in both sexes. Reference values in men and women are available for routine clinical measurement tests.[9] For example, testosterone ranges from 6.9 to 34.7 nmol/l in men and only from 0.7 to 2.8 nmol/l in women. Progesterone and estradiol in men are <0.3 to 1.3 nmol/l and <37 to 210 pmol/l, respectively. Similar levels are found in women during the follicular phase of their menstrual cycle. During the luteal phase, these two steroids vary within the range of 19 to 45 nmol/l and 699 to 1250 pmol/l, respectively. Estradiol can be as high as 2830 pmol/l at the time of ovulation. Sex steroids are associated with sex determination only during fetal life. In adults, a change in the endocrine sex will not lead to body sex reversal. Sexual development and steroids will be discussed in Chapter 2.

Because of our recent understanding of the interactions between the endocrine and nervous systems, the role of the neuroendocrine system should also be considered in the discussion of endocrine sex. Since the pituitary gland is intimately involved in the internal secretions directly or indirectly related to sexually specific reproductive functions, endocrine sex includes the interplay between neural hormones and steroids (see Chapter 3).

G.   GONADAL SEX

In addition to the differences in their endocrine functions, there are structural differences between the ovary and testis. Tissue preparations or cross sections of either an ovary or testis can readily be distinguished histologically. Amazingly, their structures are quite consistent across different vertebrate groups (see Chapters 5 and 6).

The ovary consists of primary follicles developing into mature follicles. Oocytes are released during ovulation, after which the follicles become corpus lutea responsible for preparing the uterus for pregnancy. In the testis, sperms are produced continuously from spermatogonia at the periphery of the seminiferous tubule and are passed through the lumen. All these processes require specialized structures that make the ovary and testis unique to each other.

H. GERM CELL SEX

In normally developed gonads, germ cells are also sexually differentiated. Follicles carrying oocytes are found in the ovary, while all developmental stages of spermatogonia to sperms are found in the testis. Surprisingly, the presence of germ cells in the gonad does not determine gonadal sex. For example, in mutant mice carrying homozygous atrichosis genes with deficiency in germ cells, the somatic cells in the gonad can organize into a testis devoid of germ cells.[10] In normal developing chicks and rats, drug-induced loss or surgical removal of germ cells does not inhibit gonadal development.[11,12]

In a recent study on sex reversal in mouse fetal ovaries,[13] female somatic cells transplanted into ovarian bursa in ovariectomized nude mice without germ cells formed testis cords and differentiated into Sertoli cells. These cells in the transplant did not differentiate into other testis components or ovarian tissues. If aggregates of both female and male somatic cells are transplanted, they differentiate into well-developed testes containing Leydig cells and tunica albuginea as well as Sertoli cells. In contrast, aggregates of both female germ cells and female somatic cells develop into ovaries but not testicular tissues. These results suggest that testicular differentiation is independent of germ cells, but ovarian development involves the interaction between female germ cells and somatic cells. The subsequent steps in testis development require the contributions of some male somatic cells.

I. CHROMOSOMAL SEX

This is determined on the basis of chromosomal constitution of the individual. With some exceptions, the sex chromosomes can be distinguished by their unequal size. The phenomenon is known as heterochromatic. Since chromosomal structures can now be easily observed, heterochromatism is based on structural differences. Chromosomal sex is thus a type of phenotypic sex instead of a conceptual sex difference in genetics. Therefore, chromosomal sex is strictly at the level of chromosomal structures without considering the genes inside.

In humans and other mammals, the male is heterogametic (XY) and the female is homogametic (XX). In birds and some other vertebrates, the male is homogametic (ZZ) and the female is heterogametic (ZW). Both cases are found in reptiles, amphibians, and teleosts. Examples include *Rana pipiens* (frog) and *Drosophila melanogaster* (fruit fly) with XX and XY, while *Xenopus laevis* (toad) and *Gallus domesticus* (chicken) have ZW and ZZ. There are abnormal cases such as infertile XO females with Turner's syndrome in humans. Similar XO female mice are, however, fertile.

The infertility of XO humans is explained by the absence of a process called dosage compensation in germ cells. Since a female has X chromosomes, she has a double dose of X-linked genes as compared to males with XY. With the dosage compensation device, one of the two X chromosomes is inactivated. X activation is discernible at a cellular level; the inactivated X appears as small and densely packed chromatin materials called Barr body. In humans, if one of the X chromosomes is defective, it is preferentially inactivated only in somatic cells. Although the individual still survives, she is infertile.

J.   GENETIC SEX

Although chromosomal sex is regarded by some authors to be equivalent to genetic sex, a distinction between the two needs to be clarified. Chromosomal sex is a determination method based on the presence of sex chromosomes, while genetic sex is based on the presence of a sex-determining gene. This is necessary because an individual carrying a Y chromosome without the sex-determining gene is still not a genetic male.

The sex-determining gene has been located within the interval 1A on the short arm of the Y chromosome. It is called the testis-determining factor (TDF) gene in humans and is also known as the testis-determining region of the Y chromosome (Tdy) in mice. One of the candidates for the TDF is a region called the zinc finger on Y (ZFY). The ZFY is later suspected to play a role in growth regulation only. A new region of 35 kb distal to ZFY has been identified in recent studies. It is termed as the sex-determining region on Y (SRY) and is likely to be the true TDF.[14] Figure 1.3 shows the location of the TDF gene on the Y chromosome. Using the single-strand conformation polymorphism assay and subsequent DNA sequencing, mutations were found in the SRY gene of sex-reversed XY human females.[15] In later studies on another family,[16] all XY individuals had a single basepair substitution, resulting in a conservative amino acid change in the conserved domain of the SRY open reading frame. Three of these individuals are XY sex-reversed females, and two are XY males.

Fetal expression of SRY is limited to the initial period of testicular differentiation. This expression is confined to gonadal tissues and does not require the presence of germ cells in males.[15] Ovarian differentiation requires the presence of both X chromosomes as well as normal female germ cells.[13] Genes controlling ovarian differentiation are suspected to be present on both arms of X chromosomes. Ovary-determining genes and autosomal genes have been proposed to be necessary for normal gonadal differentiation.[17] Ovary-determining genes have to be inactivated in developing testis.

According to the current concept,[18] mammalian sex determination is mediated via the lineage of somatic cells in the fetal gonad. During initial gonadal development, the fate of the supporting cell population is determined by the TDF gene expression. If this gene fails to express at an appropriate temporal sequence in a

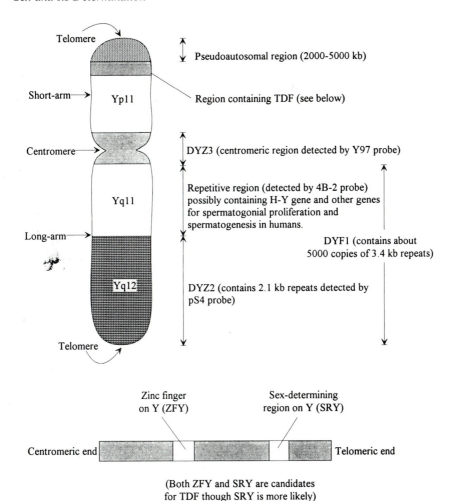

FIGURE 1.3. Proposed location of the TDF gene on the Y chromosome.

sufficient number of supporting cells, both XX and XY supporting cells differentiate as prefollicle cells and develop along the female direction. If there are sufficient supporting cells with the TDF gene expressed in a timely manner, they will differentiate into pre-Sertoli cells, followed by the formation of testis cords and the development of the gonad in a male direction. If XX supporting cells are also present, a few may be recruited into the pre-Sertoli population and participate in testis cord formation. The subsequent fate of prefollicle cells depends critically on interaction with the germ cell population in the developing gonad. If germ cells are absent, the gonad may be partially masculinized and/or the supporting cell component may become degenerated. The presence of an appropriate population of germ cells is thus crucial in completing the process of gonad sex determination.

In a recent review by Mittwoch,[19] it was concluded that male sex determination was not driven only by a single TDF gene. There are multiple Y-chromosomal genes associated with a single X chromosome in a fertile male. The genes involved in testis differentiation may act as growth regulator genes in the tissues where they are expressed. Recent studies have shown that the SRY protein binds to linear duplex DNA containing a specific target sequence AACAAAG that is structurally unique with a sharp bend.[20] The ability to recognize a kink in DNA has important regulatory functions such as DNA repair, folding of DNA segments for transcription, and other tissue-specific gene expression switches.

The ultimate sex determination is genetic sex, which governs all types of phenotypic sex. The expression of phenotypic sex, however, depends on how and when these sex-specific processes at all levels respond to environmental impacts (see Figure 1.2). The body sex of an individual is determined by the sex of the gonad that creates an appropriate endocrine environment for sexual differentiation of reproductive structures and the brain. Phenotypic sex can be considered to include gonadal sex and body sex. Brain sex, which is beyond phenotypic sex, governs behavioral sex and eventually, through the evolutionary process, contributes to the development of social sex. It is reasonable that legal sex should be based on the consideration of all these levels of sex determination.

III. GAMETOGENESIS

In a normal individual with properly determined sex and well-differentiated gonads, gametogenesis is a repetitive process occurring in the gonad throughout the reproductive life span. Gametogenesis is defined as the formation of gametes from primordial germ cells (PGCs) which differentiates into oocytes through oogenesis or into spermatozoa through spermatogenesis. The origin of these PGCs is extragonadal in fetal gonads (see Chapter 2). The fate of a PGC of undergoing oogenesis or spermatogenesis is determined, at least in the mouse, by whether it enters meiotic prophase before birth. This depends not on its chromosomal sex, but on its gonadal sex. A germ cell in or near normal testis cords developed from Sertoli cells is inhibited from entering meiosis until after birth; one that escapes this inhibition will develop into an oocyte, even if it is in a male animal and is itself XY in chromosome constitution.[21]

A. OOGENESIS

In the developing ovary, PGCs differentiate into oogonia and form primordial follicles. The oogonia enter a slow process of meiosis and reach the dictyate stage of prophase in the first meiotic division shortly after birth. An oocyte remains developmentally arrested until ovulation. It completes its first meiotic division just before ovulation and reaches metaphase II after ovulation; this transition is called meiotic maturation with the production of the first polar body. The ovulated egg becomes arrested again at metaphase II until fertilization. Upon the entry of the sperm, the process of oogenesis is said to end when the prolonged meiosis is completed with the emission of the second polar body. The whole sequence is summarized in Figure 1.4 and discussed in detail below.

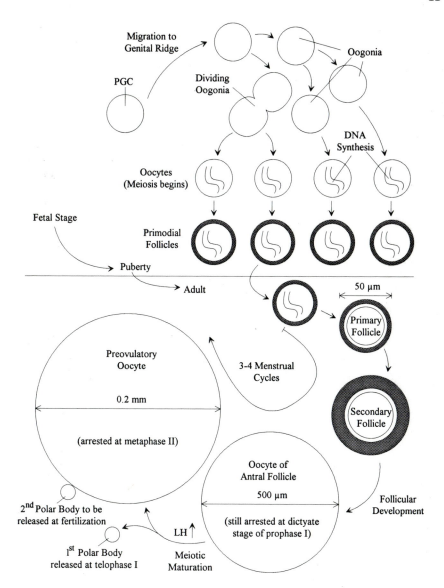

FIGURE 1.4. Oogenesis.

1. Formation of Primordial Follicles

The migration of PGCs from extragonadal sites to the genital ridge is completed on day 13 in the mouse or weeks 5 to 7 in human embryos. The ovary in a female fetus is differentiated by that time, and almost all PGCs differentiate into oogonia in the sex cords. Oogonia have a high mitotic rate so that intercellular bridges are often seen. At this time, a few oogonia proceed to meiosis in response to a factor from the rete ovarii. Oogonia are said to become oocytes when DNA synthesis occurs during the preleptotene stage shortly before the leptotene stage of the first meiotic division.[22]

A primordial follicle is formed when an oocyte is surrounded by a layer of granulosa cells. By week 20 of gestation in humans, there are over 6 million primordial follicles. In each of these follicles, the oocyte progresses through different stages of prophase in a prolonged fashion. In the mouse fetal ovary, it takes nearly 4 days to reach the pachytene stage, and almost all oocytes enter the dictyate stage late, just prior to parturition. Many follicles undergo a degenerative process called atresia, leading to the formation of atretic follicles. Therefore, the number of functional primordial follicles reduces to less than 1 million at puberty.

2.   Follicular Development

When a normal human female reaches puberty, the menstrual cycle starts to operate with an average period of 28 days (see Chapter 4). Primordial follicles are found lining the germinal epithelium of the ovary and are ready to continue their development. One of these primordial follicles takes about three to four menstrual cycles to develop into a matured follicle ready for ovulation. With an initial diameter of 50 μm, a few primordial follicles at a time start to expand as their granulosa cells become mitotic. Primary follicles are formed when the oocyte is surrounded by an acellular layer called the zona pellucida, secreted by both the oocyte and granulosa cells.[23]

With a rapid increase in the number of granulosa cells, the follicle continues to develop and becomes a secondary follicle. When the outermost layer of granulosa cells differentiates into theca cells, fluid starts to accumulate between layers of the granulosa cells, leading to the formation of a fluid-filled cavity called the antrum. At this stage, it is called an antral follicle with a diameter of 500 μm.

The oocyte volume is also increased tremendously with the follicular growth, showing an increase in metabolic activity and marked ultrastructural changes in the oocyte. In the oocyte nucleus, also known as germinal vesicle, there are one large and two small nucleoli, which also enlarge because of increased ribosomal RNA synthesis. The number of mitochondria is also increased up to 10^5 per oocyte.

In addition, the Golgi complex in the oocyte changes dramatically, indicative of increased activity. It participates in the synthesis of the protein component for the zona pellucida. Some small spherical lysosomal structures known as cortical granules are found in the cortical region of the oocyte. They are also thought to be produced by the Golgi complex and are important for the fertilization process.

All these processes contribute to the continual expansion of the antral follicle to a giant follicle with a diameter of 0.2 mm. The fully developed oocyte is surrounded by the corona radiata, and the whole structure is suspended in the large antrum on a stalk called the oophorus. Both of these new structures are derived from granulosa cells. At this stage, a matured follicle is large enough to be observed by examining the ovary from the outside. It is named the Graafian follicle, after the Dutch physician DeGraaf, who first described it in 1672.

3.   Meiotic Maturation

The final stage of follicular development before ovulation is the conversion of the oocyte in the Graafian follicle to the unfertilized egg. After the preovulatory surge of follicle-stimulating hormone (FSH) and luteinizing hormone (LH), the oocyte proceeds from the dictyate stage of meiosis I to metaphase II. This can also happen *in vitro* without hormonal stimulation.[24] This conversion is mandatory for subsequent ovulation and fertilization.

The first step of this conversion is the germinal vesicle breakdown, which is the dissolution of the nuclear membrane, and the progression to metaphase I. Under *in vitro* conditions, it takes a mean time of 11 min for the nuclear envelope of a mouse oocyte to disintegrate.[25] At the same time, there are chromosome condensation and spindle formation, which require an average time of 6 to 9 h. The second step is the progress from metaphase I to metaphase II, during which the first polar body is released. In the mouse, the oocyte takes about 30 min to go through anaphase I and telophase I.

The first polar body can be recognized by late anaphase I and is totally separated by late telophase I. Unlike the typical meiosis, the division is unequal, so that the polar body is much smaller than the oocyte. As a daughter cell of meiosis, the first polar body contains a half set of the chromosomes, mitochondria, ribosomes, and cortical granules. Since these chromosomes degenerate by late telophase I as the first polar body is eventually discarded, there is a 50% loss of genetic materials.

The oocyte is ovulated as soon as it becomes arrested at metaphase II. It remains at this stage in the oviduct and is now called an unfertilized egg. Figure 1.5 shows a mouse oocyte with a mass of granulosa cells surrounding it. Because

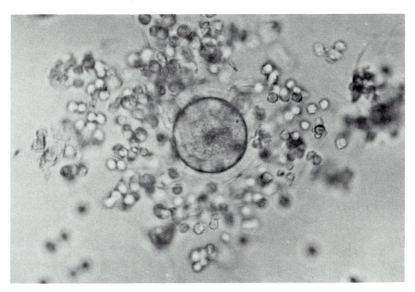

FIGURE 1.5.   Mouse oocyte with cumulus oophorus.

of its shape, this cell mass is known as cumulus oophorus, or simply cumulus. In humans and some species such as sheep and cattle, another layer of these cells, corona radiata, can be found between the cumulus and the zona pellucida. In other species, such as hamsters, the corona radiata is indistinguishable from the cumulus.

The oocyte is the only useful product after a successful oogonial meiosis. The appearance of this product also marks the end of oogenesis. The unfertilized egg is the female gamete well prepared for fertilization. It is furnished with macromolecules and organelles for fertilization, as well as RNA and protein reserves for the early development of the preimplantation zygote.

B.   SPERMATOGENESIS

In contrast to oogenesis, the whole process of spermatogenesis occurs in the seminiferous tubule of an adult testis. In the developing testis, PGCs differentiate into stem cells known as spermatogonia for the production of spermatozoa (or called sperms in short). Spermatogonia are highly mitotic so that a continuous supply of these cells is guaranteed throughout the reproductive life span of a normal male. Spermatogenesis begins when a spermatogonium enters meiosis to produce four haploid daughter cells called spermatids. These spermatids differentiate into mature sperms through spermiogenesis. X and Y chromosomes are duplicated and segregated equally among the four haploid daughter cells. The sex ratio of the offspring is 1:1 if sperms carrying X or Y are equally likely to fertilize an egg. Apart from sampling errors and statistical variations, this type of Mendelian segregation seems true and faithful.[26,27]

Figure 1.6 summaries the sequence of events in spermatogenesis involving the following cell types (see also Chapter 6). The two major processes are the reduction division of spermatogonia and the differentiation of spermatids.[28]

1.   Meiosis

As with the transition of oogonia to oocytes, spermatogonia are said to become spermatocytes when they enter the preleptotene stage shortly before meiosis. With the condensation of chromatin materials, DNA synthesis occurs during this period. There are two types of spermatocytes: those before the first meiotic division are primary and those after are secondary. According to meiotic events, primary spermatocytes are equivalent to oocytes before the emission of the first polar body, while the secondary spermatocytes correspond to unfertilized eggs.

Both secondary spermatocytes and unfertilized eggs have a haploid number of chromosomes but diploid DNA content. While unfertilized eggs remain arrested at metaphase II, secondary spermatocytes continue to complete the meiosis and become spermatids. In contrast to the increase in the oocyte volume, there is a steady decrease in size from spermatogonia to spermatids, though one spermatogonium produces four spermatids. As spermatocytes, spermatids are still spherical and appear undifferentiated before entering spermiogenesis.

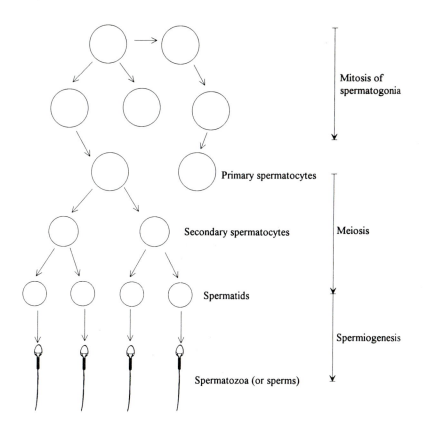

Primary spermatocytes

Secondary spermatocytes

Spermatids

Spermatozoa (or sperms)

Mitosis of spermatogonia

Meiosis

Spermiogenesis

FIGURE 1.6. Spermatogenesis.

2. Spermiogenesis

This is a complex process leading to the formation of a highly differentiated sperm. In a typical human sperm (see Figure 1.7), the head is mainly the nucleus capped by the acrosome. The tail consists of three portions: the middle, principal, and tail pieces. The middle piece contains an array of densely packed mitochondria. The transformation is obviously a drastic process of differentiation from a spherical spermatid to an elongated motile entity.

The acrosome has long been known to develop from the Golgi complex[29] and has been confirmed in mice[30] and humans[31] by electron microscopy. Proacrosomal granules derived from the Golgi complex fuse to form a single cap-like structure covering over half of the nuclear surface. At the same time, the nucleus moves from the central position to the periphery, where the acrosome first contacts the plasma membrane of the differentiating spermatid. As the cytoplasm rearranges itself to form the middle piece, the greater nuclear membrane comes into close contact with the plasma membrane.

The nucleus decreases in volume due to chromatin condensation and the loss of materials through the nuclear pores. There are redundant folds of the nuclear

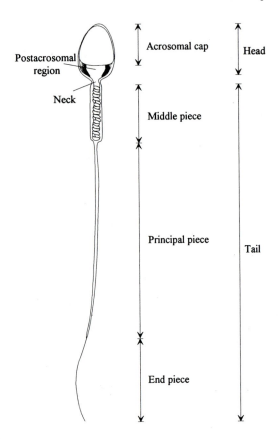

FIGURE 1.7. Whole sperm.

membrane, especially conspicuous at the tip, the abacrosomal pole of the nucleus. The degree of chromatin condensation and rearrangement varies greatly among species so that there are different shapes of the sperm head. The human sperm is symmetrical and rounded.

The origin of the sperm tail was studied by German scientists in the last century. The view that it develops from the centrioles was substantiated by investigators early in this century.[32] The centriolar complex consists of proximal (or transverse) and distal (or longitudinal) centrioles. The complex moves to the pole opposite to the acrosome, which is the caudal end. The axial filament develops from the distal centriole and elongates. The axial filament is a typical flagellum with the 9 + 2 arrangement of microtubules (see Figure 1.8). The complex eventually stops at the posterior pole where the middle piece is formed.[28]

The middle piece consists of the connecting piece and principal piece. The connecting piece is attached to the basal plate of the head and is modified to contain the proximal and distal centrioles. The proximal centriole forms the centriolar adjunct from its distal end. Later, the mitochondrial sheath is formed from rearranging the cytoplasm. It forms 5 to 14 spirals in the human sperm with

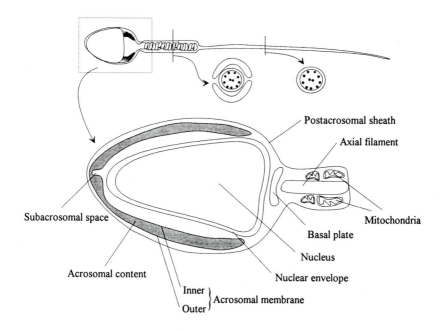

FIGURE 1.8. Sperm head.

a collection of microtubules, while the mitochondria inside come close to each other and form helical arrays. This part of the middle piece is called the principal piece, with a collection of microtubules extending from the annulus to the fibrous sheath. With the subsequent elongation of the axial filament and caudal migration of the annulus, the microtubules disappear with the formation of a complete tail.

All these developmental processes occur sequentially in close association with Sertoli cells. The Sertoli cell is a nongerminal component of the seminiferous epithelium originally reported by Italian physiologist Enrico Sertoli in 1865. The differentiating spermatids are embedded in a giant Sertoli cell; they are actually engulfed by cytoplasmic processes of the cell. Sertoli cells provide anchorage and a nutrient supply for the developing sperm. There are no cytoplasmic connections between the developing spermatids with these cells, though tight junctions are found among Sertoli cells. These junctions create a barrier dividing the epithelium into basal and adluminal compartments. The basal compartment contains spermatogonia and primary spermatocytes, while the adluminal compartment has secondary spermatocytes and differentiating spermatids. These junctions in the Sertoli cell also provide a blood-testis barrier so that the developing male gametes are protected from the general extracellular fluid.

Sertoli cells are also capable of orienting the forming sperms with their tails suspended in the lumen of the seminiferous tubule. Differentiated sperms are moved by cytoplasmic contractions of the Sertoli cell. With bulk remains of the spermatid cytoplasm in the cell, the mature sperms are released at the apex. Spermatogenesis is completed at this time. The whole developmental process from a spermatogonium to a mature sperm takes about 53 days in humans.

IV. FREEMARTIN AND H-Y ANTIGEN

In cattle, there is a case called freemartin syndrome described by Hunter in the 18th century.[33] It is an XX/XY twin in which vascular anastomosis occurs between the placentas. As a result of the "blood connection," some factors pass between the two fetuses. Interestingly, despite the genotypes, both XX and XY cells are found in the tissues of freemartins. The syndrome is characterized mainly by the presence of testicular tissues, the absence of oviducts and uterus, and an enlarged clitoris.

In 1955, a male-specific transplantation antigen in mice was identified. In the same strain of mice, females rejected skin grafts from males, while males did not reject skin grafts from females or males. This transplantation antigen was deduced to be present in the male only. In 1960, the antigen was proposed to be produced by a histocompatibility gene on the Y chromosome (H-Y gene; see Figure 1.3).[34] In 1976, Ohno et al.[35] reported the presence of the H-Y antigen in the ovotestes of the XX twin of freemartins with similar concentrations as in the XY twin's testis. Obviously, the H-Y antigen is secreted by the XY fetus and transferred to the XX fetus through the vascular anastomosis. The XX cells of the female apparently have H-Y receptors, causing the development of XY-like cells.

At that time, immunological assays were developed using antibodies raised against the H-Y antigen. The cross-reactivity of the antibodies with H-Y antigens from many species shows a phylogenetic conservation of the H-Y gene. It was also found that the presence of a testis was highly correlated with serological H-Y$^+$ results and that the H-Y gene was expressed in the male mouse embryo as early as the eight-cell stage of development. The notion that the H-Y gene product was a single molecular species responsible for triggering the indifferent gonad to differentiate into the testis became a widely accepted hypothesis. Current data, however, suggest that although H-Y is a male-specific factor and may play a role in male sex determination, it is not the primary inducer of testis differentiation.[36]

First, the transplantation H-Y antigen defined by graft rejection and by cytotoxic T-cell action appears to be different from the serological H-Y antigen which is characterized by antibodies. The gene for the transplantation H-Y is on the centromeric region of the human Y chromosome, while a regulatory gene for serological H-Y seems to be located in a distal region of the Y short arm. The serological H-Y has a 19-kDa protein that may be involved in gonadal differentiation of heterogametic vertebrates, while transplantation H-Y may be required for normal spermatogenesis.[37] In a recent review,[38] a more general role of serological H-Y as a growth regulator has been proposed.

Other findings against the "H-Y hypothesis" include the presence of H-Y antigens in female chickens, the change from H-Y$^-$ to H-Y$^+$ in ZZ male chickens induced by estradiol administration, and the detection of H-Y antigens in some 45,X women with gonadal dysgenesis. Recently, there were some minor histo-compatibility antigens found, and the genes encoding them were scattered throughout the genome, including the Y chromosome.[39] The TDF gene recently sequenced on the Y chromosome has been shown to be separate from the H-Y gene. Perhaps, H-Y antigens are involved in normal testicular development including spermatogenesis. The phenomenon may be an effect instead of a cause of sex determination.

V. THE SEX RATIO

Several efforts have been made to artificially change the primary sex ratio. Obviously, their success would have a significant impact on science, agriculture, ethics, culture, and social problems. So far, none has been successful in altering the sex ratio significantly. Most of the efforts are geared toward selection of X and Y sperms. It is known that some properties of X and Y sperms are different, e.g., mass and motility. Therefore, there are several methods tested.

1. Separation by gravity or centrifugation.
2. Exposure of semen to reduced atmospheric pressure.
3. Separation by electrophoresis based on different electrical charges on X and Y sperms.
4. In genetic selection, Y sperms are less motile in low pH. Therefore, special diets were tried to change blood pH, but were ineffective in changing the sex ratio.
5. Selective destruction of Y sperms is successful in mice, but the method requires artificial insemination and changes in the sex ratio are minimal.

Recent clinical and laboratory attempts to alter the sex ratio have been made using improved identification of Y-bearing sperm through chromosome evaluation rather than by F-body identification. Several tentative conclusions were made:[40]

1. The timing of intercourse in relation to ovulation and subsequent fertilization appears to influence the sex ratio. More females are conceived when coitus occurs close to ovulation, and more males are conceived when the sperm or egg is in the reproductive tract for a relatively longer time before conception. The influence of coital timing on the sex ratio is quite subtle overall and is not a practical method to alter the sex ratio for individual couples.
2. The use of ovulation-inducing medications slightly favors female offspring. A decrease in the sex ratio of 5 to 10% has been shown in multiple studies.
3. Artificial insemination with fresh donor or homologous spermatozoa results in more male births with a reported 7 to 10% increase in the sex ratio. It appears that ovulation induction combined with artificial insemination cancels the respective influences of each on the sex ratio.

4. Sperm separation techniques using albumin (for selection of Y-bearing sperm) or Sephadex column filtration (for selection of X-bearing sperm) are the only techniques that have been reported to alter the sex ratio to a degree that is clinically relevant. Although clinical birth data are just beginning to accumulate, these methods appear to have a 70 to 80% success rate for selection of assumed Y-bearing sperm. The validity of these results will remain questionable until fully detailed accounts are published and successfully repeated. Free-flow electrophoresis appears to achieve significant separation; however, the depressed postprocedure spermatozoa motility presently limits the usefulness of this procedure.

A recent report has shown that cryopreservation does not affect the frequencies of chromosomal abnormalities or alter the sex ratio in human sperm, provided that an adequate cryoprotective buffer and freezing system are employed.[41] There is a potential to combine clinical and laboratory methods to maximize the efficiency of sex selection for interested couples. Modern methods to identify ovulation (e.g., urinary LH kits and ultrasonography) may help the timing of coitus for sex selection. Clomiphene citrate may enhance female sex preselection when Sephadex column filtration is also employed.

Though it is not yet within our capacity to engineer the sex of a human fetus prior to conception, recent technological advances have enabled earlier and earlier detection of the sex of a fetus *in utero.* Where an embryo has been fertilized *in vitro,* detection of sex can be carried out much earlier still. These developments make it possible for couples to decide whether to continue with a pregnancy where a fetus is not of the preferred sex. To give couples such an option would raise difficult ethical issues. Careful considerations must be made before one is allowed to use expensive technology in the service of such private decision-making.[42]

VI.   EVOLUTION OF THE SEX CHROMOSOME

As stated in the beginning of this chapter, genes involved in sexual reproduction are being selected during evolution. These genes are mostly on the sex chromosomes. Logically, the ancestor of heterogametic animals must be hermaphroditic with no differences among individuals. The ancestral diploid sex chromosomes were perfectly homologous to each other. A mutation occurred and led to structurally distinct X and Y chromosomes that remain homologous to each other. Therefore, the evolution of sexual reproduction is the change from cosexuality to dioecy. Essentially, it is the evolution of the sex chromosome from homogametry to heterogametry.

Dimorphism of gametes is almost universal in eukaryotes. As reviewed earlier, some are male heterogametry (XY), while others are female heterogametry (ZW). If we consider only the case of male heterogametry (XY), the first mutant in the hermaphroditic ancestral population can be a female or male. Before understanding the evolution of the sex chromosome, we need to note some features of heterogametry:

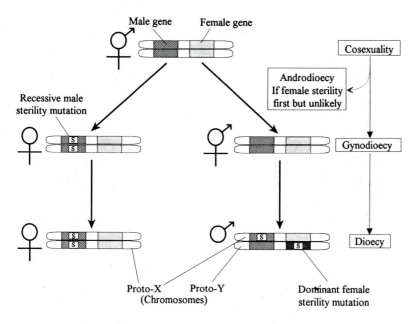

FIGURE 1.9. The evolution of sex chromosomes. (After Charlesworth, B., *Science*, 251, 1030, 1991.)

1. Since X and Y chromosomes in humans lack homology, no genetic exchange between them can be observed.
2. Highly repetitive DNA sequences are similar to transposable elements and satellite sequences. This is a condition known as heterochromatic.
3. Since there is a lack of functional loci on Y, adjustment of X activity is needed in the heterogametic sex; this is known as dosage compensation, e.g., mammals — inactivation of one X in females, and *Drosophila* — higher transcription rate on X in males.

According to Charlesworth,[43] there are at least two steps in the evolution from cosexuality to dioecy (Figure 1.9). Male sterility is suggested to happen first, followed by female sterility. For example, in plants, the access of male gametes to female gametes is restricted by self-fertilization. The primitive sex chromosomes are called proto-Y and proto-X. Mutant genes for female fertility and male sterility are on proto-X, while genes for male fertility and female sterility are on proto-Y. So the first step is a restriction of recombination between genes controlling male and female sex function. Both retain a sex-determining region and secondary sexual characteristics.

Based on an old theory, a chromosomal region that is maintained as permanently heterozygous without exchange will accumulate lethal recessive mutations. In the light of new theories based on Y degeneration and dosage compensation, this old theory is incorrect.[43] Increased X activity and decreased Y activity are found in cases showing dose compensation. The inactivation, however, does not affect genes involved in sexual expression. In addition, deleterious alleles happened to be present on Y so that individuals carrying the alleles were eliminated.

Moreover, repetitive DNA sequences on Y are transposable elements which are self-replicating and insertable into new sequence sites. Since Y activity is reduced, insertions and duplication are more tolerable. The lack of recombination provides less chance to generate deleterious segments. This hypothesis seems to explain the drastic difference in size between X and Y chromosomes.

REFERENCES

1. **Williams, G.C.,** *Sex and Evolution,* Princeton University Press, Princeton, NJ, 1975.
2. **Bancroft, J.,** *Human Sexuality and Its Problems,* Churchill Livingstone, New York, 1989.
3. **Taitz, J.,** The legal determination of the sexual identity of a post-operative transsexual seen as a human rights issue, *Med. Law,* 7(5), 467, 1989.
4. **Imperato-McGinley, J., Miller, M., Wilson, J.D., Peterson, R.E., Shackleton, C., and Gajdusek, D.C.,** A cluster of male pseudohermaphrodites with 5α-reductase deficiency in Papua New Guinea, *Clin. Endocrinol.,* 34, 293, 1991.
5. **Holden, C.,** The brain as "sexual organ" (news and comment), *Science,* 253, 957, 1991.
6. **Forger, N.G. and Breedlove, S.M.,** Sexual dimorphism in human and canine spinal cord: role of early androgen, *Proc. Natl. Acad. Sci. U.S.A.,* 84, 8026, 1986.
7. **Fattorini, P., Caccio, S., Gustincich, S., Wolfe, J., Altamura, B.M., and Graziosi, G.,** Sex determination and species exclusion in forensic samples with probe cY97, *Int. J. Legal Med.,* 104, 247, 1991.
8. **van Tienhoven, A.,** *Reproductive Physiology of Vertebrates,* 2nd ed., Cornell University Press, New York, 1983.
9. **O'Malley, B.W. and Strott, C.A.,** Steroid hormones: metabolism and mechanism of action, in *Reproductive Endocrinology: Physiology, Pathophysiology and Clinical Management,* 3rd ed., Yen, S.S.C. and Jaffe, R.B., Eds., W.B. Saunders, Philadelphia, 1991, 156.
10. **Handel, M.A. and Eppig, J.J.,** Sertoli cell differentiation in the testes of mice genetically deficient in germ cells, *Biol. Reprod.,* 20, 1031, 1979.
11. **McCarrey, J.R. and Abbott, U.K.,** Chick gonad differentiation following excision of primordial germ cells, *Dev. Biol.,* 66, 256, 1978.
12. **Merchant, H.,** Rat gonadal and ovarian organogenesis with and without germ cells. An ultrastructural study, *Dev. Biol.,* 44, 1, 1975.
13. **Hashimoto, N., Kubokawa, R., Yamazaki, K., Noguchi, M., and Kato, Y.,** Germ cell deficiency causes testis cord differentiation in reconstituted mouse fetal ovaries. *J. Exp Zool.,* 253, 61, 1990.
14. **Koopman, P., Munsterberg, A., Capel, B., Vivian, N., and Lovell-Badge, R.,** Expression of a candidate sex-determining gene during mouse testis differentiation, *Nature (London),* 348, 450, 1990.
15. **Berta, P., Hawkins, J.R., Sinclair, A.H., Taylor, A., Griffiths, B.L., Goodfellow, P.N., and Fellous, M.,** Genetic evidence equating SRY and the testis-determining factor, *Nature (London),* 348, 448, 1990.
16. **Vilain, E., McElreavey, K., Jaubert, F., Raymond, J.P., Richaud, F., and Fellous, M.,** Familial case with sequence variant in the testis-determining region associated with two sex phenotypes, *Am. J. Hum. Genet.,* 50, 1008, 1992.
17. **Eicher, E.M. and Washburn, L.L.,** Genetic control of primary sex determination in mice, *Annu. Rev. Genet.,* 20, 327, 1986.
18. **McLaren, A.,** Development of the mammalian gonad: the fate of the supporting cell lineage, *Bioessays,* 13, 151, 1991.

19. **Mittwoch, U.**, Sex determination and sex reversal: genotype, phenotype, dogma and semantics, *Hum. Genet.*, 89, 467, 1992.

20. **Ferrari, S., Harley, V.R., Pontiggia, A., Goodfellow, P.N., Lovell-Badge, R., and Bianchi, M.E.**, SRY, like HMG1, recognizes sharp angles in DNA, *EMBO J.*, 11, 4497, 1992.

21. **McLaren, A.**, Somatic and germ-cell sex in mammals, *Philos. Trans. R. Soc. London Ser. B*, 322, 3, 1988.

22. **George, F.W. and Wilson, J.D.**, Sex determination and differentiation, in *The Physiology of Reproduction*, Knobil, E. and Neill, J., Eds., Raven Press, New York, 1988, 3.

23. **Adashi, E.Y.**, The ovarian life cycle, in *Reproductive Endocrinology: Physiology, Pathophysiology and Clinical Management*, 3rd ed., Yen, S.S.C. and Jaffe, R.B., Eds., W.B. Saunders, Philadelphia, 1991, 181.

24. **Pincus, G. and Enzmann, E.**, The comparative behavior of mammalian eggs *in vivo* and *in vitro*. I. The activation of ovarian eggs, *J. Exp. Med.*, 62, 665, 1935.

25. **Sorensen, R.**, Cinemicrography of mouse oocyte maturation utilizing Normorski differential-interference microscopy, *Am. J. Anat.*, 136, 265, 1973.

26. **Werren, J.H. and Charnov, E.L.**, Facultative sex ratios and population dynamics, *Nature (London)*, 272, 349, 1978.

27. **Crow, J.F.**, Why is Mendelian segregation so exact?, *Bioessays*, 13, 305, 1991.

28. **de Kretser, D.M. and Kerr, J.B.**, The cytology of the testis, in *The Physiology of Reproduction*, Knobil, E. and Neill, J., Eds., Raven Press, New York, 1988, 837.

29. **Bowen, R.H.**, On the acrosome of the animal sperm, *Anat. Rec.*, 28, 1, 1924.

30. **Gardner, P.**, Fine structure of the seminiferous epithelium of the Swiss mouse. The spermatid, *Anat. Rec.*, 155, 235, 1966.

31. **Holstein, A.F.**, Ultrastructural observations on the differentiation of spermatids in man, *Andrologia*, 8, 157, 1976.

32. **Gatenby, J.B. and Beams, H.W.**, The cytoplasmic inclusions in the spermatogenesis of man, *Q. J. Microsc. Sci.*, 78, 1, 1936.

33. **Burns, R.K.**, Role of hormones in the differentiation of sex, in *Sex and Internal Secretions*, Young, W.C., Ed., Williams & Wilkins, Baltimore, 1961, 76.

34. **Billingham, F. and Silvers, W.K.**, Studies on tolerance of the Y chromosome antigen in mice, *J. Immunol.*, 85, 14, 1960.

35. **Ohno, S., Christian, L.C., Wachtel, S.S., and Koo, G.C.**, Hormone-like role of H-Y antigen in bovine freemartin gonad, *Nature (London)*, 261, 597, 1976.

36. **Goldberg, E.H.**, H-Y antigen and sex determination, *Philos. Trans. R. Soc. London Ser. B*, 322, 73, 1988.

37. **Muller, U. and Lattermann, U.**, H-Y antigens, testis differentiation, and spermatogenesis, *Exp. Clin. Immunogenet.*, 5, 176, 1988.

38. **Heslop, B.F., Bradley, M.P., and Baird, M.A.**, A proposed growth regulatory function for the serologically detectable sex-specific antigen H-Ys, *Hum. Genet.*, 81, 99, 1989.

39. **Simpson, E.**, Minor histocompatibility antigens, *Immunol. Lett.*, 29, 9, 1991.

40. **Zarutskie, P.W., Muller, C.H., Magone, M., and Soules, M.R.**, The clinical relevance of sex selection techniques [see comments], *Fertil. Steril.*, 52, 891, 1989.

41. **Martin, R.H., Chernos, J.E., and Rademaker, A.W.**, Effect of cryopreservation on the frequency of chromosomal abnormalities and sex ratio in human sperm, *Mol. Reprod. Dev.*, 30, 159, 1991.

42. **Young, R.**, The ethics of selecting for fetal sex, *Baillieres Clin. Obstet. Gynaecol.*, 5, 575, 1991.

43. **Charlesworth, B.**, The evolution of sex chromosomes, *Science*, 251, 1030, 1991.

2 Sexual Development

CHAPTER CONTENTS

I.   INTRODUCTION

The genetic sex of an organism is determined immediately after the union of female and male gametes. Thus, genetic sex determination is the first event that triggers sexual development. The developmental program is the gene expression of an organism's sexuality. The normal endpoint is the emergence of a fully fertile individual ready to initiate new reproductive process(es). The whole continuum can be divided into a series of sequential events: (1) genetic sex determination, (2) gonadal differentiation, (3) differentiation of secondary sex organs, (4) sexual differentiation of the brain, (5) prepubertal somatic growth, (6) puberty with the initiation of spermatogenesis and ovulation, and (7) sexual maturation involving the development of secondary sex characteristics and sexual behavior. Sexual development in humans takes more than 10 years from the time of conception to puberty. In contrast to other mammals, over 90% of the time is spent on postnatal sexual maturation. As in other vertebrates, however, the most critical event of human sexual development, gonadal differentiation, occurs during the embryonic stage.

II. GONADAL DIFFERENTIATION

In most vertebrates, the first observable process of gonadal differentiation is the migration of primordial germ cells (PGCs) or gonocytes from a certain location to the genital ridge where the gonad is formed. PGCs migrate by ameboid movement along the wall of hindgut and dorsal mesentery. They often pass through the vascular system to the genital ridges ventral to the fetal kidney. It is still uncertain why it is necessary to have such a long expedition. The process may serve as a way to select the best, active, correctly programmed PGCs to form the gonad for the next generation.

In humans, fetal gonadal development begins around 4 to 5 weeks of gestation. As shown in Figure 2.1, a bilateral pair of genital ridges is formed ventral to the mesonephric ridge, the developing fetal kidney. The genital ridges are thickenings of the coelomic epithelium suspended on either side of the dorsal mesentery in the hindgut area. The primitive gonad is "indifferent" at this stage. Outside the gonad, the genital ducts are also undifferentiated. The Müllerian and Wolffian ducts are the future oviduct in the female and vas deferens in the male, respectively.

A. THE INDIFFERENT GONAD

Within 1 to 2 weeks, the genital ridge develops into the primitive gonad. In almost all vertebrates studied, the undifferentiated gonad is identical histologically in both sexes, despite the committed genetic sex. Differences in the sex chromatin of the indifferent gonad are the apparent exception. The primitive gonad is divided into cortical and medullary regions, the sex of which will become clear within several days of development.

It is almost universal that vertebrate gonadal differentiation starts only after the appearance of PGCs in the genital ridge. PGCs originate extragonadally in an area close to the endoderm of yolk sac. PGCs are first recognizable in very young human embryos near the caudal end of the primitive streak. They appear in the hindgut entoderm of embryos only a few millimeters in length. In humans, this occurs between 5 and 7 weeks, during which the primitive gonad

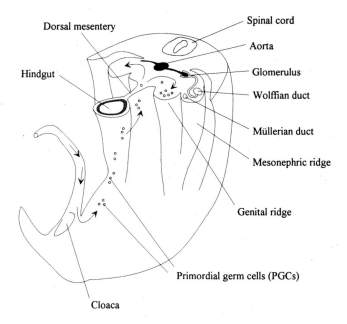

Dorsal mesentery

Hindgut

Spinal cord

Aorta

Glomerulus

Wolffian duct

Müllerian duct

Mesonephric ridge

Genital ridge

Primordial germ cells (PGCs)

Cloaca

FIGURE 2.1.   Migration of PGCs.

is formed at the genital ridge. PGCs move through the tissues and reach the genital ridges mostly because of their ameboid movement. They can destroy cells and membranes that block their way. There are several suggested theories for explaining the precisely controlled mechanism directing these cells. There are three types of mechanisms: ameboid movement, contact guidance, and differential adhesion.

PGCs can be stained histochemically for alkaline phosphatase activity in brown color. When the cells are still associated with the hindgut epithelium, they show pronounced morphological changes and can migrate actively. These cells are elongated with an irregular outline and have pseudopodia stretching out. After entering the genital ridge, they begin to lose their pseudopodia. It is still uncertain if such a loss of motility is due to the confined environment created by the surrounding cells or whether they are programmed to do so.

Contact guidance is a passive mechanism through which PGCs are transported to their destination. The route is predetermined by endodermal and mesodermal tissues. PGCs can also phagocytize materials along their paths. In differential adhesion, PGCs move by dynamically changing their adhesive contacts with the tissues along their paths. So far, we still do not have convincing experimental data showing this.

At present, the ameboid movement theory is the most plausible one with supporting experimental evidence. Microfilaments important for the contractile property of the PGC are present in the cytoplasmic processes. There is both light and electron microscopic evidence showing the attachment of the cells to the substratum at various points. This propels the whole cell forward. Another line of strong evidence is from cell culture studies. PGCs are actively migratory even *in vitro* and for at least several days. Chemotaxis may occur in all three mechanism cases. A substance is postulated to be responsible for attracting the PGCs. This is thought to be the control of timing and route.

During the migration, PGCs continue to proliferate. As shown in mice, the number increases from 50 to 5000 PGCs by the time they reach the genital ridge. They still continue dividing after settling down, but then they become mitotically arrested. DNA synthesis by the germ cells can still be detected in mouse embryos by days 12 to 14 but not afterwards. They resume mitosis 3 to 4 days after birth. The regulatory mechanism of these mitotic events is uncertain.

Studies on avian embryos indicate that the gonad primordium is the source of a soluble and diffusible agent that attracts the PGCs. Similar chemotactic mechanisms may operate in mammalian embryos. Those PGCs that are unable to differentiate into somatic elements and fail to reach the gonadal primordia degenerate and disappear.

After reaching the gonadal blastema, PGCs lose many of their characteristic features and are difficult to distinguish from nongerminal elements. Surprisingly, some PGCs die without achieving their anticipated differentiation. Other PGCs, with the incorporation of cells originally in the genital ridges, form discernible structures.

A sufficient number of active PGCs is necessary for the primitive genital ridges to initiate a proper gonad differentiation. They have to arrive at the correct position within an optimal time window to allow the gonads to develop. An unexpected event occurring during the process, such as environmental insults or genetic defects, would result in gonadal maldevelopment.

The most striking features are cortical and medullary regions that can easily be identified in the primitive gonad. Depending on the genetic sex determination factors, the cortex will develop into an ovary, while the medulla regresses. In a male fetus, the medulla will develop into a testis, while the cortex regresses.

B.   TESTIS

In an XY human fetus, the medulla of the primitive gonad develops, while the cortex regresses after the arrival of PGCs. From 7 to 8 weeks, primitive sex cords are formed and will become Sertoli cells of the testicular tubules. Between adjacent medullary cords, proliferating cells will become gonadal stromal cells or interstitial Leydig cells. Around the ninth week, the interstitial cells begin to secrete testosterone, dehydroepiandrosterone, and Müllerian-inhibiting substance (MIS).[1] Testosterone and its derivatives are grouped as androgens, which stimulate the differentiation of the Wolffian duct into seminiferous tubules, epididymis, and accessory glands. Under the influence of MIS, the Müllerian duct regresses.[2]

Testosterone synthesis and secretion are initially induced by human chorionic gonadotrophin (hCG) from the placenta. In the middle of the second trimester, testosterone production by the fetal testis is regulated by fetal LH and FSH, which are maximally produced around this time. The fetal testis is fully developed at this time. It is essentially a package of convoluted seminiferous tubules where sperms are produced. The tubules converge to form the rete testis before reaching the epididymis. As the gonadal differentiation is completed, fetal LH and FSH begin to fall to low levels at birth.

C. OVARIES

In an XX human fetus, the cortex of the primitive gonad develops, while the medulla regresses. In contrast to the male fetal testis, androgens and MIS are absent and the Müllerian duct also starts to differentiate. After the arrival of the female germ cells, epithelial cells at the border of the cortex proliferate and migrate toward the PGCs. Primordial follicles are formed with a single epithelial cell layer surrounding the PGCs. These epithelial cells later develop into granulosa cells. Early during the second trimester, primordial follicles are discernible. The theca cells also start to develop, forming a cell layer surrounding the granulosa cells but separated by a basal lamina.

The number of primordial follicles can be up to 7 million by the middle of the second trimester. Some of them, however, undergo a degenerative process called atresia, forming atretic follicles. The number decreases to 1 or 2 million at birth and about 0.3 to 0.4 million at puberty, though only 300 to 400 oocytes will be ovulated during the fertile period of a normal woman. The rest of the primordial follicles never develop or become atretic follicles. In contrast to the male, all primordial follicles are formed before birth instead of being produced on demand. Nevertheless, the oocytes in the primordial follicles are not fully differentiated. Their development is arrested at the prophase of the first meiotic division and will resume shortly before ovulation.

D. GENITAL DUCTS

Around the time of PGC migration, both the Müllerian and Wolffian ducts are well formed (Figure 2.2). In parallel with gonad differentiation, these genital ducts develop according to the genetic sex. If the gonad is a testis, the Wolffian duct becomes the epididymis, vas deferens, seminal vesicles, prostate glands, and urethra. In a recent study on the mouse, both testosterone and dihydrotestosterone can induce Wolffian development in urogenital ridges *in vitro*. The induction can be mimicked by coculturing with fetal testes.[3] If the gonad is an ovary or absent, the Müllerian duct develops to form the oviducts, uterus, cervix, and upper vagina. In the absence of testosterone stimulation, the Wolffian duct regresses. This passiveness of Müllerian development led to the suggestion that the female is a neutral sex, which is the default destiny of sexual development.

In the male fetus, the Müllerian duct regresses in response to MIS produced by the Sertoli cells in the fetal testis. MIS has been characterized as a 140-kDa glycoprotein, and its genes have been cloned in cattle and humans.[1,2] For a long time, it has been known that large doses of androgens, which are responsible for Wolffian development, cannot induce Müllerian atrophy.[4] In transgenic mice carrying a DNA sequence of human MIS, chronic expression of the gene leads to

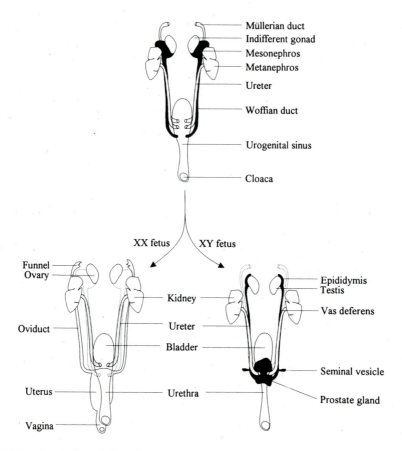

FIGURE 2.2.   Differentiation of gonads and genital ducts.

the inhibition of Müllerian duct differentiation.[5] The ovaries of these neonatal females have an abnormally low number of germ cells with the blind vagina and without uterus or oviduct. Interestingly, some somatic cells form structures like seminiferous tubules. Although most transgenic males can develop normally, some with high levels of MIS expression show feminization of external genitalia, impairment of Wolffian duct development, and undescended testes. Observations that both high and low MIS activities can cause cryptorchidism contradict earlier studies.[6] As explained by Donahoe et al., high MIS levels may downregulate MIS receptor sensitivity on cells controlling testicular descent.

E.   EXTERNAL GENITALIA

The undifferentiated external genitalia are identical in both sexes up to the eighth week. It consists of the urogenital groove, dorsal anus, and ventral genital tubercle. The opening is surrounded by bilaterally symmetrical paraurethral folds, followed by the labioscrotal folds (Figure 2.3).

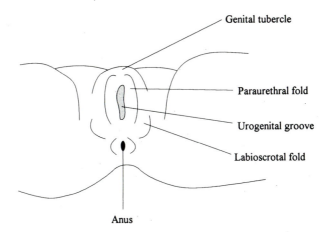

FIGURE 2.3. Undifferentiated external genitalia.

The paraurethral folds remain separate as the labia minora in the female, while they fuse to form the corpus spongiosum in the male. The labioscrotal folds also remain separate and become the labia majora in the female, but they fuse to form the scrotum in the male. The sex differences are conspicuous by weeks 12 to 14. In the male, the urogenital groove develops into the urethra surrounded by the corpus spongiosum. In the female, the same opening forms both the urethra and lower vagina. The lower vagina is continuous with the upper vagina derived from the Müllerian duct.

As in Müllerian development, the differentiation of the external genitalia occurs without androgens in the female. The presence of a testis induces its development to the male external genitalia. The steroid responsible for the induction is dihydrotestosterone, which is derived from testosterone by the enzyme 5α-reductase present in the urogenital sinus and genital tubercle.

III. STEROIDS

Previously, testosterone had been believed to be the sex-determining factor from the Y chromosome.[4] Although steroids play crucial roles in sexual development, we now understand that they are not the prime factors for sex determination as discussed in Chapter 1. In fish, amphibians, and some birds, treatment with steroid hormones can lead to sex reversal of the gonads.[4] In humans, steroids are factors derived from the developing gonad as a consequence of genetic sex determination, and they participate in gonadal differentiation.

A. BIOSYNTHESIS AND METABOLISM

As shown in Figure 2.4, the precursor of steroids is cholesterol, a 27-carbon (C_{27}) sterol mainly derived from low-density lipoproteins (LDL) from the blood

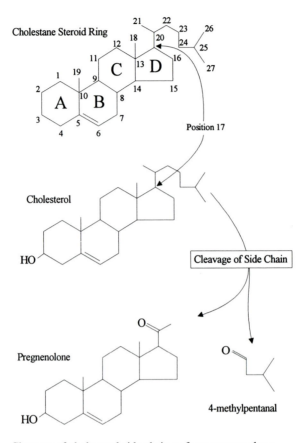

FIGURE 2.4. Cleavage of cholesterol side chain to form pregnenolone.

circulation.[7] LDL particles with cholesterol ester bind to membrane receptors on steroidogenic cells and are internalized as endocytotic vesicles. The vesicles fuse with lysosomes, and the lipoproteins are degraded by proteases and esterases, liberating cholesterol and amino acids. In rodents, however, high-density lipoproteins (HDL) are a more important cholesterol source. Alternatively, cholesterol can be synthesized *de novo* from acetate (see Figure 2.5).

Intracellular free cholesterol is either esterified and stored as lipid droplets or transported to mitochondria where it is converted to pregnenolone by the cleavage of the side chain at position C-17 (see Figure 2.4). The removal of a C_6 fragment depends on a multienzyme system, cytochrome P-450, and flavin adenine dinucleotide (FAD)-containing flavoprotein. This conversion occurs in all steroidogenic tissues and is possibly rate limiting. The C_{21} pregnenolone is the immediate key for the synthesis of three major classes of steroids: progestins, androgens, and estrogens. Progesterone and pregnenolone are progestins. Androgens are structurally similar to progestins, except that two more carbons are lost at position C-17 so that they are C_{19} steroids. Estrogens are derived from androgens by the aromatization of ring A.

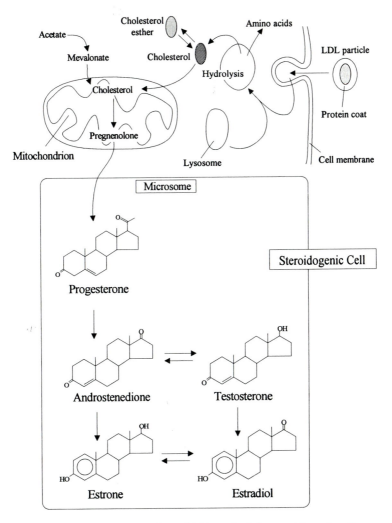

FIGURE 2.5. Cholesterol uptake and steroid biosynthesis by steroidogenic cells.

Figure 2.6 is an integrated diagram of pathways involved in steroid biosynthesis and metabolism. In different tissues with specific cell types, the variation in enzymes and receptors contributes to different steroidogenic properties and regulatory mechanisms. There are essentially two types of steroidogenic cells: LH or FSH responsive. For example, thecal and interstitial cells in ovarian follicles and Leydig cells of the testis are LH-responsive cells. Follicular granulosa cells and Sertoli cells in the testis are FSH-responsive cells.

1.   Biosynthesis of Progestins in Luteal Cells

Luteal cells are differentiated granulosa cells in the corpus luteum after ovulation. This cell type is the major source of progesterone that is synthesized from its

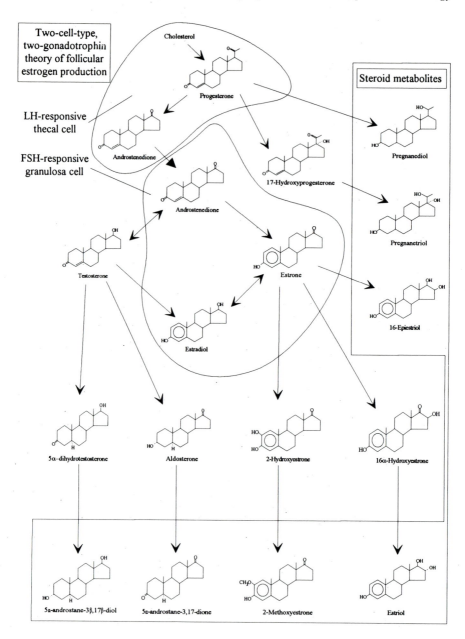

FIGURE 2.6.   Integrated pathways of steroid biosynthesis and metabolism.

immediate precursor pregnenolone by 3β-ol-dehydrogenase Δ⁵⁻⁴-isomerase in
the smooth endoplasmic reticulum. Just before ovulation, granulosa cells contribute only 50% of blood progesterone, while the other 50% is mostly secreted by
the adrenal gland. Besides ovulatory induction, the LH surge also leads to the

formation of the corpus luteum. With an increased production rate of progesterone at 25 to 40 mg/day, the corpus luteum becomes the main source of this hormone in the blood circulation.

2. Biosynthesis of Androgens in Leydig Cells

Leydig cells are the major cell type producing testosterone. According to the biochemical pathway, progesterone is synthesized first from pregnenolone. It is further converted to 17-hydroxyprogesterone by 17α-hydroxylase and then to androstenedione by desmolase. Alternatively, 17α-hydroxylase can act on pregnenolone directly to form 17-hydroxypregnenolone, which is then converted to dehydroepiandronsterone by desmolase. 17-Hydroxypregnenolone is isomerized to androstenedione by 3β-ol-dehydrogenase Δ^{5-4}-isomerase, the same enzyme that converts pregnenolone to progesterone. Testosterone and androstenedione are interconvertible by 17β-hydroxysteroid dehydrogenase.

3. Biosynthesis of Estrogens in Granulosa Cells

Granulosa cells of the preovulatory follicle are the major source of estrogens, though the supply of androstenedione from the theca cells is crucial. This is known as the "two-cell-type, two-gonadotrophin" theory of follicular estrogen production as shown in Figure 2.6. In response to LH, the conversion of cholesterol to androstenedione by theca cells is enhanced. Androstenedione is transported through the circulation to the adjacent granulosa cells where it is converted to estradiol. Since granulosa cells are responsive to FSH, the production of estrogens is very much increased in the presence of both LH and FSH. The two androgens, androstenedione and testosterone, can be aromatized by the aromatase enzyme system to estrone and estradiol, respectively. Estrone and estradiol are also interconvertible by 17β-hydroxysteroid dehydrogenase.

B. Secretion, Transport, and Metabolism

Since steroids are highly lipophilic, they are readily diffusible through the cell membrane immediately after synthesis. The rate of secretion by steroidogenic cells is regulated by the rate of steroidogenesis. Once steroids are secreted into the blood circulation, 99% of the molecules are bound by a carrier protein called sex hormone-binding globulin, a type of β-globulin. Some of them are also loosely bound with serum albumin. The remaining 1% are free steroids, which may bind with receptors, exerting their biological effects.

In the blood, the steroids can be metabolized. Progesterone can be converted to pregnanediol or pregnanetriol and excreted as monogluosiduronated forms. Androgens can be metabolized to 17-ketosteroids called androsterone and etiocholanolone, while estrogens are irreversibly converted to estriol, 16-epiestriol, or 2-methoxyestrone. These metabolites are then conjugated to glucuronoside or sulfated forms in the liver, kidney, and intestinal mucosa for excretion.

C. Steroid Receptors

Specific receptors are present in target cells for steroid actions. It is a unique class of cytoplasmic receptors that are not membrane bound, but are mobile

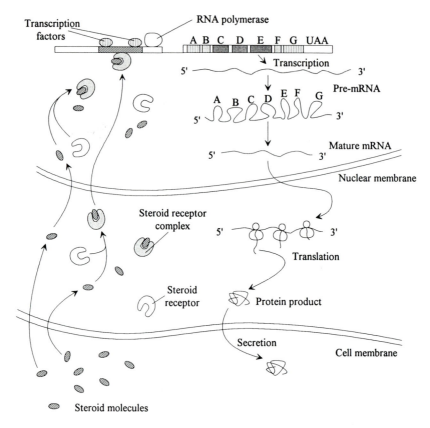

FIGURE 2.7. The molecular mechanism of steroid actions.

between the nucleus and cytoplasm (Figure 2.7). A sequence of steps is necessary for a steroid hormone to exert its effects.

1. Steroid uptake
2. Formation of receptor-steroid complex
3. Translocation of the complex from cytosol to nucleus
4. Binding of the complex to DNA
5. Activation of the transcription process
6. Protein synthesis

Briefly, a steroid molecule enters the target cell by passive diffusion through the cell membrane. At physiological temperature, the uptake of estradiol is linearly proportional to concentration.[8] The cytoplasmic receptor binds with the molecule to form the receptor steroid complex, which is then translocated to the nucleus. Recent studies have shown that the journey to the nucleus is a well-controlled process involving specific microsomal acceptor sites for the complex.[9] After entering the nucleus, the receptor-steroid complex binds to specific DNA sequences on the chromatin, resulting in gene expression. Alternatively, some steroid molecules may diffuse directly into the nucleus and bind with unoccupied receptor proteins. In addition to sex steroids, this receptor type is also found in other hormones such as aldosterone, glucocorticoids, thyroid hormone, retinoic acids, and vitamin D3.[10-13]

Within the same class of steroid receptors, there are differences among receptors for progesterone, estrogens, and androgens. For example, estrogen receptors from mammalian breast cancer cells (MCF-7) is a 4.5S and 65-kDa protein,[14] while progesterone receptors from the same cell type have two 4S subunits of 80- and 108-kDa proteins.[15] However, there are variable results in molecular weight determinations. It seems to depend on conditions and cell types.

To produce an effect, the receptor-steroid complex must interact with the target genes. In the past two decades, the molecular pathways involved have been elucidated.[16] The complex usually binds to the 5′-flanking region of target genes, leading to the induction or repression of specific sets of genes. There are specific interactions between the complex and the DNA sequences of target genes. It is part of the gene regulation by steroid hormones.[17]

Free testosterone enters a target cell such as the prostate cell by diffusion and is converted to dehydrotestosterone (DHT). DHT binds with its receptor to form a complex and enters the nucleus. The receptor-DHT complex binds to the nuclear matrix where changes in DNA topology can be detected, such as DNA loops of about 60 kb pairs. In an active cell, there are 20,000 DNA loops, and about 10% of them are bound by receptor-DHT complexes.[18]

D. EFFECTS OF PROGESTERONE, TESTOSTERONE, AND ESTRADIOL

Progesterone is mainly responsible for the maintenance of pregnancy. In the luteal phase of the menstrual cycle, the endometrium is induced by progesterone to grow as preparation for pregnancy. It also has effects on breast development and the decrease in pulse frequency of gonadotrophin-releasing hormone (GnRH) secretion. Deficiency in progesterone production leads to abnormal sexual development. In a recent study, mifepristone (RU486), a progesterone receptor antagonist, significantly advanced the onset of the vaginal opening in females and attenuated defeminization of the lordosis response measured in males castrated as adults.[19]

Testosterone is found in both males and females. In the female, it is secreted in minuet quantities and it counters the estrogen-induced follicular development so that follicular atresia is enhanced in the presence of high testosterone levels. In the male, the testis provides high levels of testosterone which sustain sperm production. Sexual development is severely affected by the lack of androgen. This can be caused by deficiency in 5α-reductase or defects in the androgen receptor.[20] 5α-Reductase deficiency is a rare autosomal recessive disorder in males who exhibit a defect in virilization most evident as impairment of the virilization of the external genitalia and urogenital sinus. Disorders of the androgen receptor in genetic males cause a spectrum of developmental abnormalities that vary from phenotypic females to men with mild defects in virilization.

Estrogens are not only important for reproductive functions, but they are also involved in general metabolic processes. Gonadotrophin synthesis depends on circulating estrogens with a well-defined negative feedback mechanism. In the ovary, estrogens stimulate granulosa cell proliferation. They also induce the growth of endometrium, production of cervical mucus, and maintenance of the vaginal epithelium. According to the idea of estrogen-induced "sexual differentiation of the brain", the action of estrogen on the rat brain is lifelong. Processes responsive to estrogen effects include neurogenesis in the fetus, synaptogenesis in the newborn, and synaptic remodeling in the adult. Estrogen produces sex differences in the rat brain by shaping synaptology, postsynaptic membranes, and glia within the arcuate nucleus. These estrogen effects on the arcuate nucleus play a crucial role in sexual maturation of both sexes and the development of constant estrus in senescent females.[21]

IV. SECONDARY SEX CHARACTERISTICS AND THE BRAIN

The expression of secondary sex characteristics is an important part of sexual development. Puberty is the transition from childhood to adulthood, during which profound changes can be observed. Normal pubertal development is characterized by major physical alterations: sexual maturation, changes in body composition, and rapid skeletal growth. The brain also plays an important role in the development of sexual behaviors. The sexual differentiation and development of the nervous system are continual processes from prenatal through puberty and beyond.

A. FEMALE PUBERTY

The interactions between the ovary with the nervous systems and other associated organs during female sexual maturation are summarized in Figure 2.8. The development of female reproductive structures and the onset of menstruation are two crucial events during female puberty.

1. Breast Development

Breast development is the first manifestation of puberty in approximately 85% of girls; the normal age for initial breast development is 8 to 13 years.[22] The breast starts to develop initially as a bud. Estrogens stimulate the growth of the ductal epithelium. The connective tissues around these ducts increase in size and elasticity with an accumulation of fatty tissues. The vascular supply also develops rapidly at this stage. Although progesterone alone does not show significant effect on breast development experimentally, the combination of estrogens and progesterone produces full enhancing effects on the maturing mammary glands.

2. Menarche

Menarche is the onset of menstruation; it occurs in American girls at a mean age of 12.8 years.[22] One or two years before this time, pubic hair begins to grow

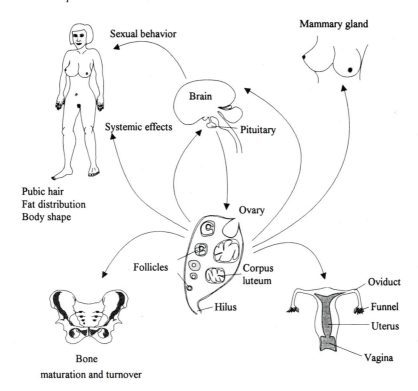

FIGURE 2.8. Interactions of the ovary with the nervous system and associated structures during female sexual maturation.

in response to adrenarche, an increased production of adrenal androgens, dehydroepiandrosterone sulfate, and androstenedione. Although the hypothalamo/pituitary/gonadal axis is functional before puberty, FSH and LH concentrations in the blood circulation are low. The sensitivity of the hypothalamus to estrogens increases after reaching puberty.

3. External Genitalia

There are conspicuous changes in the female external genitalia during puberty. Pubic hairs grow on the top of the mons veneris. Both the labia majora and minora develop into conspicuous folds of adipose tissues. The color, texture, and shape of these folds vary greatly among different individuals. They are supplied with blood vessels and covered with mucus membrane. The outer surface of the labia majora is usually hairy and is different from its inner surface. The clitoris also develops and elongates out of the prepuce at the anterior junction of the labia majora (see also Chapter 5).

B. MALE PUBERTY

The first manifestation of puberty is testicular enlargement; the normal age for initial signs of puberty is 9 to 14 years in males. Pubic hair in boys generally appears 18 to 24 months after the onset of testicular growth and is often conceived as the initial marker of sexual maturation by male adolescents. Skeletal growth is one of the most striking characteristics of puberty. Linear-growth velocity begins to increase in males at genital stage III and pubic-hair stage II, but peak height velocity is not attained until age 14 in boys. Lean body mass, which primarily reflects muscle mass, begins to increase during early puberty (see also Chapter 6).

C.   THE BRAIN

There are two aspects of sexual differentiation of the brain. First, the sexual development of the hypothalamo-pituitary-gonadal axis is differentiated between two sexes. Second, the controversial sexual dimorphism in behaviors, including sexual preferences, gender differences, cognition, and other brain activities, may exist. We are, however, certain that the hypothalamo-pituitary-gonadal axis is sexually differentiated, resulting in differences in secondary sex characteristics such as voice quality, body figure, etc. In view of sexual differences in gonadal differentiation, developing brains exposed to different hormonal environments are likely to be different. The differences may not be sexual only but also individual. This contributes to both gender and individual differences.

V.   ABNORMAL SEXUAL DEVELOPMENT

Developmental failure at any time produces malformed sexual structures at varying degrees. The abnormality ranges from mild cases of deviant sexual behavior to severe cases of irreversible sterility. Abnormal sexual development of the brain is particularly difficult to evaluate, especially in humans. For example, homosexuality was previously regarded as an aberrant sexual behavior. New evidence suggests that homosexuality may be a normal type of sexual orientation with a possible genetic origin (see Chapters 7 and 12). However, distinct clinical entities with conspicuous symptoms are not rare. The following diseases are common clinical cases.

A.   TURNER'S SYNDROME

Turner's syndrome occurs in 0.02-0.05% of neonatal females with a variety of chromosomal karyotypes and clinical phenotypes.[23] Many are apparently normal but others have major clinical manifestations such as short stature and gonadal failure. Growth hormone treatment has been suggested to be helpful in some patients with stunted growth. For patients with gonadal malfunction, the severity varies from one case to another. Some may have spontaneous puberty with potentials for normal fertility, while others suffer from complete gonadal failure. In a few rare cases, mothers with Turner's syndrome may deliver normal babies.

Using a series of polymorphic DNA probes, the origin of the normal X chromosome was investigated in 34 families having children or fetuses with Turner's syndrome.[24] Based on the pattern of restriction enzyme sites on the X chromosome, it is possible to determine whether the X chromosome is maternal.

The observed X in each of the 4 fetuses and 12 live births from 16 families with 45,X karyotype was maternal, suggesting a preferential loss of paternal sex chromosome. The remaining 18 families with other karyotypes also showed a strong tendency to have normal maternal X, especially those with a child having an isochromosome of Xq or a ring X. The authors did not find any evidence for the incidence of abnormality being associated with paternal age.

B. KLINEFELTER SYNDROME

Klinefelter syndrome (XXY syndrome) of testicular dysgenesis is the most common form of male hypogonadism.[25] Other kinds of testicular dysgenesis include Kallman syndrome and idiopathic hypogonadotropic hypogonadism. In a world-wide cytogenetic survey,[26] a population of XXY males of different races with records from the newborn period through adolescence has been identified. XXY individuals may have specific physical signs at all ages. These phenotypic features are attributed to a sex chromosome complement that includes two or more X chromosomes and one or more Y chromosomes. In addition to physical signs, XXY individuals often have language deficits, neuromaturational lag, academic difficulties, and psychological distress. Early identification, anticipatory guidance, and proper medical management may be helpful in treating these deficiencies.

C. HERMAPHRODITES

An interesting case of hermaphroditism showing an apparent 46,XX karyotype in blood and testis cultures with a hypoplastic penis and polyorchidism has recently been reported.[27] Exploratory laparotomy and bilateral gonadal biopsy showed the presence of two right testes and one left. Histologically, testicular tissues were hypoplastic and uncultured testis smears showed Y chromatin in approximately 20% of the cells. Using Southern blot and polymerase chain reaction, some Y chromosome-derived DNA sequences were detected in the perineal skin but not in lymphocytes. This patient had a small population of Y chromosome-containing cells with mosaicism in some tissues, such as the testes and perineal skin. It is possible that these Y fragments are responsible for testicular genesis in some XX patients, true hermaphrodites or male pseudohermaphrodites with 46,XX karyotype.

In another study, three XX males, two XX true hermaphrodites, and an XY female were studied for possible deletions using probes for the recently characterized SRY gene and the pseudoautosomal boundary. One of the XX males was sibling with one of the two XX true hermaphrodites. The XX males and true hermaphrodites showed negative response to the probes, while the XY female was positive. In a previous study, a sibling pair of XX male and XX true hermaphrodite had also been shown to be positive for Y chromosomal material near the pseudoautosomal boundary. Therefore, different deletions might have occurred in individuals with similar phenotypes; some mutations may involve the SRY gene but not in others.[28] Figure 2.9 shows the external genitalia of a true hermaphrodite. Despite their XX karyotypes, most hermaphrodites are reared as males because of their conspicuous phallic structures.[29]

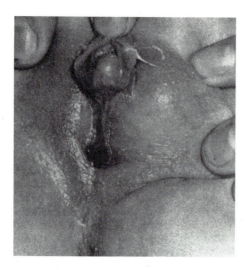

FIGURE 2.9. External genitalia of a true hermaphrodite. (From Dewhurst, J., *Practical Pediatric and Adolescent Gynecology,* Marcel Dekker, New York, 1980. With permission.)

D.   PSEUDOHERMAPHRODITES

In contrast to true hermaphroditism attributed to XY chromosomal aberrations, pseudohermaphrodites are mostly caused by defects in steroidogenic enzymes. A group of male pseudohermaphrodites from the Simbari Anga linguistic group in the Eastern Highlands of Papua New Guinea has recently been reported.[30] They have rudimentary penises and pseudovaginal perineoscrotal hypospadias. At puberty, the clitoral-like penis enlarges, while pubic and axillary hairs are growing. Although there are significant muscular development and facial hair growth, the extent is less than that of their normal male siblings or other male relatives. All subjects had high urinary aetiocholanolone/androsterone ratios, and C_{19}- and $C_{21}5\beta/5\alpha$-metabolite ratios. Four of them showed elevated testosterone levels, low to normal dihydrotestosterone levels, and elevated testosterone/dihydrotestosterone ratios in the blood plasma. Cultured fibroblasts from genital tissues had lower 5α-reductase activity. This phenotypic and biochemical profile is similar to that in subjects from the Dominican Republic, except for more facial and body hair. The differences may be associated with variations in familial expression and the degree of enzyme deficiency. Infants previously thought to be females at birth were reared as girls. In accord with the physiologic changes at puberty, a switch of gender roles was instituted socially. Some Muniri, Dunkwi and northern Simbari hamlets are able to identify these individuals early as males and rear them as boys. To distinguish these individuals socially from normal males, they call them "kwalatmala" and accept them as intersexual individuals who will later assume male adult roles.

Male pseudohermaphrodites (MPHs) have a general defect in 5α-metabolism affecting both C_{19} androgen metabolism and C_{21} steroid metabolism.[31] The

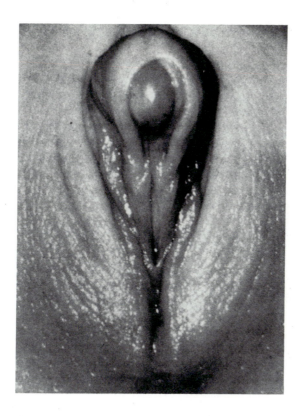

FIGURE 2.10. External genitalia of an XY child reared as a girl. (From Dewhurst, J., *Practical Pediatric and Adolescent Gynecology,* Marcel Dekker, New York, 1980. With permission.)

genetic defect is the deficiency in the enzyme 5α-reductase, leading to a decrease in 5α-reduction of testosterone to dihydrotestosterone. Only this impaired steroid conversion leads to clinical consequences such as ambiguous genitalia, impaired prostate differentiation and development, and decreased facial and body hair. In normal male patients with benign prostatic hyperplasia treated with finasteride, a potent inhibitor of both C_{19} androgen and C_{21} 5α-steroid metabolism affecting both hepatic and peripheral 5α-metabolism, the profile of 5α-steroid metabolites was similar to that of MPHs with inherited 5α-reductase deficiency.

Another possibility is that differentiating tissues are insensitive to androgens during prenatal sexual development in some genetic males. As in MPHs, these individuals appear to be females. However, the sensitivity to androgens may be restored, at least partially, during puberty. An apparent "spontaneous sex change" is also witnessed in these individuals. Figure 2.10 shows the external genitalia of an XY child reared as a girl because of insensitivity to androgen. Masculinization is in progress and may be more pronounced later at puberty.[29]

REFERENCES

1. **Cate, R.L., et al.,** Isolation of the bovine and human genes for Müllerian inhibiting substance and expression of the human gene in animal cells, *Cell,* 45, 685, 1986.
2. **Josso, N.,** Antimüllerian hormone: new perspectives for a sexist molecule, *Endocr. Rev.,* 7, 421, 1986.
3. **Tsuji, M., Shima, H., and Cunha, G.R.,** *In vitro* androgen-induced growth and morphogenesis of the Wolffian duct within urogenital ridge, *Endocrinology,* 128, 1805, 1991.
4. **Burns, R.K.,** Role of hormones in the differentiation of sex, in *Sex and Internal Secretions,* Young, W.C., Ed., Williams & Wilkins, Baltimore, 1961, 76.
5. **Behringer, R.R., Cate, R.L., Froelick, G.J., Palmiter, R.D., and Brinster, R.L.,** Abnormal sexual development in transgenic mice chronically expressing Müllerian inhibiting substance, *Nature (London),* 345, 167, 1990.
6. **Donahoe, P.K., Hutson, J.M., Fallat, M.E., Kamagata, S., and Budzik, G.P.,** Mechanism of action of Müllerian inhibiting substance, *Annu. Rev. Physiol.,* 46, 53, 1984.
7. **Gwynne, J.T. and Strauss, J.F., III,** The role of lipoproteins in steroidogenesis and cholesterol metabolism in steroidogenic glands, *Endocr. Rev.,* 3, 299, 1982.
8. **Peck, E.J., Jr., Burgner, J., and Clark, J.H.,** Estrophilic binding sites of the uterus. Relation to uptake and retention of estradiol *in vitro, Biochemistry,* 12, 4596, 1973.
9. **Muldoon, T.G., Watson, G.H., Evans, A.C., Jr., and Steinsapir, J.,** Microsomal receptor for steroid hormones: functional implications for nuclear activity, *J. Steroid Biochem.,* 30, 23, 1988.
10. **Dahlman-Wright, K., Wright, A., Carlstedt-Duke, J., and Gustafsson, J.A.,** DNA-binding by the glucocorticoid receptor: a structural and functional analysis, *J. Steroid Biochem. Mol. Biol.,* 41, 249, 1992.
11. **Norman, A.W., Nemere, I., Zhou, L.X., Bishop, J.E., Lowe, K.E., Maiyar, A.C., Collins, E.D., Taoka, T., Sergeev, I., and Farach-Carson, M.C.,** 1,25(OH)2-vitamin D3, a steroid hormone that produces biologic effects via both genomic and nongenomic pathways, *J. Steroid Biochem. Mol. Biol.,* 41, 231, 1992.
12. **Horisherger, J.D. and Rossier, B.C.,** Aldosterone regulation of gene transcription leading to control of ion transport, *Hypertension,* 19, 221, 1992.
13. **Rees, J.,** The molecular biology of retinoic acid receptors: orphan from good family seeks home, *Br. J. Dermatol.,* 126, 97, 1992.
14. **Greene, G.L.,** Immunochemical studies of estrogen receptor, in *Gene Regulation by Steroid Hormones, Vol. II,* Roy, A.K. and Clark, J.H., Eds., Springer-Verlag, New York, 1984, 191.
15. **Lessey, B.A., Alexander, P.S., and Horwitz, K.B.,** The subunit structure of human breast cancer progesterone receptors: characterization by chromatography and photoaffinity labeling, *Endocrinology,* 112, 1267, 1983.
16. **O'Malley, B.W. and Tsai, M.J.,** Molecular pathways of steroid receptor action, *Biol. Reprod.,* 46, 163, 1992.
17. **Truss, M., Chalepakis, G., Pina, B., Barettino, D., Bruggemeier, U., Kalff, M., Slater, E.P., and Beato, M.,** Transcriptional control by steroid hormones, *J. Steroid Biochem. Mol. Biol.,* 41, 241, 1992.
18. **Coffey, D.S.,** Androgen action and the sex accessory tissues, in *The Physiology of Reproduction,* Knobil, E. and Neill, J., Eds., Raven Press, New York, 1988, 1081.
19. **Weinstein, M.A., Pleim, E.T., and Barfield, R.J.,** Effects of neonatal exposure to the antiprogestin mifepristone, RU486, on the sexual development of the rat, *Pharmacol. Biochem. Behav.,* 41, 69, 1992.
20. **Wilson, J.D.,** Syndromes of androgen resistance, *Biol. Reprod.,* 46, 168, 1992.
21. **Naftolin, F., Garcia-Segura, L.M., Keefe, D., Leranth, C., Maclusky, N.J., and Brawer, J.R.,** Estrogen effects on the synaptology and neural membranes of the rat hypothalamic arcuate nucleus, *Biol. Reprod.,* 42, 21, 1990.

22. **Wheeler, M.D.,** Physical changes of puberty, *Endocrinol. Metab. Clin. North Am.,* 20, 1, 1991.

23. **Lippe, B.,** Turner syndrome, *Endocrinol. Metab. Clin. North Am.,* 20, 121, 1991.

24. **Loughlin, S.A., Redha, A., McIver, J., Boyd, E., Carothers, A., and Connor, J.M.,** Analysis of the origin of Turner's syndrome using polymorphic DNA probes, *J. Med. Genet.,* 28, 156, 1991.

25. **Schwartz, I.D. and Root, A.W.,** The Klinefelter syndrome of testicular dysgenesis, *Endocrinol. Metab. Clin. North Am.,* 20, 153, 1991.

26. **Mandoki, M.W., Sumner, G.S., Hoffman, R.P., and Riconda, D.L.,** A review of Klinefelter's syndrome in children and adolescents [published erratum appears in *J. Am. Acad. Child Adolesc. Psychiatry,* 1991 May;30(3):516], *J. Am. Acad. Child Adolesc. Psychiatry,* 30, 167, 1991.

27. **Yoshida, M., Kakizawa, Y., Moriyama, N., Minowada, S., Higashihara, E., Aso, Y., Nakagome, Y., Nakahori, Y., Nagafuchi, S., and Tanae, A.,** Deoxyribonucleic acid and cytological detection of Y-containing cells in an XX hypospadiac boy with polyorchidism, *J. Urol.,* 146, 1356, 1991.

28. **Pereira, E.T., de Almeida, J.C., Gunha, A.C., Patton, M., Taylor, R., and Jeffery, S.,** Use of probes for ZFY, SRY, and the Y pseudoautosomal boundary in XX males, XX true hermaphrodites, and an XY female, *J. Med. Genet.,* 28, 591, 1991.

29. **Dewhurst, J.,** *Practical Pediatric and Adolescent Gynecology,* Marcel Dekker, New York, 1980.

30. **Imperato-McGinley, J., Miller, M., Wilson, J.D., Peterson, R.E., Shackleton, C., and Gajdusek, D.C.,** A cluster of male pseudohermaphrodites with 5α-reductase deficiency in Papua New Guinea, *Clin. Endocrinol.,* 34, 293, 1991.

31. **Imperato-McGinley, J.,** 5α-Metabolism in finasteride-treated subjects and male pseudohermaphrodites with inherited 5α-reductase deficiency. A review, *Eur. Urol.,* 20 (Suppl. 1), 78, 1991.

3 Reproductive Neuroendocrinology

CHAPTER CONTENTS

I. INTRODUCTION

During sexual differentiation, the gonad acquires the ability to synthesize steroids and a set of appropriate responses to regulatory factors from the brain. Both steroid biosynthesis and responsiveness to brain factors may not be required for early stages of the developmental program. Later in the fetal life, the developing reproductive system becomes dependent on the interaction between the gonad and the brain. Coupled with the sexual differentiation of the brain, this interactive mechanism becomes established during puberty. There are two components in this interactive regulatory mechanism: the brain response to hormones from the gonad and the gonadal response to neural hormones from the brain.

Evidently, the nervous system is involved in the regulation of the endocrine system. These two systems interact with each other to maintain and coordinate with other systems, creating an integrative control of the general function. Historically, the nervous and endocrine systems were considered to have separate controls working independently. The concept of integrative control was first recognized in lower animals because some of them have brains and ganglia acting as endocrine organs.

This type of integrative control is not limited to reproduction. It includes almost all functions involving the nervous and endocrine systems. Hormones, neural hormones, and neurotransmitters are found similar in their functions. The reproductive system represents an elaborated example of neuroendocrine feedback control systems involving the brain, gonads, and target tissues. Such an extensive integration also allows the system to respond to environmental changes as discussed in Chapter 11.

There are two possible ways of interactions between the nervous and endocrine systems. First, hormones can exert effects on the nervous system. A hormone can alter synaptic transmission and neuronal conductance of action potentials. This can be observed in certain endocrine diseases showing abnormal reflex activity and behavioral changes. Second, factors from the nervous system can affect endocrine functions. When endocrine cells are innervated, their secretory functions can be altered by local actions of neurotransmitters.

II. THE BRAIN AS A SEXUAL ORGAN

In recent years, the concept of the brain being a sexual organ has been strongly advocated mainly because of the identification of sexual dimorphism in the nervous system.[1] The control of sexual behavior by the brain evolved well before the emergence of humans. Lesion and electrical stimulation studies have been performed to delineate neural pathways and areas responsible for specific behavior such as male and female sexual responses.[2,3] In addition, as one of the sexual organs, these areas in the brain are under the influence of steroids secreted by the gonads. In other words, the control of motor and sensory functions of the brain related to sexual behavior is linked with neural centers that are responsive to gonadal factors. Such an interaction also exists during sexual differentiation of the brain.

Figure 3.1 summarizes the regional specialization of the brain related to its role as a sexual organ to achieve reproduction. The pituitary and pineal glands are included to underscore the importance of the coordination of the whole system with internal and external environmental factors. It should be noted that species variations are significant and the figure is mainly based on humans. In addition, individual variation is also considerable, so that a generalization of brain centers correlated with behavior is inaccurate. The use of animal data to interpret human brain functions is even less reliable. There is, however, one commonality across different mammalian species: differences can be found between male and female brains. The difference may be anatomical, functional, and behavioral. Sexual differences in the human brain still need further verification.

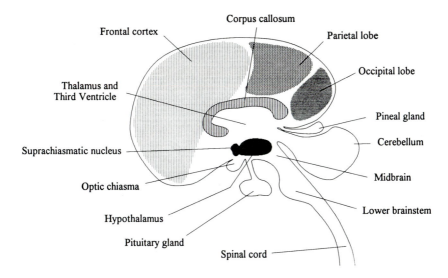

FIGURE 3.1. Regional specialization of the human brain.

Even if it is not sexually different, the brain can still be classified as a sexual organ. It is well established that the brain is the target organ of gonadal steroids.[4] Through a feedback mechanism, gonadal steroids influence the synthesis and release of neural hormones from the hypothalamus and pituitary. Endogenous opioid peptides play a regulatory role in LH secretion by inhibiting hypothalamic neurons that produce gonadotrophin-releasing hormone (GnRH), modulating the activity of sex steroids on the hypothalamus-pituitary-gonadal axis. Considering the sexual differences in steroid secretion, the brain is responsive to a sexually specific endocrine environment. This is a characteristic feature of a sexual organ. Most importantly, the fact that the brain governs our sexual behavior is a sufficient condition for it to be a sexual organ.

As we shall discuss in Chapter 7, sexual behavior is the prerequisite for successful sexual reproduction. The brain, being responsive to gonadal steroids, can modify sexual behavior with reference to gonadal maturity, cyclicity, and responsiveness. Reciprocally, the brain exerts effects on gonadal development and activity, coordinating with other inputs to the brain. This suggests that the brain is a major sexual organ with a significant regulatory role. It should be noted, however, that castrated individuals do show a drastically reduced copulatory behavior in mammals.[5] Therefore, the gonad is still central to reproductive physiology.

III. THE HYPOTHALAMO-HYPOPHYSEAL COMPLEX

The pituitary gland, or hypophysis, occupies a central but ventral position of the brain and lies within the sella turcica at the base of the skull. It is a pendulous structure suspended below and posterior to the optic chiasm where the two optic nerves intersect with each other. The gland weighs from 500 to 900 mg and has a volume of about 0.7 cm³. There are two major portions: anterior and posterior. The

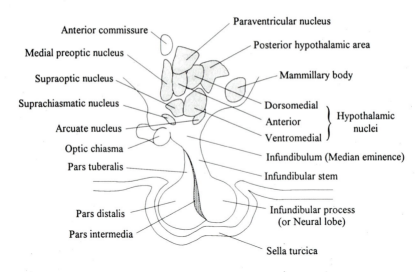

FIGURE 3.2.   The hypothalamo-hypophyseal complex and associated nuclei.

anterior pituitary is also called adenohypophysis, which is derived from the ectoderm of the roof of the developing pharynx, the Rathke's pouch. The posterior pituitary, or neurohypophysis, is differentiated as a pocket from the floor of the brain.

According to Galen (130 to 200 A.D.), the pituitary was a sump for phlegm (Latin: *pituita),* which is the waste product excreted from the brain as a result of distillation of the spirit. The phlegm was then filtered though the ethmoid into the nasal passages. This view was accepted for centuries — until 1655, when Schneider found that fluids could not pass from the cranial cavity into the nose. Later, the dual embryonic origin of the pituitary was suggested by Rathke in 1838. With the advent of microtome and hematoxylin dye at that time, the histology of the pituitary was studied. In 1912, its structures had been reported in detail by Harvey Cushing, though he saw the pituitary as a neural organ with an epithelial portion lying in the sella turcica.[6] At that time, this bilobed structure was still thought to be a vestigial organ.

As shown in Figure 3.2, there is another structure between the anterior and posterior lobes, called the pars intermedia. All these structures are tightly packed together. The whole pituitary gland and its stalk can easily be removed from a dissected brain. The gland, however, should also include part of the floor of the third ventricle. This part where the stalk is rooted is called the median eminence. The ceiling of the third ventricle is the thalamus, below which is the hypothalamus. Lateral to the third ventricle on both sides, there are bilaterally symmetrical hypothalamic nuclei.[7]

A.   ADENOHYPOPHYSIS

Adenohypophysis is the glandular lobe including the pars tuberalis, pars distalis, and pars intermedia. The pars intermedia, which is also called the intermediate lobe, is distinct from the other two structures. The major portion of the anterior lobe is the pars distalis, which is a tapering process attached to the infundibular stem of the posterior pituitary and forms the stalk of the gland.

All these structures in the adenohypophysis are derived from the Rathke's pouch, which is part of the development oral cavity, instead of neural tissues. The anterior portion of the pouch grows massively to form the pars distalis, and the posterior portion becomes the pars intermedia. In humans, however, the pars intermedia is absent except in pregnant women and developing fetuses.

B. NEUROHYPOPHYSIS

The whole neurohypophysis is derived from neural tissues. It consists of the infundibulum, infundibular stem, and infundibular process (or the neural lobe). The deeply rooted infundibulum is also called the median eminence and is the floor of the third ventricle. The infundibular stem is the major part of the pituitary stalk and is connected to the infundibular process commonly known as the neural lobe. The whole structure is the posterior pituitary gland. However, the term "posterior lobe" refers to the neural lobe and pars intermedia.

It receives axons of neurons originated from the hypothalamus. In the neural lobe, there are glial cells called pituitcytes and capillaries that are fenestrated. There are five types of pituitcytes. First, major pituitcytes are typical astrocytes with processes usually found in the perivascular space of capillaries. More electron-dense variants of these pituitcytes are the second type called dark pituitcytes. Another two types called ependymal and oncocytic pituitcytes are those having cilia and numerous mitochondria, respectively. The last type is called granular pituitcytes showing many electron-dense cytoplasmic granules.

In the infundibular stem, there are axons of the magnocellular (large) and parvicellular (small) neurons. The magnocellular neurons are peptidergic because they produce the peptide hormones oxytocin and vasopressin, which are stored in dense-core vesicles. The paricellular neurons are both peptidergic and aminergic.

C. HYPOTHALAMUS

The hypothalamus is a collection of nuclei in an area at the base of the brain above the pituitary but below the thalamus (see Figure 3.2). Each nucleus is a bundle of nerve cell bodies. As shown in Figure 3.3, most of the nuclei are bilaterally symmetrical about the third ventricle except the suprachiasmatic nucleus (SCN) and arcuate nucleus. The lateral hypothalamic area is a bundle of nerve cells connecting the hypothalamic nuclei with the rest of the brain.

The preoptic nucleus (PON), arcuate nucleus, and anterior hypothalamic nucleus are involved in reproduction. The SCN is a circadian generator responsible for maintaining endogenous rhythms associated with reproductive cycles (see Chapters 4 and 11). In addition, a sexually dimorphic nucleus (SDN) has been identified in humans and laboratory animals to be related to sexual behavior.

Some authors include the median eminence in the hypothalamus. The neurohypophysis is actually an extension of the hypothalamus. It serves as an area for

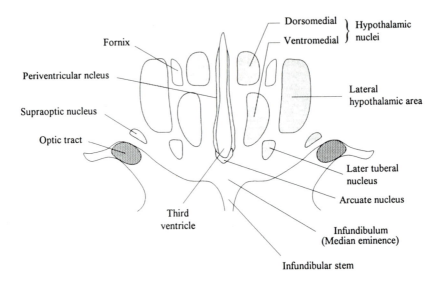

Dorsomedial ⎫ Hypothalamic
Ventromedial ⎰ nuclei

Fornix

Periventricular ncleus

Supraoptic nucleus

Optic tract

Lateral
hypothalamic area

Later tuberal
nucleus

Arcuate nucleus

Third
ventricle

Infundibulum
(Median eminence)

Infundibular stem

FIGURE 3.3. Bilateral symmetry of hypothalamic nuclei.

integrating neural and humoral stimuli. Others, however, still consider it to be part of neurohypophysis in the pituitary gland. It has a close relationship with the neural lobe and also a structurally distinct capillary plexus in this area (see next section).

D. VASCULAR PORTAL SYSTEM OF THE PITUITARY

As shown in Figure 3.4, there is an elaborated vascular system extending from the median eminence and infundibular stem to the adenohypophysis. It is a portal system with a characteristic portal blood vessel having capillaries at both ends. The whole system consists of one long and one short portal vessel. The long portal vessel connects between the median eminence and adenohypophysis, while the short portal vessel relays from the adenohypophysis to neurohypophysis.

Therefore, the blood in the arterial system flows from internal carotid artery to the primary capillary plexus in the median eminence and infundibular stem. It drains through the long portal vessel to secondary adenohypophyseal capillary plexus (not sinusoids) in which the capillaries are fenestrated and interposed between epithelial cells. The plexus also receives blood from the inferior hypophyseal artery in the neurohypophysis via the short portal vessel. All combine to form the hypophyseal veins before going to the superior vena cava. Another branch of the inferior hypophyseal artery joins the capillary plexus in the neural lobe before returning to the venous system.

Obviously, such a system is necessary for the transfer of humoral signals from the hypothalamus to the pituitary. These include hypothalamic releasing and inhibiting factors. For releasing factors, there are GnRH, thyrotropin-releasing hormone (TRH), corticotropin-releasing hormone (CRH), and growth-hormone-releasing hormone (GHRH). There are two inhibiting factors, somatostatin and prolactin-inhibiting factor (PIF).

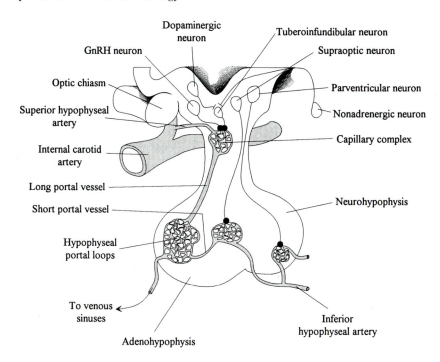

FIGURE 3.4. Vascular portal system of the pituitary and associated neurons.

IV. THE PINEAL GLAND

The human pineal gland, which is also known as epiphysis, occupies a central location between the two cerebral hemispheres and in front of the cerebellum at the posterodorsal area of the diencephalon. It develops as a small invagination from the roof of the thalamus, the epithalamus. The first documented discussion of pineal function was probably by Galen, who previously described the pituitary gland. He claimed that the pineal was the seat of soul. In contrast to Aristotle, Galen placed the seat of the soul in the brain instead of the heart. Although Galen was not the discoverer of the pineal gland, he was the first to write about its location, structure, form, and function.[8]

In the late 17th century, anatomists critically examined and became skeptical about Descartes' claim that the pineal gland was the seat of the soul. Based on later morphological and comparative studies, the pineal gland was thought to be a vestigial gland in the brain without significant functions. The pineal gland was rarely studied until the late 1950s. A new substance, called melatonin, was isolated and identified from bovine pineal glands in 1958. Now, melatonin is known to be the major hormone of this gland with a major influence on the reproductive system, modulating the neuroendocrine-reproductive axis.

A. DISCOVERY OF MELATONIN

In 1958, Lerner et al.[9] successfully isolated a substance from bovine pineal extracts which had been shown to lighten the skin color of tadpoles, frogs, toads, and fish.[10,11] As dermatologists, Lerner et al. hoped to identify a factor for regulating skin pigmentation in humans. They performed bioassays using isolated frog *(Rana pipiens)* skin darkened with caffeine and measured the lightening effect photometrically. They also showed that melatonin had neither adrenaline nor noradrenaline-like activity on the rat uterus and no serotonin-like effect on the clam heart. Later, Lerner and co-workers[12,13] elucidated the structure of melatonin and further characterized its lightening ability.

B.   MELATONIN BIOSYNTHESIS

Melatonin is synthesized from the amino acid tryptophan, which is first converted to serotonin and then *N*-acetylserotonin (NAS). Serotonin is derived from the amino acid tryptophan (TRP) through 5-hydroxytryptophan (5HTP) as the intermediate. The conversion of TRP to 5HTP is catalyzed by tryptophan hydroxylase (TH; EC 1.14.16.4). 5HTP is then oxidized to serotonin by 5-hydroxytryptophan decarboxylase (5HTPD; EC 4.1.1.28).

Weissbach et al.[14] demonstrated that the conversion of serotonin to NAS is performed by acetylation catalyzed by an enzyme *N*-acetyltransferase (NAT; EC 2.3.1.5).[15] The final conversion of NAS to melatonin was also found to be an enzymatic process; an enzyme called hydroxyindole-*O*-methyltransferase (HIOMT; EC 2.1.1.4) responsible for the *O*-methylation step of NAS was purified and characterized by Axelrod and Weissbach in 1961.[16] They found that this enzyme was highly localized in the pineal gland, so melatonin biosynthesis was thought to be carried out solely in this organ. In 1965, Quay reported HIOMT activity in other tissues including the retina.[17] These findings led to the suggestion that the neural retina can synthesize and regulate its own melatonin independent of the pineal gland.[18] Since the notion of melatonin biosynthesis in extrapineal tissues is relatively new, an understanding of melatonin biosynthesis is based primarily on studies on the pineal. The pathway of melatonin biosynthesis was recently reviewed[19] and is summarized in Figure 3.5.

C.   REGULATION OF MELATONIN BIOSYNTHESIS

In darkness, melatonin biosynthesis in the pineal is increased by electrical signals originating from neurons in the SCN.[20] These neurons receive inputs from the lateral eyes and send inputs via the paraventricular nucleus (PVN). The fibers go through the spinal cord to the superior cervical ganglia (SCG) of the sympathetic nervous system (Figure 3.6) and terminate adjacent to pinealocytes. Some central fibers with an unexplained role have also been found entering the pineal via the stalk.[21]

The neurotransmitter at the postganglionic sympathetic nerve terminal is norepinephrine (NE), which is synthesized from tyrosine with the conversion being catalyzed by TH. A combination of increased impulse frequency[22] and TH activity at night[23,24] results in an increased NE release into the synaptic cleft. NE binds to α_1- and β-adrenergic receptors on the pinealocyte membrane and triggers a series of intracellular responses through specific signal transduction processes (Figure 3.6).

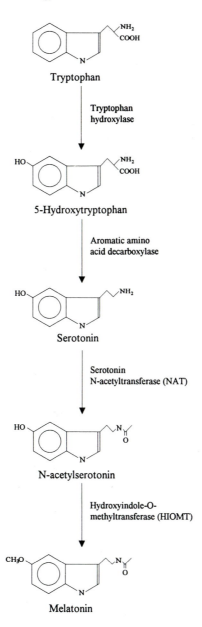

Tryptophan

Tryptophan hydroxylase

5-Hydroxytryptophan

Aromatic amino acid decarboxylase

Serotonin

Serotonin N-acetyltransferase (NAT)

N-acetylserotonin

Hydroxyindole-O-methyltransferase (HIOMT)

Melatonin

FIGURE 3.5. Melatonin biosynthesis.

A NE molecule binds to a membrane-bound receptor on pinealocytes and triggers the signal transduction. The β-adrenergic receptor is the predominant receptor type for NE, and their density in the rat pineal is highest at night.[25,26] NE also binds to α-receptors, resulting in an enhanced response when both α- and β-receptors are stimulated. Other receptors responding to other neurotransmitters

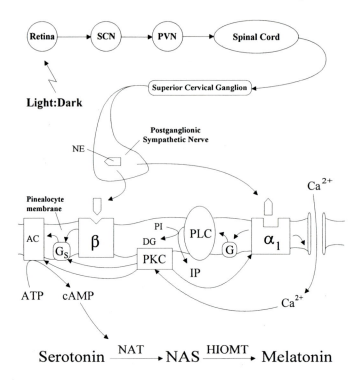

FIGURE 3.6. Proposed neural pathway of photic input through the eye to the pineal gland where pinealoctyes are innervated by sympathetic nerve endings. The lower part of the diagram shows a model of the signal transduction at the pinealocyte membrane. (AC) adenylate cyclase, (DG) diacylglycerol, (G) guanine nucleotide-binding protein (G-protein), (G_s) stimulatory G-protein, (HIOMT) hydroxyindole-*O*-methyltransferase, (IP) inositol phosphate, (NAS) *N*-acetylserotonin, (NAT) *N*-acetyltransferase, (NE) norepinephrine, (PI) phosphotidylinositol, (PKC) protein kinase C, (PLC) phospholipase C, (PVN) paraventricular nuclei, (SCN) suprachiasmatic nuclei, (α_1) α_1-adrenergic receptor, and (β) β-adrenergic receptor. (From Yu, H.S. and Reiter, R.J., Eds., *Melatonin: Biosynthesis, Physiological Effects, and Clinical Applications,* CRC Press, Boca Raton, FL, 1993. With permission.)

are also present on the pinealocyte membrane, but their functions are not clear at present.[27] For example, σ-receptor has been found highly concentrated in the rat pineal gland.[28]

When the β -receptor is activated, there is a separation of the stimulatory guanine nucleotide-binding protein (stimulatory G-protein, G_s) subunit that stimulates adenylate cyclase.[29] When ATP is hydrolyzed, intracellular cAMP levels rise. The increased intracellular cAMP enhances a cAMP-dependent protein kinase which activates mRNA expression for the synthesis of the NAT enzyme protein or of a regulatory protein enhancing NAT activity.[30,31] In parallel with the rise in cAMP levels and NAT activity at night, there is a peak activity of a phosphodiesterase, which hydrolyzes cAMP.[32] Although a rise in NAT activity is usually accompanied by increased melatonin biosynthesis in the rat pineal, this is less apparent in some other species such as Syrian hamster.[33,34]

Activated α-receptors initiate a G-protein-linked phosphotidylinositol cascade process involving phospholipase C (PLC), diacylglycerol (DG), and protein kinase C (PKC).[35] PKC, in turn, activates adenylate cyclase and enhances NAT activity and melatonin synthesis (Figure 3.6). cAMP rise by β-adrenergic stimulation may be amplified by phosphorylating G_s or adenylate cyclase. Since β-adrenergic stimulation is associated with the expression of protooncogene c-*fos*,[36,37] the entire network of signal transduction pathways may be linked with gene expression in the nucleus. Recently, a marked rise in c-*fos* expression at night was demonstrated in the rat pineal.[38]

An alternative regulatory mechanism of melatonin biosynthesis directly dependent on the light:dark cycle may exist in addition to the major β -adrenergic regulation control. Rhodopsin-like photosensitivity has been reported in the chick pineal,[39] which can convert 11-*cis* retinal to all-*trans* retinal.[40] These results probably explain why NAT activity is directly sensitive to light[41] and its circadian rhythm persists in cultured chick pineals.[39] Interested readers should also refer to a recent book on melatonin.[42]

V. NEUROENDOCRINE SYSTEMS

A neuroendocrine system has two components: neuronal and hormonal. When the origins of the two components are traced back to developmental stages, the hormonal component may also be derived from the nervous system such as the adrenal medulla. In other systems, the two components develop from separate origins and involve a wide variety of tissues.

A. NEUROSECRETORY NEURONS AND PARANEURONS

The neurons shown in Figure 3.7 have axonal and dendritic processes, are innervated by other neurons, and have polarized membranes for conducting action potentials. They do not innervate and secrete neural hormones directly into the blood. An ordinary neuron also secretes products such as NE. The product of a neurosecretory neuron, however, acts on target tissues over a long distance as a hormone instead of the small synaptic cleft.

Pinealocytes are classified as paraneurons. The concept of paraneurons began in the early 1970s. The term "paraneuron" was first proposed by Fujita at an "International Symposium on Chromaffin, Enterochromaffin, and Related Cells" (1975) held in Japan. According to Fujita et al.,[43] a paraneuron produces substances identical or related to neuronal secretions that are stored in neurosecretion-like and/or synaptic vesicle-like granules which are released by the cell in response to stimuli. Paraneurons are variable in structure and function. Examples include basal-granulated bipolar cells in the gut, chemoreceptors, melanocytes, mast cells, etc. Pinealocytes are typical paraneurons.

Pinealocytes are the principal cellular components of the pineal gland. They have cytoplasmic organelles such as synaptic ribbons and spherules, annulate lamellae, subsurface cisterns, and the several types of synaptic arrangements seen in relation to the pinealocyte soma and its processes.[44] Recent ultrastructural

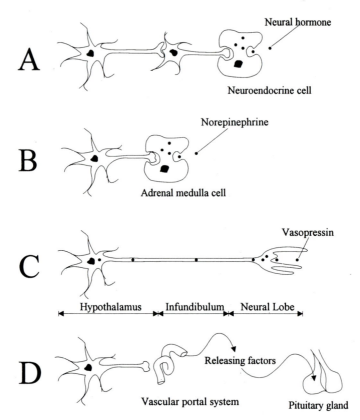

FIGURE 3.7. Neurosecretory neurons and paraneurons.

studies on monkey pinealocytes demonstrated that they receive direct synaptic contacts of nerve fibers with cholinergic terminal morphology.[45] Therefore, it is similar to other neurosecretory neurons innervated and regulated by neurons.

B.   ADRENAL MEDULLA

This is the oldest known endocrine gland developed from the nervous system. The secretory cells are differentiated postganglionic cells of the sympathetic nervous system. They secrete epinephrine and NE into the blood when their preganglionic nerve fibers are stimulated. Since this system is not directly related to reproductive physiology, it is discussed as a model of the neuroendocrine system for comparison.

C.   HYPOTHALAMO-ADENOHYPOPHYSEAL SYSTEM

There are groups of neurons in the hypothalamus, synthesizing and releasing neural hormones into the portal system. The neural hormones regulate the hormonal secretion of the anterior lobe of the pituitary. The adenohypophysis includes both the anterior and intermediate lobes of the pituitary.

The link between the hypothalamus and the adenohypophysis is the vascular portal system as shown in Figure 3.4. The long and short portal vessels are in continuation with the superior and inferior hypophyseal arteries, respectively. Neural hormones are secreted by neurons in different regions in the hypothalamus, and they terminate at the median eminence where the portal vessels originate. Since the releasing and inhibiting hormones are peptides, these neurons are called peptidergic neurons. They are, in turn, innervated by other neurons from higher centers of the brain.[46]

D. HYPOTHALAMO-NEUROHYPOPHYSEAL SYSTEM

There is a group of neurons in the anterior hypothalamus. Their cell bodies are located in supraoptic and paraventricular nuclei (SON and PVN) with axons extending to the posterior pituitary or neurohypophysis. Two major hormones secreted are vasopressin for antidiuretic function and oxytocin for inducing milk ejection. Oxytocin induces contraction of myoepithelial cells of the alveolus to eject the milk. Oxytocin is also involved in causing uterine contractions during labor.

As shown in Figure 3.8, the biosynthesis of vasopressin or oxytocin involves three steps.[47]

1. Transcription of the vasopressin or oxytocin genes
2. mRNA expression of the polypeptide precursor (prepropressin or preprooxyphysin) in rough endoplasmic reticulum (RER) and vesicles formed in the Golgi complex
3. Posttranslational cleavage to form the hormones during axonal transport of the vesicles to the nerve ending

The oxytocin gene as shown in Figure 3.8 consists of three exons, A, B, and C, as well as two introns. Exon A is mainly coded for the neural peptide, while exons B and C are for the carrier protein, neurophysin. Neurophysin is the major 10-kDa protein core carrying the hormone. Neurophysin I for oxytocin and neurophysin II for vasopressin are slightly different; the latter has an extra glycoprotein chain.[48]

Although the entire gene is transcribed to produce a full-length mRNA including both the exons and introns, transcriptional splicing results in a mature mRNA containing only a sequence coded by the exons. The mature mRNA is transported from the nucleus to RER where translation is initiated. The vasopressin gene is similar to the oxytocin gene except that exon A has 163 bp and exon C has 210 bp. Exon C for vasopressin is longer, containing an extra sequence for the glycoprotein which is later cleaved before secretion.

For oxytocin, the immediate translated protein precursor is preprooxyphysin with its amino terminal attached by a signal peptide (SP) which is mandatory for transport into the lumen of RER. During its transport from RER to the Golgi complex, the SP is removed. Vesicles are formed in the Golgi complex of the cell body and transported through the long axon in the infundibulum to its terminal in the neural lobe.

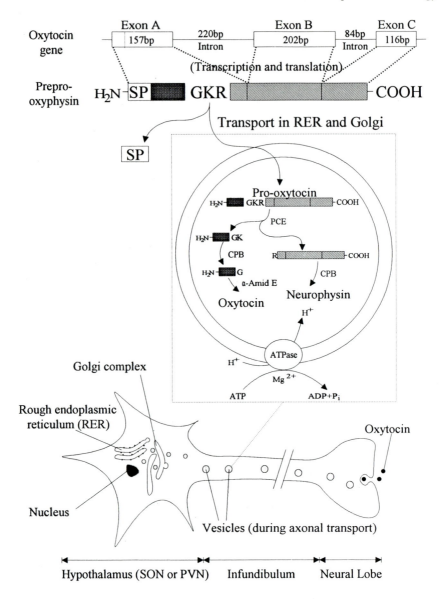

FIGURE 3.8.   Gene expression, biosynthesis, and secretion of oxytocin (see text for abbreviations).

Posttranslational processing is thought to occur in the membrane-bound secretory vesicle during axonal transport (see insert in Figure 3.8). Between the sequences of oxytocin and neurophysin I, there are three amino acids, glycine (G), lysine (K), and arginine (R), specific for the action of prohormone-converting enzyme (PCE), a dibasic residue specific endopeptidase. PCE results in the cleavage of the K-R bond so that the oxytocin sequence is separated from the neurophysin. By another two enzymes, carboxypeptidase-B-like enzyme (CPB) and α-peptidyl glycine-amidating monooxygenase (α-Amid-E), the lysine and glycine are removed, respectively. The arginine attached to the neurophysin is removed by CPB. For vasopressin, an extra step to cleave the glycoprotein from neurophysin II is necessary.[48]

The final secretory process at the nerve terminal involves membrane depolarization and Ca^{2+} influx. The entire sequence of events is initiated by depolarization of the neuron, resulting in the increased Ca^{2+} permeability which induces exocytosis. The secretory activity is determined by the frequency, number, and pattern of the incoming nerve impulses. Neurophysin is also secreted during exocytosis. In addition to being a carrier protein, neurophysin II for vasopressin has also been suggested to be a prolactin-releasing factor.[49] The role of neurophysin as a carrier protein appears to be too simple. Oxytocin and vasopressin are the two unique cases showing a gene having an exon for the carrier protein, and the gene products are transcribed and translated together. The neuropeptide and neurophysin are cotransported and cosecreted.[50] Interestingly, the exon C for the neurophysin is highly conserved throughout different vertebrates, showing its evolutionary significance.

E. PINEAL-REPRODUCTIVE SYSTEM

The system acts as a neuroendocrine transducer, conveying messages from the environment, such as the light-dark cycle, to the endocrine system. Since the circadian control mechanisms are extremely important in seasonal animals, this neuroendocrine system plays a vital role in regulating reproduction in these types of animals. Recent studies have shown presumptive melatonin receptors in neural and extraneural tissues, but the most important one is the pars tuberalis.

In recent years, the use of $2\text{-}^{125}\text{I}$-melatonin as a ligand has made studies on melatonin-binding sites more reproducible. Melatonin-binding sites have been demonstrated in cells of pars tuberalis where melatonin inhibits the forskolin-induced elevation of cAMP concentration.[51–54] In the chick retina, the specific binding of this radioligand has been found in the outer and inner plexiform layers[55,56] and in the retinal pigment epithelium.[57] These findings provide a strong indication that melatonin's physiological effects are at a cellular level via these binding sites. At the present time, the physiological relevance of these binding sites requires a parallel demonstration of melatonin actions. Melatonin agonists and antagonists with high specificity[58,59] are required to prove that these binding sites are, indeed, melatonin receptors. The definitive evidence will be the isolation of the receptor protein and the eventual sequencing of the gene.

VI. THE ENDOCRINE ORCHESTRA

All endocrine and neuroendocrine systems in a normal individual must be orchestrated and integrated to function holistically. Endocrine systems are glands without neural components; they secrete hormones into the blood circulation, e.g., the secretion of the hormones insulin and glucagon by the pancreas. Although some systems may not participate directly in reproductive processes, they must be well coordinated with the neuroendocrine systems involved in reproduction. In order to understand the interactions among different components, an analogy of an orchestra is used to visualize this complicated coordination.

The assignment of hierarchical order is arbitrary because it depends on the point of reference. If the gonad is considered as the central control of reproductive physiology, the other systems play the roles of providing regulatory signals and information. As part of the reproductive-neuroendocrine system, the endocrine orchestra is conducted by the pituitary gland that is, in turn, under the higher hierarchy of the neural components. The main players are the gonads, which help coordinate other players to respond to the signals from the conductor.

A.   THE CONDUCTOR AND PLAYERS

If the endocrine component of the neuroendocrine system is considered an orchestra, the pituitary gland plays the conductor's role in response to signals from the higher hierarchy and to feedbacks from the target tissues. It secretes ACTH, GH, LH, FSH, TSH, MSH, prolactin, vasopressin, and oxytocin as signals to the players.

Target reproductive organs are the players including the gonad, accessory sexual structures, and structures associated with secondary sex characteristics. In the female, the ovary is the main player, while the uterine structures and mammary glands are also being targeted. In addition, estrogen and progesterone secreted by the ovary have influences on fat distribution, bone maturation and turnover, and other physiological processes leading to feminine sex characteristics.

In the male, the testis is the main player. The penis, prostate gland, and seminal vesicles are the other reproductive structures involved. Hair distribution, muscle development, and sexual behavior are influenced. It should be emphasized that the testis, being the main player, also participates in regulating other players through testosterone.

B.   THE HIGHER HIERARCHY

The hypophysis is under the influence of higher centers in the hypothalamus, the gonad, and possibly the pineal gland. Hypophysiotropic hormones are signals given to the hypophysis by hypothalamic nuclei; they are releasing or inhibiting factors. They are TRH, CRH, GnRH, GHRH, somatostatin (or growth hormone-inhibiting hormone, GHIH), prolactin-releasing factor (PRF), and dopamine (or PIF).

PVN is an important hypothalamic center. It has magnocellular neurons, 20% of which project to the neural lobe for neuropeptide secretion. Another pathway of the magnocellular neuron is to the median eminence. Parvicellular neurons in PVN also project to the brainstem. Interestingly, most of these neurons contain oxytocin and vasopressin, though they are not the same neuronal type.

PVN is also a source of TRH, a tripeptide (p-Glu-His-Pro-NH$_2$) derived from a 30-kDa peptide.[48] The TRH-producing neurons terminate at the arcuate nucleus and median eminence. TRH is primarily responsible for stimulating the release of

TSH from thyrotropes in adenohypophysis. However, it also enhances prolactin and GH release. There are other effects, such as increased NE turnover, leading to the possible antidepressive action of TRH. Interestingly, TRH has also been postulated to play a role, with serotonin, in the control of male sexual behavior in rats.[60]

CRF is also produced in PVN; it is mainly found in parvicellular neurons and is colocalized with oxytocin and vasopressin. It is a peptide with 41 amino acids and is derived from a precursor molecule of 196 amino acids. The major function of CRF is to induce the release of hormones derived from proopiomelanocortin (POMC). POMC is the precursor for ACTH and β-lipotropin produced in corticotropes of adenohypophysis. As shown in Figure 3.6, PVN is also a relay station for the signals from the retina to the pineal gland. PVN also has a pathway to the third ventricle, secreting into CSF.

SON has magnocellular neurons, and up to 90% of them project to the neural lobe, as in PVN, for the secretion of oxytocin and vasopressin. As the name implies, SON is above the optic tract on both sides. There are two nuclei laterally symmetrical to each other at approximately the same level as the floor of the third ventricle.

The arcuate nucleus is situated in the mediobasal hypothalamus just beneath the floor of the third ventricle. It is an important nucleus for reproductive functions such as menstrual cyclicity,[61] primarily responsible for GnRH and dopamine. This is a neuronal oscillator responsive to many endogenous factors; one of them has been shown to be estrogen.[62] As demonstrated in the rat brain, estrogen is possibly involved in fetal neurogenesis, shaping sex differences in synaptology, postsynaptic membranes, and glia within the arcuate nucleus.

The gonad and the pineal gland appear to be the two ends of this hypothalamo-hypophyseal-gonadal axis. Environmental light-dark information is fed to the pineal gland, mostly through the retina, and is transduced into neuroendocrine signals acting at various levels. The gonad, as the ultimate target organ, responds to a set of these signals from the entire hierarchy. The ultimate effect expressed holistically is simply a timed developmental program of the gonad. In this way, gonadal development is orchestrated with environmental changes.

C. THE SIGNALS

There are specialized cell types responsible for producing the signals from the pituitary gland.[3] Known signals from the conductor include ACTH, prolactin, dopamine, oxytocin, vasopressin, and gonadotrophins. Although it is generally thought that most of the endocrine signals originate from the pituitary, recent data suggest that signals generated by the hypothalamus and pineal gland may act directly on reproductive target organs.

ACTH is secreted by chromophobe cells in the pars distalis of the adenohypophysis. The release is regulated by CRH from PVN in the hypothalamus. ACTH is a signal to the adrenal gland, regulating androgen and corticosteroid production. As part of the ACTH molecule in the precursor POMC, α-MSH is also secreted with a function in regulating skin pigmentation. Like MSH, β-endorphin or enkephalin is also found in POMC with an inhibitory effect on LH release, but a stimulatory effect on prolactin secretion.[63]

Prolactin is secreted by lactotrophs found in the pars distalis, and the release is regulated by a factor called PHI27 from PVN. Enkephalin is also produced in PVN and inhibits dopamine release in neighboring neurons. Dopamine is a PIF that downregulates prolactin production. Prolactin is a signal to the mammary gland for milk production. In association with oxytocin, prolactin is secreted by the anterior pituitary for stimulating milk secretion by alveolar epithelial cells.

Oxytocin is secreted by oxytocin neurons originated from both PVN and SON. It is a signal to the uterus for inducing smooth muscle contraction (oxytocic effect) and also to the mammary gland for milk ejection (galactogogic effect). The oxytocic effect of neurohypophyseal extracts on mammalian uteri was first discovered and confirmed by Dale nearly a century ago.[64,65] The oxytocic effect is important for the induction of labor, and the neuropeptide was named with reference to this effect as oxytocin.

Vasopressin is secreted by vasopressin neurons originated from both PVN and SON. It is an antidiuretic hormone with two main effects: pressor effect (V_1 receptor linked) and antidiuresis (V_2 receptor linked). The pressor effect is the induction of vascular smooth muscle contraction, and the antidiuresis is the enhanced water retention in the kidney. There are membrane-bound V_2 receptors on epithelial cells lining the lumen of distal tubules and collecting ducts. The receptor is linked with adenylate cyclase that converts ATP to cAMP, leading to activation of a protein kinase. The protein kinase phosphorylates some membrane proteins, causing an increase in water permeability. Since the lumen of tubules and ducts is hypotonic to the extracellular fluid, water flows from the lumen to the blood. V_1 receptors mediating a different effect are less defined; they are linked to Ca^{2+} instead of cAMP. Vasopressin is crucial for osmoregulation. Its secretory process is regulated by the neuron with osmoreceptors responsive to blood osmolality.

Recently, a new protein called pituitary adenylate cyclase-activating polypeptide (PACAP) has been found in a high concentration in the central nervous system (CNS), adrenal medulla, and testis.[66] cDNAs encoding its precursor have also been cloned in sheep, human, and rat. Immunohistochemical localization has shown PACAP-containing neural fibers in the median eminence, SON, and PVN. In addition, there are four types of high-affinity PACAP receptors demonstrated in CNS, pituitary, adrenal medulla, and germ cells. A recent study has shown that PACAP stimulates cAMP accumulation in cultured Sertoli cells of the rat.[67] It also stimulates the secretion of lactate, estradiol, and inhibin in a dose-response fashion. Therefore, PACAP may be a new member of hypothalamic signals with a direct action on the gonad.

The ultimate function of the endocrine orchestra is to provide a balanced control of all physiological processes in harmony with the neural component. The entire neuroendocrine system must allow the individual to interpret environmental signals and act accordingly to adapt. As shown in Figure 3.6, the pineal gland acts as a neurotransducer to interpret light:dark signals through the retina. It sends a series of melatonin signals through the blood circulation, orchestrating diversely expressed biorhythms at different levels.[19] As part of the system, the reproductive-neuroendocrine component drives a well-coordinated reproductive process responsive to environmental changes.

REFERENCES

1. **Gibbons, A.,** The brain as "sexual organ" (news and comment), *Science,* 253, 957, 1991.
2. **Sachs, B.D. and Meisel, R.L.,** The physiology of male sexual behavior, in *The Physiology of Reproduction,* Knobil, E. and Neill, J., Eds., Raven Press, New York, 1988, 1393.
3. **Pfaff, D.W. and Schwartz-Giblin, S.,** Cellular mechanisms of female reproductive behaviors, in *The Physiology of Reproduction,* Knobil, E. and Neill, J., Eds., Raven Press, New York, 1988, 1487.
4. **Genazzani, A.R., Gastaldi, M., Bidzinska, B., Mercuri, N., Genazzani, A.D., Nappi, R.E., Segre, A., and Petraglia, F.,** The brain as a target organ of gonadal steroids, *Psychoneuroendocrinology,* 17, 385, 1992.
5. **van Tienhoven, A.,** *Reproductive Physiology of Vertebrates,* 2nd ed., Cornell University Press, New York, 1983.
6. **Cushing, H.,** *The Pituitary Body and Its Disorders,* Lippincott, Philadelphia, 1912.
7. **Page, R.B.,** The anatomy of the hypothalamo-hypophyseal complex, in *The Physiology of Reproduction,* Knobil, E. and Neill, J., Eds., Raven Press, New York, 1988, 1161.
8. **Reiter, R.J. and Vaughan, M.K.,** Pineal gland, in *Endocrinology: People and Ideas,* McGann, S. M., Ed., American Physiological Society, New York, 1988, 215.
9. **Lerner, A.B., Case, J.D., Takahashi, Y., Lee, T. H., and Mori, W.,** Isolation of melatonin, the pineal gland factor that lightens melanocytes, *J. Am. Chem. Soc.,* 80, 2587, 1958.
10. **McCord, C.P. and Allen, E.P.,** Evidences associating pineal gland function with alterations in pigmentation, *J. Exp. Zool.,* 23, 207, 1917.
11. **Kitay, J.O. and Altschule, M.D.,** *The Pineal Gland,* Harvard University Press, Cambridge, 1954, 56.
12. **Lerner, A.B., Case, J.D., and Heinzelman, R.V.,** The structure of melatonin, *J. Am. Chem. Soc.,* 81, 6084, 1959.
13. **Lerner, A.B. and Case, J.D.,** Pigment cell regulatory factors, *J. Invest. Dermatol.,* 32, 211, 1959.
14. **Weissbach, H., Redfield, B.G., and Axelrod, J.,** Biosynthesis of melatonin: enzyme conversion of serotonin to N-acetylserotonin, *Biochem. Biophys. Acta,* 43, 352, 1960.
15. **Weissbach, H., Redfield, B.G., and Axelrod, J.,** The enzymic acetylation of serotonin and other naturally occurring amines, *Biochim. Biophys. Acta,* 54, 190, 1961.
16. **Axelrod, J. and Weissbach, H.,** Purification and properties of hydroxyindole-O-methyl transferase, *J. Biol. Chem.,* 236, 211, 1961.
17. **Quay, W.B.,** Retinal and pineal hydroxyindole-O-methyltransferase activity in vertebrates, *Life Sci.,* 4, 983, 1965.
18. **Yu, H.S.,** Melatonin in the eye: functional implications, in *Melatonin: Biosynthesis, Physiological Effects, and Clinical Applications,* Yu, H.S. and Reiter, R.J., Eds., CRC Press, Boca Raton, FL, 1993, 365.
19. **Yu, H.S., Tsin, A.T.C., and Reiter, R.J.,** Melatonin: history, biosynthesis, and assay methodology, in *Melatonin: Biosynthesis, Physiological Effects, and Clinical Applications,* Yu, H.S. and Reiter, R.J., Eds., CRC Press, Boca Raton, FL, 1993, 1.
20. **Moore, R.Y. and Klein, D.C.,** Visual pathways and the central neural control of a circadian rhythm in pineal serotonin *N*-acetyltransferase activity, *Brain Res.,* 71, 17, 1974.
21. **Reiter, R.J.,** The pineal gland, in *DeGroot's Endocrinology,* Vol. 2, 2nd ed., DeGroot, L.J., Ed., W.B. Saunders, Philadelphia, 1989, 240.
22. **Taylor, A.N. and Wilson, R.W.,** Electrophysiological evidence for the action of light on the pineal gland of the rat, *Experientia,* 26, 267, 1970.
23. **McGeer, E.G. and McGeer, P.L.,** Circadian rhythm in pineal tyrosine hydroxylase, *Science,* 153, 73, 1966.
24. **Craft, C.M., Morgan, W.W., and Reiter, R.J.,** 24-Hour changes in catecholamine synthesis in rat and hamster pineal glands, *Neuroendocrinology,* 38, 193, 1984.
25. **Deguchi, T. and Axelrod, J.,** Control of circadian change of serotonin *N*-acetyltransferase activity in the pineal gland by the β-adrenergic receptor, *Proc. Natl. Acad. Sci. U.S.A.,* 69, 2547, 1972.

26. **Pangerl, B., Pangerl, A., and Reiter, R.J.,** Circadian variations of adrenergic receptors in the mammalian pineal gland: a review, *J. Neural Transm.,* 81, 17, 1990.

27. **Ebadi, M. and Govitrapong, P.,** Orphan transmitters and their receptor sites in the pineal gland, in *Pineal Research Reviews,* Vol. 4, Reiter, R.J., Ed., Alan R. Liss, New York, 1986, 1.

28. **Jansen, K.L.R., Dragunow, M., and Faull, R.L.M.,** Sigma receptors are highly concentrated in the rat pineal gland, *Brain Res.,* 507, 158, 1990.

29. **Spiegel, A.M.,** Receptor-effector coupling by G-proteins: implications for endocrinology, *Trends Endocrinol. Metab.,* 1, 72, 1989.

30. **Klein, D.C.,** Photoneural regulation of the mammalian pineal gland, in *Photoperiodism, Melatonin and the Pineal,* Evered, D. and Clark, S., Eds., Pitman Medical, London, 1985, 38.

31. **Binkley, S.A.,** Circadian rhythms of pineal function in rats, *Endocrinol. Rev.,* 4, 255, 1983.

32. **Minneman, K.P. and Iversen, L.C.,** Diurnal rhythm in pineal cyclic nucleotide phosphodiesterase activity, *Nature (London),* 260, 59, 1976.

33. **Nilsson, K.J. and Reiter, R.J.,** *In vivo* stimulation of Syrian hamster pineal melatonin levels by isoproterenol plus phenylephrine is not accompanied by a commensurate large increase in N-acetyltransferase activity, *Neuroendocrinol. Lett.,* 11, 63, 1989.

34. **Menendez-Pelaez, A., Buzzell, G.R., Nonaka, K.O., and Reiter, R.J.,** *In vivo* administration of isoproterenol of forskolin during the light phase induces increase in the melatonin content of the Syrian hamster pineal gland without a commensurate rise in N-acetyltransferase activity, *Neurosci. Lett.,* 110, 314, 1990.

35. **Ho, A.K., Thomas, T.P., Chik, C.L., Anderson, W.B., and Klein, D.C.,** Protein kinase C: subcellular redistribution by increase Ca^{2+} influx, *J. Biol. Chem.,* 263, 9292, 1988.

36. **Yeh, C.K., Locus, J.M., and Kousvelari, E.E.,** β-adrenergic regulation of c-*fos* gene expression in an epithelial cell line, *FEBS Lett.,* 240, 118, 1988.

37. **Gubits, R.M., Smith, T.M., Fairhurst, J.L., and Hong, Y.,** Adrenergic receptors mediate changes in c-*fos* mRNA levels in brain, *Mol. Brain Res.,* 6, 39, 1989.

38. **Carter, D.A.,** Temporally defined induction of c-*fos* in the rat pineal, *Biochem. Biophys. Res. Commun.,* 166, 589, 1990.

39. **Deguchi, T.,** Rhodopsin-like photosensitivity of isolated chicken pineal gland, *Nature (London),* 290(5808), 702, 1981.

40. **Sun, J.I.H., Reiter, R.J., Nathan, M., and Tsin, A.T.C.,** Identification of 11-cis retinal and demonstration of its light-induced isomerization in the chicken pineal gland, *Neurosci. Lett.,* 133, 97, 1991.

41. **Wainwright, S.D. and Wainwright, L.K.,** Regulation of the cycle in chick pineal serotonin N-acetyltransferase activity *in vitro* by light, *J. Neurochem.,* 35(2), 451, 1980.

42. **Yu, H.S. and Reiter, R.J., Eds.,** *Melatonin: Biosynthesis, Physiological Effects, and Clinical Applications,* CRC Press, Boca Raton, FL, 1993.

43. **Fujita, T., Kanno, T., and Kobayashi, S.,** *The Paraneuron,* Springer-Verlag, Tokyo, 1988.

44. **Bhatnagar, K.P.,** The ultrastructure of mammalian pinealocytes: a systematic investigation, *Microsc. Res. Techniq.,* 21, 85, 1992.

45. **Ichimura, T.,** The ultrastructure of neuronal-pinealocytic interconnections in the monkey pineal, *Microsc. Res. Tech.,* 21, 124, 1992.

46. **Kupfermann, I.,** Hypothalamus and limbic system I: peptidergic neurons, homeostasis, and emotional behavior, in *Principles of Neural Science,* 2nd ed., Kandel, E.R. and Schwartz, J.H., Eds., Elsevier, New York, 1985, 46.

47. **Hedge, G.A., Colby, H.D., and Goodman, R.L.,** *Clinical Endocrine Physiology,* W.B. Saunders, Philadelphia, 1987.

48. **Weiner, R.I., Findell, P.R., and Kordon, C.,** Role of classic and peptideneuromediators in the neuroendocrine regulation of LH and prolactin, in *The Physiology of Reproduction,* Knobil, E. and Neill, J., Eds., Raven Press, New York, 1988, 1235.

49. **Shin, S.H., Obonsawin, M.C., and Vincent, S.,** The major prolactin releasing activity from bovine posterior pituitary is identified as neurophysin II, in *Prolactin: Basic and Clinical Correlates,* MacLeod, R.M., Thorner, M.O., and Scapagnini, U., Eds., Liviana Press, Padova, 1985, 95.

50. **Neill, J.D.,** Prolactin secretion and its control, in *The Physiology of Reproduction,* Knobil, E. and Neill, J., Eds., Raven Press, New York, 1988, 1379.

51. **Williams, L.M., Morgan, P.L., Hastings, M.H., Lawson, W., Davidson, G., and Howell, H.E.,** Melatonin receptor sites in the Syrian hamster brain and pituitary: localization and characterization using [^{125}I]iodomelatonin, *J. Neuroendocrinol.,* 1, 315, 1989.

52. **Morgan, P.J., William, L.M., Davidson, G., Lawson, W., and Howell, H.E.,** Melatonin receptors on ovine pars tuberalis: characterization and autoradiographical localization, *J. Neuroendocrinol.,* 1, 1, 1989.

53. **Morgan, P.J., Lawson, W., Davidson, G., and Howell, H.E.,** Melatonin inhibits cyclic AMP production in cultured ovine pars tuberalis cells, *J. Mol. Endocrinol.,* 3, R5, 1989.

54. **Morgan, P.J., Lawson, W., Davidson, G., and Howell, H.E.,** Guanine nucleotides regulate the affinity of melatonin receptors on the ovine pars tuberalis, *Neuroendocrinology,* 50, 359, 1989.

55. **Dubocovich, M.L. and Takahashi, J.S.,** Use of 2-[^{125}I]iodomelatonin to characterize melatonin binding sites in chicken retina, *Proc. Natl. Acad. Sci. U.S.A.,* 84, 3916, 1987.

56. **Laitinen, J.T. and Saavedra, J.M.,** The chick retinal melatonin receptor revisited: localization and modulation of agonist binding with guanine nucleotides, *Brain Res.,* 528, 349, 1990.

57. **Chong, N.W.S. and Sugden, D.,** The nucleotides regulate 2-[^{125}I]iodomelatonin binding sites in chick retinal pigment epithelium but not in neuronal retina, *J. Neurochem.,* 57, 685, 1991.

58. **Dubocovich, M.L.,** Luzindole (N-0774): a novel melatonin receptor antagonist, *J. Pharmacol. Exp. Therap.,* 246(3), 902, 1988.

59. **Dubocovich, M.L.,** Pharmacology and function of melatonin receptors, *FASEB J.,* 2, 2765, 1988.

60. **Hansen, S., Svensson, L., Hökfelt, T., and Everitt, B.J.,** 5-Hydroxytryptamine-thyrotropin releasing hormone interactions in the spinal cord: effects on parameters of sexual behavior in the male rat, *Neurosci. Lett.,* 42, 299, 1983.

61. **Krause, B. and Moller, S.,** Menstrual cycle, opioids and hypothalamic amenorrhea: from physiology to pathology, *Zentralbl. Gynakol.,* 112, 725, 1990 (in German).

62. **Naftolin, F., Garcia-Segura, L.M., Keefe, D., Leranth, C., Maclusky, N.J., and Brawer, J.R.,** Estrogen effects on the synaptology and neural membranes of the rat hypothalamic arcuate nucleus, *Biol. Reprod.,* 42, 21, 1990.

63. **Mastroianni, L., Jr. and Coutifaris, C.,** Reproductive physiology, in *The F.I.G.O. Manual of Human Reproduction,* Vol. 1, Rosenfield, A. and Fathalla, M.F., Eds., Parthenon Publishing Group, Park Ridge, NJ, 1990.

64. **Dale, H.H.,** On some physiological actions of ergot, *J. Physiol. (London),* 34, 165, 1906.

65. **Dale, H.H.,** The action of extracts of the pituitary body, *Biochem. J.,* 4, 427, 1909.

66. **Arimura, A.,** Pituitary adenylate cyclase activating polypeptide (PACAP): discovery and current status of research, *Regulatory Peptides,* 37, 287, 1992.

67. **Heindel, J.J., Powell, C.J., Paschall, C.S., Arimura, A., and Culler, M.D.,** A novel hypothalamic peptide, pituitary adenylate cyclase activating peptide, modulates Sertoli cell function *in vitro, Biol. Reprod.,* 47, 800, 1992.

4 Reproductive Cycles: The Ovarian and Endometrial Cycles

CHAPTER CONTENTS

I.   WHAT IS A REPRODUCTIVE CYCLE?

There are two types of reproductive cycles: cyclic events with alternating reproductive activity and quiescence (e.g., seasonal cycle) or cyclic events within the period of reproductive activity (e.g., menstrual cycle). These two types may share similar regulatory mechanisms involving the interactions between the internal and external environment.

Why should a species adopt a certain breeding season? There are two causes proposed: ultimate and proximate. Ultimate causes are the favorable environment for the growth of the young. Proximate causes are the favorable environment (e.g., temperature and food availability) for the parents to reproduce. However, another important factor is the photoperiod, i.e., the light-dark cycle, which acts as a proximate cause to regulate reproductive activities via the neuroendocrinology of the parents.

Although reproductive cycles are apparently driven by external causes, the cyclicity in seasonal breeders is endogenous. The animal has mechanisms to synchronize the endogenous cycles with the environmental cycle. Again, we have two types of endogenous cycles: circadian and circannual. Without external signals, a circadian rhythm has a period close to 24 h, while a circannual rhythm is nearly 365 days. The circadian rhythm is synchronized to the light-dark cycle and the circannual rhythm by the yearly changes in the light-dark cycle and/or temperature. The effect of the light-dark cycle and circadian rhythms will be discussed in Chapter 11.

As in other vertebrates, there are well-defined circadian rhythms in humans associated with reproduction. Most of these rhythms are hormonal, and our internal environment is responsive to changes in daylength. In spite of this, human reproduction is apparently nonseasonal, though yearly reproductive patterns do exist in some of the population studied. Mostly, the reproductive cycle correlates with the pattern of their activities. The only rigorous reproductive cycle is the menstrual cycle in women with well-defined hormonal profiles and physiological changes.

II.   THE MENSTRUAL CYCLE

Menstruation has long been known to occur in humans and some other primates, and its possible control by the ovary was postulated by a Dutch physician, Lambert van Velthuysens (1622–1685), and was experimentally tested in the 17th century. The other primates having menstruation include the great apes (Pongidae), the gibbons (Hylobatidae), and the Old World monkeys (Cercopithecidae). Interestingly, almost all New World monkeys (Callithrichidae and Cebidae) such as marmosets and tamarins do not menstruate.[1] In other mammalian species with the placenta (Eutheria), they have equivalent cycles known as the estrous cycle.

The menstrual cycle, in contrast to the estrous cycle, involves endometrial bleeding (i.e., menstruation or the shedding of menses). The start of bleeding is

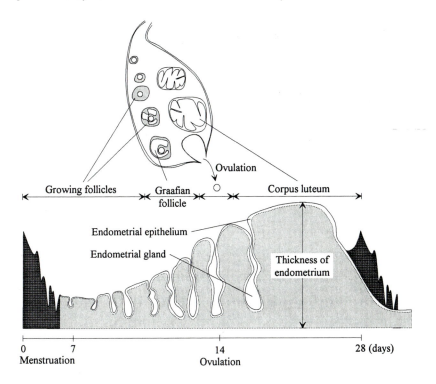

FIGURE 4.1. The ovarian and endometrial cycles.

designated as day 1 of the menstrual cycle. Since estrous animals have no noticeable bleeding, the demonstration of estrous behavior (i.e., estrus or "in heat") is a sign showing the onset of the estrous cycle. In humans, the occurrence of similar behavioral changes is questionable. Both the menstrual and estrous cycles are coupled with the ovarian cycle that is, in turn, regulated by LH and FSH from the hypothalamo-adenohypophyseal system.

Despite the great variation in the expression of the cycles, the basic theme is almost identical. Cyclic hormonal changes are precisely timed and monitored to synchronize ovulation with the preparation of the uterine for pregnancy. The hypothalamo-adenohypophyseal neuroendocrine system secretes LH and FSH to signal the cyclic changes in the ovary where estrogens and progesterone are produced to regulate the activity of hypothalamic nuclei involved. Follicular development is the major event of the ovarian cycle and is synchronized with endometrial growth as summarized in Figure 4.1.

The mean period of the menstrual cycle is 28 days with a typical ovulation time at day 14 in response to an LH surge 36 h before the release of the ovum. The preovulatory period is called the follicular phase starting from the first day of menses, while the postovulatory period is the luteal phase ending with the onset of menstruation. Figure 4.2 shows the different phases of the human menstrual cycle. The timing appears to be imposed by the luteinizing hormone-releasing

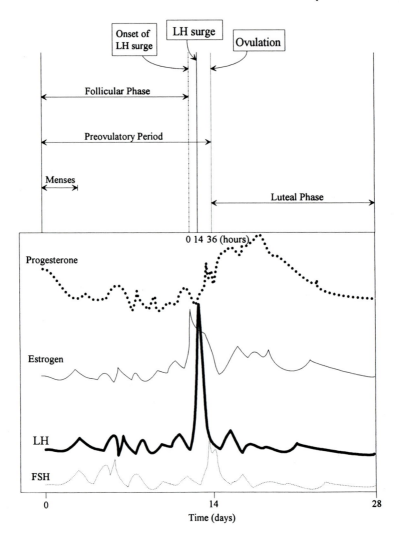

FIGURE 4.2.   The human menstrual cycle.

hormone (LHRH) pulse generator in the mediobasal hypothalamus where the arcuate nucleus and periventricular structures are found, at least in the rhesus monkey. The rhesus monkey has been a widely accepted animal model for studying the human menstrual cycle.[2]

A.   OVARIAN CYCLE

In humans, the mean time for a primary follicle to become a Graafian follicle just before ovulation is 85 to 90 days.[3] In other words, when a primary follicle is given a signal to develop, it will be scheduled to be ovulated 3 to 4 cycles later if it can form a Graafian follicle successfully. Since the number of primary follicles remains constant in a normal ovary, the recruitment of primordial follicles seems to occur frequently. These early stages of follicular development are often considered independent of LH and FSH influences. Perhaps, the follicular developmental program allows a supply of a sufficient number of antral follicles in each cycle to provide at least one Graafian follicle suitable for ovulation. Other antral follicles undergo atresia, while the "privileged" follicle becomes dormant.

On day 1 of the menstrual cycle, such a dominant follicle is not readily discernible. During the early follicular phase, a high level of FSH induces an increase in the number of LH receptors on the theca cells of the dominant follicle. By days 6 to 10, the dominant follicle becomes distinguishable by its enormous size; it reaches a diameter of up to 13 mm. The next healthy follicle is usually smaller than half of its size. With more LH receptors, the theca cells are more responsive to LH and begin synthesizing an increasing amount of androstenedione and testosterone. According to the "two-cell-type, two-gonadotrophin" theory (see Chapter 2), these androgens are transported to the granulosa cells where aromatases are present for converting them to estrogens. This leads to a rapid increase in the blood estradiol level.

Estradiol has dual effects on LH and FSH releases; it is inhibitory at low concentrations, but stimulatory when its plasma level exceeds 150 pg/ml for 36 h. This sudden reversal of estradiol effects brings about an enormous LH surge and a smaller FSH surge, leading to ovulation. Estradiol mainly acts at the level of pituitary as a gonadotrophin-inhibiting or -releasing hormone. Recent studies have also suggested its direct effects on the LHRH pulse generator possibly located within the LHRH neuronal network. Cultured LHRH neurons are capable of pulsatile LH secretion into the medium.[4]

Just before the gonadotrophin surge, there is a rise in serum progesterone that may play a role in causing ovulation. A recent study[5] has demonstrated the effects of a low dose (1 mg/day, orally) of the antiprogesterone RU486 on the timing of the gonadotrophin surge and ovulation in women with normal menstrual cycles. The drug treatment delays the preovulatory rise in progesterone, gonadotrophin surge, and ovulation. Later progesterone administration (5 to 10 mg/day, intra-muscular, for 2 days) to a 5-day course of RU486 induced LH and FSH surges and completely reversed the effects of RU486 at midcycle. The authors suggested that progesterone may be the ultimate ovarian signal to the estrogen-primed hypothalamic-pituitary unit to trigger the gonadotrophin surge that leads to ovulation.

Subsequent to ovulation, the ruptured follicle develops into a new endocrine organ, the corpus luteum, dedicated to progesterone production (see Figure 4.1). The process is called luteinization. The progesterone level continues to rise until a maximum on days 21 to 22 of the menstrual cycle. Progesterone reduces the LHRH pulse frequency, but increases the amplitude, maintaining a baseline LH necessary for the corpus luteum. FSH level is low, and the development of new follicles is suppressed until the end of the cycle. In the absence of pregnancy, the corpus luteum regresses, the LH level decreases, and the FSH level increases just before menstruation. A new ovarian cycle begins.

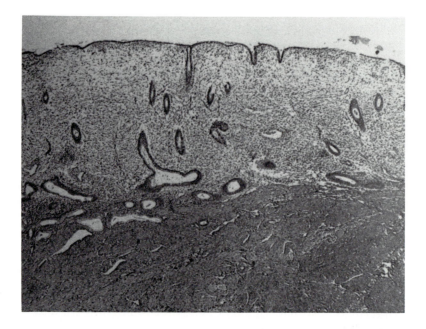

FIGURE 4.3. Human endometrium at the early follicular phase of the menstrual cycle. (From Dallenbach-Hellweg, G. and Poulsen, H., *Atlas of Endometrial Histopathology,* Munksgaard, Copenhagen, 1985. With permission.)

Synchronizing with the menstrual cycle, the ovarian cycle begins with at least one antral follicle becoming responsive to FSH when the corpus luteum loses its inhibitory effect on the follicle at the conclusion of the previous cycle. Since the development from primary follicles and the complete regression of corpus lutea require a much longer time, several generations of developing follicles and regressing corpus lutea with an ovary can be observed at one time.

B. ENDOMETRIAL CYCLE

The early concepts of the menstrual cycle were based on studies on the endometrial cycle. The endometrium is the innermost wall of the uterus lining the uterine cavity. It consists of long and narrow glandular lumina lined by columnar epithelial cells and the stroma with abundant blood capillaries. The endometrial cycle is a repetitive, alternating thickening and loss of tissues (see Figures 4.3 to 4.5). The renewal process involves proliferation and differentiation of stromal and glandular cells with extensive vascularization. These events are known to be regulated by the interplay between estradiol and progesterone.[6]

As early as 1950, a detailed study on endometrial changes based on 8000 biopsies was performed by Noyes et al.[7] On days 4 to 7 of the menstrual cycle in women, the endometrium just after menstruation is less than 3 mm in thickness, and the glands are short and straight (see Figure 4.3). As the blood estrogen concentration increases, it enters the proliferative stage, which is roughly subdivided

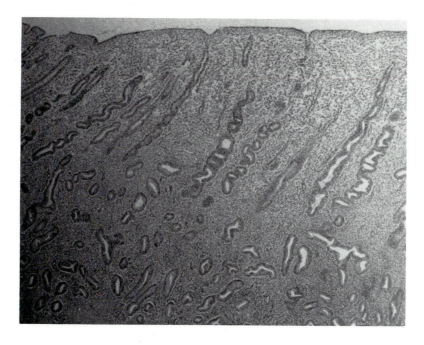

FIGURE 4.4. Human endometrium at the midfollicular phase of the menstrual cycle. (From Dallenbach-Hellweg, G. and Poulsen, H., *Atlas of Endometrial Histopathology,* Munksgaard, Copenhagen, 1985. With permission.)

into early, mid, and late phases. During the midproliferative phase from days 8 to 10, both the stroma and glandular epithelium are highly proliferative, and the tubular glands elongate and start to coil (see Figure 4.4). Under the full effect of high estrogen levels, rapid differentiation of the cells occurs during the late proliferative stage from days 11 to 14 (see Figure 4.5).

By the time of ovulation, the endometrium is fully developed with a pseudostratified epithelium and dense stroma. The stromal cells have little cytoplasm with many mitotic nuclei. Ovulation indicates the change from the proliferative to luteal phase, and rapid changes in the endometrium are discernible within 1 to 2 days. Vacuoles are formed, and more blood capillaries are developed in a spiral configuration. In response to increasing progesterone concentration, glycogen starts to accumulate in the basal side of the epithelial cell. On day 18, the glycogen deposits in the vacuoles move to the apex of the epithelial cells and are secreted into the lumen of the gland. More and more acidophilic secretory products are found in the lumen. These changes are characteristic features of ovulation for diagnosis.

In a normal uterus, the endometrium at this time is suitable for implantation of the zygote if fertilization has occurred. Even in the absence of a zygote, the endometrial secretion continues and is maintained until 1 week before menstruation. Significant changes become conspicuous by day 23; stromal cells start to enlarge and differentiate into decidual-like cells. At the same time, lymphocyte

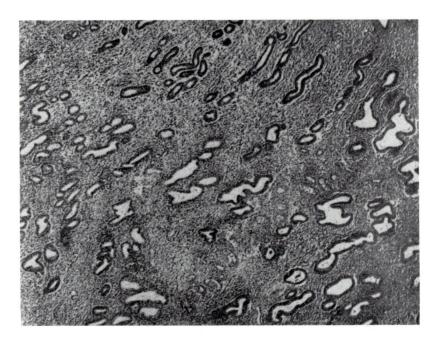

FIGURE 4.5. Human endometrium at the late follicular phase of the menstrual cycle. (From Dallenbach-Hellweg, G. and Poulsen, H., *Atlas of Endometrial Histopathology,* Munksgaard, Copenhagen, 1985. With permission.)

infiltration begins on days 24 to 25. Many polymorphonuclear leukocytes can be found in the final days.

Lymphocyte infiltration is the prelude to the endometrial breakdown on day 1 of the menstrual cycle. The extent of tissue loss varies greatly from one uterus to another. Generally, about two thirds in thickness of the stratum spongiosum are lost, while the tissues close to the basal layer remain intact at the end of menstruation. By day 4, the lumen surface of these tissue remains undergoes repair that involves extensive regeneration and rapid reorganization.[8]

C.   OVIDUCTAL CYCLE

In contrast to the endometrium, atrophy and deciliation of the oviductal epithelium occur in response to progesterone during the luteal phase, especially in the oviductal funnel (fimbriae). When the corpus luteum regresses just prior to menstruation, the oviductal epithelium enters the ciliogenic process — the regeneration of cilia on the epithelial cells. At this time, progesterone drops dramatically and its antagonistic action estrogen subsides. As the estrogen level increases in the early follicular phase, ciliogenesis continues with an enhanced secretory activity.

By the time of ovulation, the differentiation of the fully ciliated and secretory oviductal epithelium is completed, while the endometrium is still developing. The preparation of a fully functional oviduct is important for sperm transport, ovum selection, and zygote migration. There are also biochemical changes in the composition of the oviductal secretion. Using an organ culture system, the human oviduct obtained during midcycle has been shown to synthesize 120- to 130-kDa glycoproteins which were almost undetectable in oviducts from other stages of the menstrual cycle.[9] As the progesterone level increases after ovulation, the oviductal epithelium enters its degenerative phase again, while the endometrium continues to undergo hypertrophy.

III. THE ESTROUS CYCLE

According to Conaway,[10] reproductive cycles in Eutheria are classified into five types as shown in Table 4.1. Menstruating primates including humans are classified in type IA, but, as discussed in the preceding section, the menstrual cycle is substantially different from the estrous cycle, especially in the endometrial cycle. In the discussion of the human menstrual cycle, however, it is imperative to discuss the estrous cycle because two of our common laboratory animal models, the rabbit and the rat, are estrous. In addition, the rabbit is an induced ovulator, while the rat is not. With the understanding of their differences and similarities, extrapolation of animal data to human reproductive physiology would be more cautious.

Within a single type, the mechanisms involved may be different between two species (see Table 4.1). The superficial similarities may not correlate with neuroendocrine mechanisms. The diversification of the mammalian reproductive cycle may have its evolutionary advantage. Conaway has suggested an explanation based on prey-predator relationships. Type IA animals are usually prey species with a longer lifespan so that a short estrous cycle is not necessary. Types IB and IIB are large predators with low reproductive rates. In contrast, types IIA and III are small prey species of high reproductive rates that may compensate for their short lifespan and high mortality rates.[11]

A. THE RAT ESTROUS CYCLE

Like humans, the laboratory rat *(Rattus norvegicus)* is a spontaneous ovulator and nonseasonal mammal.[11] The rat ovarian cycle continues throughout the year and is apparently similar to the human cycle. The estrous cycle, however, has a short period of 4 to 5 days with a higher frequency of ovulation. Besides, the number of ovulated eggs is higher from both ovaries in each cycle, suggesting that the turnover rate of the rat ovarian cycle is higher than that in humans.

As shown in Figure 4.6, the rat estrous cycle consists of four major stages: proestrus (12 to 14 h), estrus (25 to 27 h), metestrus (6 to 8 h), and diestrus (55 to 57 h). Diestrus can be subdivided into I and II. Metestrus is a transition period between estrus and early diestrus I. As in humans, ovulation is also triggered by LH surge. The profiles of plasma LH, estradiol, and progesterone are quite similar to the human menstrual cycle, but the whole period is very much shortened. At proestrus, the rising estradiol acts on the preoptic hypothalamic area and limbic structures above the medial preoptic area. Estradiol reaches a peak on day 3 and causes LH and prolactin peaks.

TABLE 4.1.

Types of Estrous Cycles in Nonpregnant Eutheria

Type	Examples	Cycle length	Features
IA	Guinea pigs *(Cavia porcellus)*	5–18 d	Spontaneous ovulation
	Sheep *(Ovis aries)*	16 d	
	Cattle *(Box taurus)*	21 d	
	Swine *(Sus scrofa)*	21 d	
	Horse *(Equus caballus)*	21 d	
	Elephant *(Loxodonta africana)*	28–30 d	
IB	Dog *(Canis familiaris)*	60–70 d	Spontaneous ovulation
IIA	Rabbit *(Oryctolagus cuniculus)*	Induced pseudopregnancy (17 d)	Induced ovulation (9–12 h p.c.)
IIB	Cat *(Felis domesticus)* Ferret *(Mustela furo)*	Induced pseudopregnancy (1–2 months)	Induced ovulation (30–50 h p.c.)
III	Golden hamster *(Mesocricetus auratus)*	4 d	Spontaneous ovulation and induced pseudopregnancy
	House mouse *(Mus musculus)*	4–5 d	
	Rat *(Rattus norvegicus)*	4–5 d	

Note: h = hours; d = days; p.c. = postcoitus. Data from Ramirez, V.D. and Beyer, C., The ovarian cycle of the rabbit: its neuroendocrine control, in *The Physiology of Reproduction,* Knobil, E. and Neill, J., Eds., Raven Press, New York, 1988, 1873.

As in humans, rising estradiol is a result of increased secretion by the developing follicle, and progesterone is produced by the corpus luteum after ovulation. Postovulatory rise in progesterone is inhibitory to the adenohypophyseal response to LHRH. A high concentration of progesterone during metestrus and diestrus may sometimes block ovulation. This is similar to the contraceptive effect of progesterone-only pills used in humans for suppressing ovulation.

It should be noted that the cycle shown in Figure 4.6 is a typical 4-day cycle. Even in the same rat, the cycle length may sometimes be 5 days. A prolonged progesterone secretion occurs in a 5-day cycle. This hormonal change may be the cause or the result of the cycle extension. The timing of the cycle in rats has been suggested to be controlled by the clock in the CNS, such as the SCN, possibly with the involvement of the pineal gland. Activity of melatonin-synthesizing enzymes in the pineal gland changes drastically during the estrous cycle in rats under the influence of gonadal steroids.[12] Since the pineal gland is responsive to the light:dark cycle, these interactions may be part of the timing mechanism (see Chapter 3).

There are also cyclic changes in the endometrial and vaginal wall. Stages of the estrous cycle can be identified by examining the vaginal smear. This had been

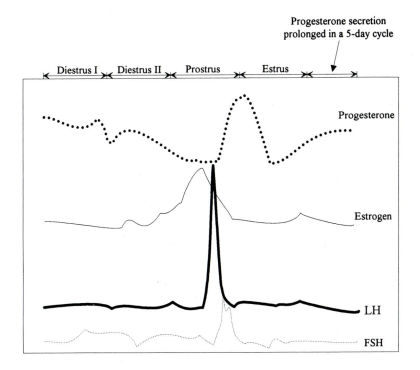

FIGURE 4.6. The rat estrous cycle.

studied by Evans and Long as early as 1921,[13] and an excellent account was provided by the classical textbook for general endocrinology by Turner and Bagnara.[14] Briefly, the characteristic cheesy masses of cornified cells are found in the vaginal smear during estrus while ovulation occurs. Metestrus is a variable transition period when leukocytes begin to infiltrate. The vaginal smear at metestrus contains many leukocytes in the presence of a few cornified cells that are absent in diestrus. Diestrus is the longest period of about 2 to 3 days. The endometrium begins to build up again, while the corpus luteum regresses. The vaginal mucosa remains thin until proestrus, during which the vaginal smear is dominated by individual or sheets of nucleated epithelial cells.

B.   INDUCED OVULATION AND PSEUDOPREGNANCY

The rat estrous cycle is an example of spontaneous ovulators. Ovulation is scheduled to occur during estrus while the female rat is "in heat" for copulation. Behavioral changes include quivering of ears and lordosis in response to approaching male rats. As in humans, if copulation is timed with ovulation, fertilization may occur. However, there is another type of ovulatory mechanism called induced ovulation. The rabbit is an excellent example.

In normal estrous rabbits, ovulation is induced by mating. Figure 4.7 shows the postcoital changes in plasma concentrations of LH, FSH, and 20α-dihydroprogesterone. LH surge is still the hormonal trigger for ovulation, but the LH

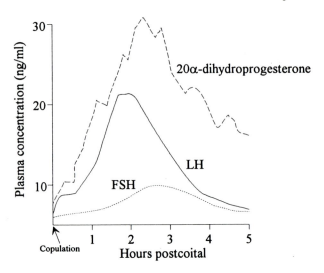

FIGURE 4.7.   Hormonal profiles in the estrous rabbit. (Data from van Tienhoven, A., *Reproductive Physiology of Vertebrates,* 2nd ed., Cornell University Press, New York, 1983.)

surge is induced within 2 h after mating. A recent study provided some data supporting that gonadotrophin-releasing hormone (GnRH) and norepinephrine (NE) releases from mediobasal and anterior hypothalamus are directly induced by mating.[15] A neural route involving NE is part of the reflex ovulatory mechanism. Wild rabbits are seasonal breeders, but laboratory rabbits can copulate throughout the year. Occasionally, ovulation may not occur in some laboratory rabbits for 1 to 2 months within a year.[11] As the rat, the rabbit has an estrous cycle with spontaneous estrus.

Ovulation in estrous rabbits is possibly induced by copulation because of physical vaginal stimulation. After fertilization, a normal pregnancy takes about 1 month. For various reasons, if fertilization does not occur, the rabbit may become pseudopregnant for about 17 days. Pseudopregnancy can also be induced by physical stimulation of the vagina and is found in many other species such as rats and mice. A pseudopregnant rat can easily be prepared by cervical stimulation with a plastic spatula. In mice, pseudopregnancy is commonly induced by mating with vasectomized males. These cases provide further evidence showing the neural involvement during induced ovulation. The onset of pseudopregnancy in rats clearly has been shown to be associated with an increase in hypothalamic neuronal activity.[16]

It should be noted that the natural induced ovulation in rabbits is different from hormonally induced ovulation in mice or humans. In contrast to rabbits, the association between cervical stimulation and ovulation is apparently lost in rats or mice though they become pseudopregnant. Pseudopregnancy in laboratory rodents has been a useful tool in reproductive biology. In embryo transfer, preimplantation zygotes injected into the uterus of pseudopregnant mice at the right time can implant successfully. In humans, ovulation can only be induced hormonally in responsive women. Although pseudopregnancy does not exist in humans, transfer of preimplantation zygotes to the uterus of a woman at the right time of the menstrual cycle also results in a successful pregnancy (see Chapter 9).

IV. OVULATION

The mechanism of ovulation has been a subject of extensive study since the discovery of the follicle in the 15th century.[17] The initial controversy was the existence of smooth muscle in the follicular wall until 1849 when von Kolliker demonstrated smooth muscle in the frog ovary[18] and, subsequently, in the human follicle where smooth muscle was found by Thomson to be less abundant than other species.[19] The dispute then shifted to the role of smooth muscle of the ovary in ovulation because it had been suggested to be responsible for the discharge of ova similar to the penis discharging semen. The contraction of smooth muscle was thought to contribute to the rise in intrafollicular pressure induced by increased arterial pressure, leading to the rupture of follicular wall. Since no increase in intrafollicular pressure can be demonstrated, the smooth muscle was later considered to be nonessential. So far, there is no known role played by the smooth muscle, though it may possibly facilitate the evacuation of follicle contents after ovulation.

In 1919, Thomson[19] had already introduced the concept of the "multifactor hypothesis of ovulation." He thought that the increase in follicular size was attributed to an increase in intrafollicular pressure and the presence of some enzymes causing thecal digestion. The search for intrafollicular enzymes was started by Schochet as early as 1916.[20] Many enzymes are now known to be present in the follicular fluid, though only plasmin and collagenase may be involved in ovulation.[21] In addition to enzymes, the roles of neural innervation and ovarian blood supply have also been studied. It is likely that the mechanism of ovulation depends on a multitude of factors.

Over the years, there have been different models proposed to explain ovulation based on either a possible rise in intrafollicular pressure or enzymatic digestion of the follicular wall. The model of intrafollicular pressure is the weakest since the rise cannot be demonstrated. In 1980, Espey hypothesized an inflammatory model of ovulation with an effort to encompass all known physical and biochemical events occurring in a periovulatory follicle.[22] As later suggested by Lipner,[21] the mechanism can be called the multifactor hypothesis of ovulation as originally conceived by Thomson.

A. THE WORKING MODEL

As recently reviewed by LeMaire,[23] the ovulatory sequence triggered by LH, with the help of FSH, is mainly mediated through adenylate cyclase, cAMP, and cAMP-dependent protein kinase (see Figure 4.8). The increased cAMP level leads to a series of four steps in the ovulatory sequence. First is the stimulation of steroidogenesis, followed by the second step of increased prostaglandin/leukotriene synthesis stimulated by cyclooxygenase/lipooxygenase. The third

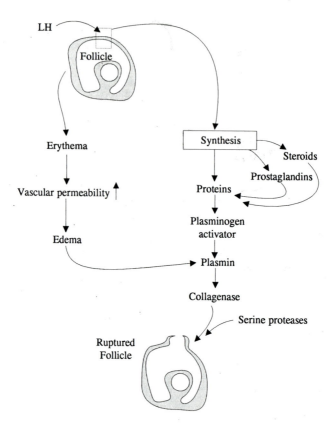

FIGURE 4.8.   Proposed mechanism of ovulation. (After Lipner, H., *The Physiology of Reproduction,* Knobil, E. and Neill, J., Eds., Raven Press, New York, 1988, 447.)

step is the conversion of plasminogen to plasmin catalyzed by plasminogen activator. The fourth step is the activation of latent collagenase and an increase in collagenase inhibitors, though the direct role of cAMP is uncertain. It is possible that leukotrienes, prostaglandins, and plasmin are involved in collagenase activation as in an inflammatory response.

Collagenase digests collagen fibers in the follicular wall, which is further attacked by plasmin and possibly other proteolytic enzymes such as proteoglycanases. As the dissociation of the collagen fibers proceeds, there is thinning of the entire follicular wall; it weakens and formation of the stigma and rupture is localized at the apex of the follicle. The intrafollicular pressure remains constant from 15 to 20 mmHg. Although smooth muscle contractions and vascular changes such as increased permeability, vasodilation, and vasoconstriction are known to be caused by prostaglandins and leukotrienes, the role of these processes in ovulation is still uncertain. The cascade reaction of enzymes to LH stimulation resulting in collagen proteolysis and the ultimate rupture of the follicular wall appears to be the main engine of the ovulatory mechanism.

B. OVARIAN INNERVATION AND VASCULATURE

The presence of innervation to the ovarian smooth muscle with the well-formed vasculature led to the description of the ovary as an erectile organ. Follicular contractions in response to hCG were first demonstrated by Lipner and Maxwell in follicles autotransplanted to the anterior chamber of the rabbit eye.[24] The role of ovarian contractibility in ovulation is uncertain.

1. Innervation

The gross anatomy of ovarian innervation was first described in 1867. The nerves arise from spinal segments T_{10} and T_{11} through the aortorenal plexus, running along with the ovarian artery into the ovary at the hilus. The parasympathetic innervation is from the vagus and also spinal segments S2 to S4, but they are nonessential as shown by denervation studies.[21] The presence of both adrenergic and cholinergic nerves in the follicular wall has been demonstrated also in humans.

Adrenergic innervation of the ovary has been suggested to play a role in follicular growth, compensatory ovarian hypertrophy, and ovulation. Autotransplantation of ovary to subcutaneous sites in rats did not affect ovulation,[25] while rabbits with one denervated ovary ovulated equally well.[26] Selective degeneration of adrenergic terminals by 6-hydroxydopamine also failed to inhibit ovulation in mice.[27]

Despite the lack of influence of innervation on ovulation, autonomic innervation to the ovary does play a role in ovarian contractility which can be demonstrated *in vitro*. Using strips of follicular wall from the human ovary, catecholamines are able to induce measurable contractions *in vitro*; the potency of NE is the highest, followed by epinephrine, phenylephrine, and isoproterenol.[28] Since ovarian contractions have not been shown to have direct effects on ovulation, neural innervation of the follicle may only modulate the process of ovulation.

2. Vasculature

The blood supply to the ovary was studied as early as 1899 by Clark.[29] The ovarian arteries are derived from the abdominal aorta inferior to the renal arteries and run through the mesovarium to the ovaries. Each ovarian artery at the hilus of each ovary divides into primary and secondary spiral arteries. Follicles are surrounded by rich capillary plexus with arterioles and venules. The venous system consists of primary and secondary veins, leaving the ovary at the hilus along the reverse path of the arterial system.

At the time of ovulation, the rupture of the follicular wall at the apex is accompanied by increased capillary permeability and the eventual dilation of the blood vessels. Before ovulation, hCG treatment does not induce such changes, though the preovulatory follicle enlarges rapidly. In contrast, LH administration causes an immediate increase in follicular blood flow as a result of decreased vascular resistance induced by arteriolar vasodilation. There is accumulating evidence showing that histamine plays a crucial role in regulating this capillary response to LH.

Mast cells, endothelial cells, basophils, and platelets are possible sources of histamine in the ovary.[30] In addition, histamine also stimulates ovarian contractility and ovulation and follicular progesterone secretion as shown in an *in vitro* system. Bradykinin is also detected in follicular fluid, and it may act on the vascular system, as histamine, leading to increased vascular permeability. These are strikingly similar to the vascular reaction in an inflammatory response.

3.   Intrafollicular Pressure

By observing the development of the Graafian follicle just prior to ovulation, it is tempting to postulate that the bulging out of the follicular wall at the stigma is caused by increased pressure from inside. The rupture is an inevitable result at the climax of the pressure increase. In the 1950s, Zachariae and Jensen performed several histochemical experiments and physicochemical studies on follicular fluids, as well as the permeability of the blood-liquor barrier in bovine follicular fluids.[31,32] They concluded that the increased colloid-osmotic pressure resulting from the enzymatic depolymerization of mucopolysaccharide components in the follicular fluid was the key in the ovulatory mechanism.

In the early 1960s, Espey and Lipner conducted a series of experiments to measure the intrafollicular pressure with an improved methodology.[33–35] They found the normal intrafollicular pressure was 17 mmHg and was almost directly proportional to the vascular pressure in the carotid artery. The pressure was not changed just prior to the rupture of the follicular wall at the time of ovulation, but it fell to 5 mmHg afterward. Their results were supported by other studies. In addition, it was also demonstrated that artificial increase in pressure exerted on the Graafian follicle could not trigger ovulation.

Therefore, the initiation of rupture should occur under constant intrafollicular pressure. If intrafollicular pressure is proportional to carotid pressure, the increased blood flow as a result of vasodilation with no rise in arterial pressure also suggests a constant intrafollicular pressure. The best hypothesis would explain the observable physical changes throughout the rupturing process under the force of a steady pressure in the antrum.

C.   Ovulation as an Inflammatory Process

The working model presented earlier is actually the elaborated version of the multifactor hypothesis conceived by Thomson in 1919 and by the inflammatory model proposed by Espey in 1980.[19,22] Inflammation is a dynamic process with a series of metabolic and cellular events which are morphologically discernible. They include vascular reaction, infiltration of leukocytes and macrophages, fibroblast proliferation, and proteolysis. Biochemically, the involvement of steroids, prostaglandins, histamine, and other inflammatory components can also be observed in the ovulatory mechanism (see Figure 4.8). These components are now well studied.

1.   Vascular Dynamics

As discussed earlier, vasodilation and increased capillary permeability are observed just prior to the rupture of the follicular wall at ovulation. These are strikingly similar to events occurring in inflamed tissues.[36] As a result of these vascular changes, the follicle becomes edematous until the stigma ruptures.

2. Leukocytes and Macrophages

In a typical inflammatory response, the first line of defense is the infiltration of polymorphonuclear leukocytes and macrophages.[36] Similar infiltration to the ovarian follicle is observed during the ovulatory process. A recent study[37] on basophil counts in capillary blood samples of 13 normal young women during the follicular and progestational phases showed the counts to be 36.6 and 39.3/ml, respectively. A significant midcycle (36%) and premenstrual (22%) fall in the counts was observed. The authors suggested that the fall might be a result of cell migration from the peripheral blood into the rupturing follicle of the ovary and into the ischemic premenstrual endometrium.[37]

Recently, peptides recovered from two fractions of the follicular wall of periovulatory ovine follicles have been sequenced.[38] Both fractions have leukocyte chemoattractant activity. One fraction contained 16 amino acid residues with repeating triplets of G-P-OHP where OHP is hydroxyproline. Since this motif is often found in α-collagens, this chemoattractant is possibly derived from the connective tissue matrix of the follicle after the degradation of thecal collagen during ovulation. Peptide isolated from the other bioactive chromatographic fraction has 15 amino acids rich in glycine.

3. Fibroblast Proliferation

Fibroblasts are found in a dense layer of thecal tissue surrounding the Graafian follicle. They migrate into the stratum granulosum at the time of ovulation. As in leukocytes, chemoattractants may be present, inducing the fibroblasts to migrate and proliferate. This is also the repair process immediately after ovulation. The major function of these fibroblasts has been suggested to be building a collagenous support for the mass of developing lutein tissues.[39]

4. Steroids and Prostaglandins

Steroidogenesis in the theca interna and granulosa cells has been discussed in Chapter 2 based on the two-cell-type two-gonadotrophin hypothesis (see Figure 2.6). In short, FSH stimulates the synthesis of LH receptors in theca cells and enhances their response to LH. This causes a shift of steroidogenesis from progesterone to androgen synthesis in these cells. Granulosa cells adjacent to theca cells are responsible for converting androgen to estrogen, which is vital to follicular development. Although the use of antitestosterone or antiprogesterone antisera has been shown to inhibit ovulation, the direct link between steroidogenesis and ovulation has not been established.

Estradiol may stimulate the synthesis of prostaglandins which, in turn, participate in the inflammation-like response during ovulation.[40] Various prostaglandins such as PGE_2, $PGF_{2\alpha}$, and prostacyclin ($PGI_{2\alpha}$) are synthesized from arachidonic acid by prostaglandin cyclooxygenase. Through an alternative pathway catalyzed by lipooxygenase, arachidonic acid is converted to leukotrienes with chemotactic effects on leukocytes and macrophages in the inflammatory reaction. Together with the actions of prostaglandins in promoting proteolytic enzymes, the activity of cyclooxygenase/lipooxygenase is crucial in the ovulatory mechanism.[23]

Indomethacin, which suppresses prostaglandin synthesis by inhibiting cyclooxygenase, also blocks ovulation. Using cultured follicles, prostaglandins have been shown to exert effects similar to LH, such as stimulating adenylate cyclase and inducing resumption of oocyte meiosis. PGE_2 appears to be more effective than $PGF_{2\alpha}$. In terms of contractility of human ovarian follicles, they have opposite effects. PGE_2 is inhibitory, while $PGF_{2\alpha}$ is stimulatory. Since the results are different from studies on animal ovarian follicles, there is no clear relationship with the ovulatory mechanism.[21]

It should be noted that nonsteroidal anti-inflammatory drugs (NSAIDs) such as aspirin, ibuprofen, piroxicam, and indomethacin are inhibitory to ovulation as a result of blocking prostaglandins by suppressing cyclooxygenase. On the other hand, dexamethasone, a potent steroidal anti-inflammatory drug, has little or no effect on ovulation. Recent studies have shown that, however, the inhibitory effect of indomethacin on ovulation may be independent of the cyclooxygenase pathway of arachidonate metabolism. Possibly, as shown in sheep, the inhibition of ovulation by indomethacin is not attributed to its suppression on follicular prostaglandin biosynthesis, but it is associated with its effects on follicular collagenolysis and leukocyte chemoattraction.[41]

5. Collagenolysis

Reich et al.[42] have demonstrated that ovulation induced by LH and hCG is accompanied by an increase in collagenolysis. Talopeptin, a metalloproteinase inhibitor known to suppress collagenase, blocks ovulation. The breakdown of collagen is a necessary step for the rupture of the follicular wall. A recent study provided additional evidence that a platelet-activating factor (PAF) antagonist, BN52021, also suppresses ovarian collagenolysis and inhibits ovulation. The inhibitory effect of BN52021 can be reversed by simultaneous administration of PAF, suggesting that PAF may be part of the cascade mechanism.[43]

A recent study on the rabbit ovary shows that hCG-induced ovulation is inhibited by prolactin, at least in part, via a suppressive mechanism on the plasmin-generating system in preovulatory follicles.[44] With reference to Figure 4.8, plasmin is produced from plasminogen through a urokinase-type plasminogen activator as part of the enzymatic cascade process. Plasmin is responsible for activation of latent collagenase, converting collagen to telopeptide-free collagen. Under a system of nonspecific serine proteases, this telopeptide-free collagen is degraded, leading to follicular rupture.

There are other substances present in the follicular fluid such as noradrenaline, dopamine, and serotonin. A recent study on human Graafian follicles in *in vitro* fertilization (IVF) patients superovulated by HMG and hCG has shown higher contents of these hormones.[45] Bodis et al. suggested that they might play an important role in the mechanism of ovulation, the regulation of postovulatory tubal motility, and the release of progesterone from granulosa cells. The elucidation of the ovulatory mechanism is crucial for understanding the pathophysiology of ovarian dysfunction and the treatment of infertility.[46]

V. COMPARATIVE ACCOUNT OF VERTEBRATE REPRODUCTIVE CYCLES

In humans, the menstrual cycle appears to be the only reproductive cycle discernible. It is, however, a unique type of cycles among vertebrates. It would be interesting to see reproductive cycles in various vertebrate groups as discussed earlier by von Tienhoven (1983).[11]

A. CYCLOSTOME

The spawning time of lampreys is probably regulated by water temperature. Since they die of gut atrophy after spawning (100,000 eggs!), there is no cyclicity within the reproductive season. They metamorphose in the fall of their 4th year of life and reproduce in the following spring. Gut atrophy starts as soon as the vitellogenetic growth of the follicles commences. The hagfish, in contrast, releases only a few eggs over several seasons. Amazingly, corpora atretica and lutea are found in the ovary without obvious functions.

B. ELASMOBRANCHS

There are three types of cycles in elasmobranchs such as sharks. Some are reproductively active throughout the year, some have a partial annual cycle, and others have an annual or biennial cycle. Most are migratory and the cycle is probably regulated by water temperature. The pattern of ovulation is still uncertain. The presence of eggs in the oviduct appears to inhibit ovulation. Again, there are corpora atretica and lutea without known functions.

C. TELEOSTS

There are oviparous and viviparous bony fishes Oviparous fishes have a reproductive cycle of two periods: gametogenesis and spawning.

1. Gametogenesis — This occurs in salmonids during the summer and fall when day length decreases, e.g., in rainbow trout *(Salmo gairdneri),* decreasing day length and water temperature at about 16°C accelerate spermatogenesis. Plasma gonadotrophins appear to correlate with testicular development. A rise in testicular weight and activity coincides with a peak in plasma gonadotrophins.
2. Spawning — There are different patterns, e.g., fall, spring and summer, spring, summer, winter, year-round, and intermittent breeding. Water temperature is also a major factor. In rainbow trout, plasma 17β-estradiol concentration at spermiation was about 1.5ng/ml, which is lower than the level (2.5 ng/ml) during the early spermatogenesis. The endocrine mechanisms are uncertain, though steroids are possibly involved.

Viviparous fishes have different patterns among different species. The difference is in the sequence and duration between ovulation, fertilization, hatching, and parturition. In the common river fish called *Gambusia,* the oocyte is fertilized in the follicle and the gestation period is about 1 month. Hatching and parturition follow quickly.

D. AMPHIBIANS

As in teleosts, there are also oviparous and viviparous types in amphibians. The first type is oviparous anura such as *Rana.* The main proximate factor is temperature. Most of them breed in spring. The second type is viviparous anura such as East African frog *(Nectophrynodies occidentalis).* The female ovulates and mates at the end of the rainy season in October. It then estivates during the dry season for 6 months. During this period, the embryonic development is retarded. In April, the pregnant mother emerges and gives birth to the young in June.

There is another type called urodeles, e.g., salamanders. The proximate causes are usually temperature, humidity, and photoperiod. They mate in the fall, and sperms are stored in spermatheca through hibernation during which vitellogenesis proceeds. Fertilization occurs in the spring and they mate again, followed by oviposition from spring to summer.

E. REPTILES

In reptiles, sperms have an unusually long survival time in the female reproductive system (e.g., it may be 7 years in some species!). Ovulation, copulation, and hormonal changes are not synchronized. In the turtle, for example, mating occurs in April to May and spermatogenesis in June to October, but plasma testosterone peaks are detected in December and April. The most famous example is the American chameleon *(Anolis carolinensis).* During winter in the southeastern U.S., they are reproductively inactive. In late January, the males build their breeding territories, waiting for the females to emerge from their hiding places in late February. Following vitellogenesis in March, yolk is deposited in one follicle for about 2 weeks until it develops up to about 8 mm in diameter. Ovulation occurs every 2 weeks, and corpora lutea are formed from ruptured follicles. These corpora lutea are thought to make the female refractory to environmental stimuli such as exogenous gonadotrophins.

F. BIRDS

There are several types of reproductive cycles in birds. The first type is continuous breeding such as Khaki Campbell ducks. They may lay more than 365 eggs a year. Some chickens can do that too. In contrast, there are opportunistic breeders such as grass parakeet; these birds are also continuous but dependent on conditions. Another type of bird with breeding cycles of less than 1 year is the sooty tern *(Sterna fuscata);* the intervals between breeding periods can be 9.6 months. This may be advantageous for birds vulnerable to predation. There are some with semiannual or annual cycles with 6- or 12-month periods, respectively; their proximate causes are photoperiod and rainfall. For the annual type, most species are in the temperate, subarctic and arctic zones. Their endogenous circannual rhythms are synchronized with the photoperiod, e.g., American goldfinch *(Carduelis* species).

G. MAMMALS

There are three types of mammalian reproductive cycles.

1. Prototeria, e.g., the duck-billed platypus *(Ornithorhynchus anatinus)* in Australia — The breeding period is from fall to winter. In the male, the testicular weight increases in May to a maximum in August and regresses in September to a minimum in December. Spermatogenesis occurs in winter. In the female, the uterus and the left ovary increases in weight, but not the right ovary. Ovulation occurs in August, and fertilization takes place in the infundibulum of the oviduct. The shell is formed when the egg is transported through the oviduct. This is an unusual egg-laying mammal.
2. Metatheria, e.g., marsupials — They have estrous cycles with varying lengths in different species. Gestation has profound inhibitory effects on the estrous cycle. The ovarian cycle is also inhibited by lactation through suppressing the development of the corpus luteum.
3. Eutheria — Sperms usually do not survive for a long time in the female (except some bats). Generally, there are three types. Estrous cycles are found in most species such as sheep, swine, cattle, and rats. The second type is induced ovulators; rabbits are a common example. The third type is the menstrual cycle that is unique to primates.

The basic function of mammalian reproductive cycles, including the menstrual cycle in humans, is to ensure the timing of ovulation. The advantage is obvious in seasonal breeders where reproductive activities must coincide with optimal environmental conditions. Seasonality of human reproduction will be discussed in Chapter 11. In short, humans are not truly seasonal though seasonality is observed in human conception rates. Human sexual behavior apparently does not fluctuate with the menstrual cycle, though anovulatory cycles may occur under erratic light-dark rhythms.

REFERENCES

1. **Hearn, J., Ed.,** *Reproduction in New World Primates,* MTP Press, Lancaster, 1983.
2. **Knobil, E. and Hotchkiss, J.,** The menstrual cycle and its neuroendocrine control, in *The Physiology of Reproduction,* Knobil, E. and Neill, J., Eds., Raven Press, New York, 1988, 1971.
3. **Greenwald, G.S. and Terranova, P.F.,** Follicular selection and its control, in *The Physiology of Reproduction,* Knobil, E. and Neill, J., Eds., Raven Press, New York, 1988, 387.

4. **Wetsel, W.C., Valenca, M.M., Merchenthaler, I., Liposits, Z., Lopez, F.J., Weiner, R.I., Mellon, P.L., and Negro-Vilar, A.**, Intrinsic pulsatile secretory activity of immortalized luteinizing hormone-releasing hormone-secreting neurons, *Proc. Natl. Acad. Sci. U.S.A.*, 89, 4149, 1992.

5. **Batista, M.C., Cartledge, T.P., Zellmer, A.W., Nieman, L.K., Merriam, G.R., and Loriaux, D.L.**, Evidence for a critical role of progesterone in the regulation of the midcycle gonadotropin surge and ovulation, *J. Clin. Endocrinol. Metab.*, 74, 565, 1992.

6. **Hisaw, F.L. and Hisaw, F.L., Jr.**, Action of estrogen and progesterone on the reproductive tract of lower primates, in *Sex and Internal Secretions,* Young, W.C., Ed., Williams & Wilkins, Baltimore, 1961, 556.

7. **Noyes, R.W., Hertig, A.T., and Rock, J.**, Dating the endometrial biopsy, *Fertil. Steril.*, 1, 3, 1950.

8. **Brenner, R.M. and Maslar, I.A.**, The primate oviduct and endometrium, in *The Physiology of Reproduction,* Knobil, E. and Neill, J., Eds., Raven Press, New York, 1988, 303.

9. **Verhage, H.G., Fazleabas, A.T., and Donnelly, K.**, The *in vitro* synthesis and release of proteins by the human oviduct, *Endocrinology*, 122, 1639, 1988.

10. **Conaway, C.H.**, Ecological adaptation and mammalian reproduction, *Biol. Reprod.,* 4, 239, 1971.

11. **van Tienhoven, A.**, *Reproductive Physiology of Vertebrates,* 2nd ed., Cornell University Press, New York, 1983.

12. **Alonso, R., Abbr, P., and Fajardo, N.**, Steroid influences on pineal melatonin production, in *Melatonin: Biosynthesis, Physiological Effects, and Clinical Applications*, Yu, H.S. and Reiter, R.J., Eds., 1993, CRC Press, Boca Raton, FL, 73.

13. **Evans, H.M. and Long, J.A.**, On the association of continued cornification of the vaginal mucosa with the presence of large vesicles in the ovary and the absence of corpus luteum formation, *Anat. Rec.,* 21, 67, 1921.

14. **Turner, C.D. and Bagnara, J.T.**, *General Endocrinology,* 5th ed., W.B. Saunders, Philadelphia, 1971.

15. **Kaynard, A.H., Pau, K.Y., Hess, D.L., and Spies, H.G.**, Gonadotrophin-releasing hormone and norepinephrine release from the rabbit mediobasal and anterior hypothalamus during the mating-induced luteinizing hormone surge, *Endocrinology*, 127, 1176, 1990.

16. **Dafny, N. and Terkel, J.**, Hypothalamic neuronal activity associated with onset of pseudopregnancy in the rat, *Neuroendocrinology*, 51, 459, 1990.

17. **Jocelyn, H.D. and Setchell, B.P.**, Translation of Regnier de Graaf. On human reproductive organs from the Latin text *Tractus de Vivorum Organis Generationi Inservientibus (1668)* and *DeMulierum Organis Generationi Inservientibus Tractatus Novus (1672)*, pp. 131–135, *Reprod. Fertil.,* 17 (Suppl.), 131, 1972.

18. **von Kolliker, A.**, Beitrage zur kenntniss der glatten Muskeln (Contribution to the knowledge of smooth muscle), *Abh. Wiss. Zool.,* 1, 48, 1949.

19. **Thomson, A.**, The ripe human Graafian follicle, together with some suggestions as to its mode of rupture, *J. Anat.,* 54, 1, 1919.

20. **Schochet, S.S.**, A suggestion as to the process of ovulation and ovarian cyst formation, *Anat. Rec.,* 10, 447, 1916.

21. **Lipner, H.**, Mechanism of mammalian ovulation, in *The Physiology of Reproduction,* Knobil, E. and Neill, J., Eds., Raven Press, New York, 1988, 447.

22. **Espey, L.L.**, Ovulation as an inflammatory reaction — a hypothesis, *Biol. Reprod.,* 23, 73, 1980.

23. **LeMaire, W.J.**, Mechanism of mammalian ovulation, *Steroids*, 54, 455, 1989.

24. **Lipner, H. and Maxwell, B.A.**, Hypothesis concerning the role of follicular contractions in ovulation, *Science,* 131, 1737, 1960.

25. **Deanesly, R.**, Cyclic function in ovarian grafts, *J. Endocrinol.,* 13, 211, 1956.

26. **Weiner, S., Wright, K.H., and Wallach, E.E.**, Lack of effect of ovarian denervation on ovulation and pregnancy in the rabbit, *Fertil. Steril.,* 26, 1083, 1975.

27. **Tranzer, J.P. and Thoenen, H.,** An electron microscopic study of selective acute degeneration of sympathetic nerve terminals after administration of 6-hydroxydopamine, *Experientia,* 24, 155, 1968.

28. **Walles, B., Falck, B., Owman, C., and Sjoberg, N.O.,** Characterization of autonomic receptors in the smooth musculature of human Graafian follicle, *Biol. Reprod.,* 17, 423, 1977.

29. **Clark, J.G.,** Origin, development and degeneration of the blood vessels of the ovary, *Bull. Johns Hopkins Hosp.,* 96, 40, 1899.

30. **Krishna, A., Beesley, K., and Terranova, P.F.,** Histamine, mast cells and ovarian function, *J. Endocrinol.,* 120(3), 363, 1989.

31. **Zachariae, F.,** Studies on the mechanism of ovulation. Permeability of the blood-liquor barrier, *Acta Endocrinol.,* 27, 339, 1958.

32. **Zachariae, F. and Jensen, C.E.,** Studies on the mechanism of ovulation. Histochemical and physicochemical investigations on genuine follicular fluids, *Acta Endocrinol.,* 27, 343, 1958.

33. **Espey, L.L. and Lipner, H.,** Measurement of intrafollicular pressures in the rabbit ovary, *Am. J. Physiol.,* 205, 1067, 1963.

34. **Espey, L.L. and Lipner, H.,** Changes in the properties of the walls of the sow Graafian follicle, *Am. Zool.,* 4, 325, 1964.

35. **Espey, L.L. and Lipner, H.,** Enzyme-induced rupture of rabbit Graafian follicle, *Am. J. Physiol.,* 208, 208, 1965.

36. **Ebert, R.H. and Grant, L.,** *The Experimental Approach to the Study of Inflammatory Process,* Academic Press, New York, 1974, 4.

37. **Rajan, P., Rao, G.S., and Walter, S.,** Blood basopenia as an indicator of ovulation, *Indian J. Physiol. Pharmacol.,* 36, 115, 1992.

38. **Murdoch, W.J. and McCormick, R.J.,** Sequence analysis of leukocyte chemoattractant peptides secreted by periovulatory ovine follicles, *Biochem. Biophys. Res. Commun.,* 184, 848, 1992.

39. **Espey, L.L.,** The distribution of collagenous connective tissue in rat ovarian follicles, *Biol. Reprod.,* 14, 502, 1976.

40. **Kuelh, F.A., Cirillo, V.J., Zanetti, M.E., and Ham, E.A.,** The regulatory role of steroid hormones on the PGF/PG ratio in target tissues, *Agents Actions,* 6, 165, 1976.

41. **Murdoch, W.J. and McCormick, R.J.,** Dose-dependent effects of indomethacin on ovulation in the sheep: relationship to follicular prostaglandin production, steroidogenesis, collagenolysis, and leukocyte chemotaxis, *Biol. Reprod.,* 45, 907, 1991.

42. **Reich, R., Tsafriri, A., and Mechanic, G.L.,** The involvement of collagenolysis in ovulation in the rat, *Endocrinology,* 116, 522, 1985.

43. **Abisogun, A.O., Braquet, P., and Tsafriri, A.,** The involvement of platelet activating factor in ovulation, *Science,* 243, 381, 1989.

44. **Yoshimura, Y., Nakamura, Y., Oda, T., Ando, M., Ubukata, Y., Koyama, N., Karube, M., and Yamada, H.,** Effects of prolactin on ovarian plasmin generation in the process of ovulation, *Biol. Reprod.,* 46, 322, 1992.

45. **Bodis, J., Bognar, Z., Hartmann, G., Torok, A., and Csaba, I.F.,** Measurement of noradrenaline, dopamine and serotonin contents in follicular fluid of human graafian follicles after superovulation treatment, *Gynecol. Obstet. Invest.,* 33, 165, 1992.

46. **Irianni, F. and Hodgen, G.D.,** Mechanism of ovulation, *Endocrinol. Metab. Clin. North Am.,* 21, 19, 1992.

47. **Dallenbach-Hellweg, G. and Poulsen, H.,** *Atlas of Endometrial Histopathology,* Munksgaard, Copenhagen, 1985.

48. **Ramirez, V.D. and Beyer, C.,** The ovarian cycle of the rabbit: its neuroendocrine control, in *The Physiology of Reproduction,* Knobil, E. and Neill, J., Eds., Raven Press, New York, 1988, 1873.

5 The Female Reproductive System

CHAPTER CONTENTS

I. INTRODUCTION

After our discussion of the neuroendocrine component of the reproductive system, we can appreciate the harmonious gonad-brain interaction performed by the endocrine orchestra. The orchestration of their communicating signals such as gonadotrophins, GnRH, and steroids is genetically determined. The genetic program is expressed during sexual development according to the schedule of gene expression. Gonadal differentiation is the earliest event, while the sexual differentiation of the brain starts later in fetal life. By weeks 12 to 14 of gestation, the external genitalia and internal reproductive structures become sexually different shortly after gonadal differentiation.

Apparently, the external genitalia and internal reproductive structures are essential parts of either the female or male reproductive system in a fertile adult human. In this chapter, we discuss the female reproductive system, which is composed only of anatomically observable structures. Therefore, the neuroendocrine component is excluded in this definition of the female reproductive system. It should be clearly understood that well-developed external and internal reproductive structures alone are not sufficient for the reproductive process. The female reproductive system requires the sex-specific neuroendocrine component and a proper sexual physiology for successful reproduction.

II.   EXTERNAL GENITALIA

The female external genitalia is an elaborated structure surrounding the only opening of the uterine cavity to the exterior. The opening of the urethra from the urinary bladder is integrated with the structure. Although the basic plan is similar, the details of the female external genitalia vary greatly among mammals. The vulva is the area of the female external genitalia including the mons veneris, labia majora and minora, clitoris, vestibule, and urethral and vaginal openings. True labia are found only in human females. There are considerable individual differences in details among women as shown in the two examples in Figure 5.1. Figure 5.2 shows a diagrammatic representation of a typical female external genitalia.

A.   LABIA MAJORA AND MINORA
The mons veneris is a thick layer of adipose tissues covering the bone symphysis pubis. It is the ventral area of confluence of two large longitudinal folds, the labia majora (major lips). Both the mons veneris and the outer surface of the labia majora are covered with hairs. The inner surface of the labia majora are hairless and moist. The posterior area of confluence is the perineum that lies between the vulva and the anus. These tissues are highly vascularized.

The labia minora (minor lips) are two thin folds inside the labia majora. The anterior confluence is the clitoris covered by the prepuce. At the other end, labia minora come together to form the posterior side of the vaginal opening. The area enclosed by the labia minora is called the vestibule.

B.   CLITORIS
The clitoris is a structure equivalent to the penis with erectile tissues that are highly vascularized and innervated. As described in Chapter 2, in some pseudohermaphrodites with XY genetic sex found in New Guinea, infants are thought to be female. The penis is clitoral-like, but enlarges at puberty, turning into adult males with a functional male reproductive system. In normal adult females, the clitoris also contains androgen receptors and is responsive to the growth stimulation by androgens.

C.   URETHRAL AND VAGINAL OPENINGS
The urethral and vaginal openings are located within the vestibule. Anterior to the vaginal opening, the urethral opening is closer to the clitoris. On its two sides, there are small, inconspicuous openings of the ducts from the Skene's glands.

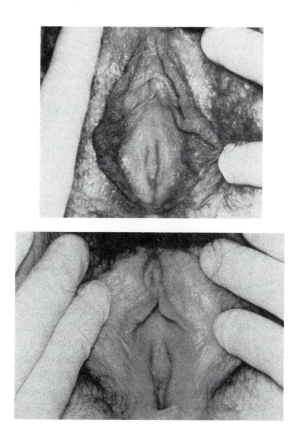

FIGURE 5.1. Two examples showing the vulva. (From McLean, J.M., *The Vulva,* Ridley, C.M., Ed., Churchill Livingstone, Edinburgh, 1988. With permission.)

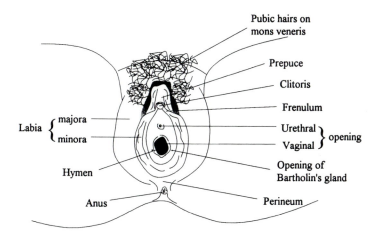

FIGURE 5.2. Diagrammatic representation of female external genitalia.

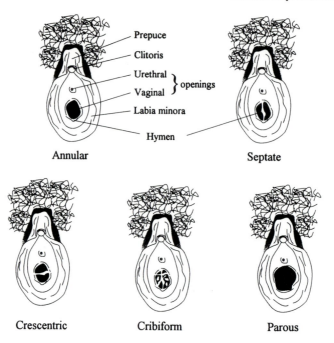

Prepuce
Clitoris
Urethral ⎱
            ⎰ openings
Vaginal ⎰
Labia minora
Hymen

Annular   Septate

Crescentric   Cribiform   Parous

FIGURE 5.3.   Different types of hymens.

Similar glands called Bartholin's glands are also found on either sides of the vaginal opening. These glands secrete lubricating mucus.

D.   HYMEN

The hymen is a thin mucus membrane covering the vaginal opening in young women. In Latin, it is known as "carunculae myrtiformes," or "little piece of flesh." The function of this delicate structure is unknown. The hymen can usually be torn during sexual intercourse, by tampons, or some types of physical exercise (e.g., biking). Breakage is very often accompanied by slight bleeding. The hymen rarely remains intact after sexual intercourse.

The morphology of the hymen varies greatly among different individuals. They can be classified into five types: annular, septate, crescentric, cribiform, and parous (see Figure 5.3). On intact hymens, there is usually an aperture of different sizes. Such an opening is required for menstrual bleeding. There is a single aperture in the parous and virginal types, though the parous type tends to be larger. In the septate type, there is a septum across the aperture, and the septum may be equatorial or longitudinal. In some rare cases, the vaginal opening is absent and surgical reconstruction is necessary to rectify the congenital anomaly.[1] This is known as an imperforate condition where the hymen is composed of firm connective tissues covered on both sides by stratified squamous epithelia.

The female external genitalia primarily provides necessary structures for penile intromission and insemination. Apparently, it also serves as a characteristic external feature for body sex determination. Some true male transsexuals develop such a

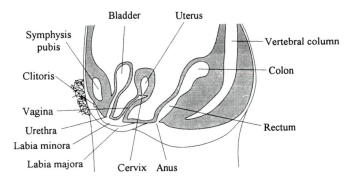

FIGURE 5.4.   The female reproductive system (sagittal section).

psychological rejection of their external genitalia that they may physically harm their own penises.[2] Successful plastic surgeries have been performed to build female external genitalia. These "sex-changed" males may perform sexual acts as a female. Without relevant female internal reproductive structures, the presence of female external genitalia only does not provide an appropriate female sexual physiology apart from the psychology of being a female at the level of external body sex.

III.   INTERNAL REPRODUCTIVE STRUCTURES

The connection between the female external genitalia and the ovary is the female reproductive tract. Two main purposes of this tract are gamete transport and embryonic development. Sperms are transported from the vagina through the uterus to the ampulla of the oviduct where fertilization takes place. The fertilized egg is transported down the oviduct to the uterus where implantation occurs. The internal reproductive structures in the female are thus crucial to the success of fertilization and pregnancy. Sperm transport and zygote implantation will be discussed in detail in Chapters 8 and 9, respectively. Figure 5.4 is a diagrammatic representation of a sagittal section of the female reproductive system.

A.   VAGINA

The vagina is a canal connecting the uterus to the exterior. Although the front part of the vagina at the entrance is sometime exposed to the exterior, most of the vagina is internal. It is lined by a stratified squamous epithelium. As described in Chapter 4, the vaginal epithelial changes during the menstrual cycle, but the change is not as well defined as in estrous rats. The cellular changes are responses to variations in estrogen and progesterone levels. This is a peak of cellular growth and maturity around the time of ovulation when estrogen level is high.

A sensitive area called the Grafenberg Spot (G-spot) has been claimed to exist in the vaginal canal, despite the lack of anatomical evidence. This area is a possible sensory point for inducing vaginal orgasm independent of clitoral stimulation.[3] Without an accurate anatomical location, the G-spot may be a sensitive area inside the vaginal canal that can be perceived by some women.

B.   CERVIX

The cervix is located between the uterus and the vagina. The cervix in humans consists of three basic components: smooth muscle, connective tissue matrix, and elastin.[4] The connective tissue matrix is composed of collagen and glycosaminoglycans. In a nonpregnant uterus, 85% of the cervical dry weight is collagen, which comprises 70% type I and 30% type II. When it is wet, 80% of its weight is water. Collagen fibril is made up of tropocollagen molecules packed in parallel. Each tropocollagen unit consists of three helical 300-kDa collagen molecules. These proteins give rigidity to the system. Elastin, on the other hand, is a protein providing elasticity to the system.

There are numerous mucous glands on the cervix, and the secretory activity varies with the menstrual cycle. With high estrogen levels during the late follicular phase, cervical mucus secretion is enhanced. This is the characteristic preovulatory mucus that subsides after ovulation when progesterone level increases. The cervical mucus contains mainly a glycoprotein rich in carbohydrates called mucin and a soluble component (e.g., salts, small peptides, carbohydrates). The main component is water (95%) at midcycle.[5]

C.   UTERUS

The uterus is highly muscular and elastic. In humans, as most other primates, the uterus is a simplex type. In Eutheria, there are four main types of uteri. First, the simplex uterus, as in humans, has one cervix and one uterine body. Second, the duplex uterus, as in rabbits, has two cervices and two uterine horns. Third, the bicornuate uterus, as in pig, mice, and rats, has one cervix and two uterine horns. The fourth type is bipartite, which is similar to the bicornuate uterus, but the uterine horns may be fused.

The uterine wall consists of two major layers, the endometrium and myometrium. As described in Chapter 4, the innermost endometrium is a dynamic layer most of which undergoes cyclic changes during the menstrual cycle. It has an epithelial layer lining the uterine lumen and an inner stromal layer with secretory glands. The myometrium, in the simplex type of uterus, is mainly made up of longitudinal and circular smooth muscle fibers. Four distinct layers can be identified: the outermost serous epithelium, then the longitudinal muscle layer, followed by the circular muscle layer, and the decidua.

Postganglionic sympathetic fibers innervating the myometrium from lumbar and mesenteric ganglia are found. Although cholinergic innervation is rare, it has been shown to be associated with blood capillaries. There are also vasoactive intestinal peptide (VIP) neurons inhibitory to myometrial contraction.[4]

D.   OVIDUCT

The oviduct or fallopian tube, discovered by Gabrielle Fallopius in 1561, is a highly differentiated tubal structure connecting the uterus with the ovaries. With reference to external features of an oviduct, there are four distinct regions: the fimbriae, ampulla, isthmus, and uterotubal junction. If the luminal structures are compared in cross-sections, the isthmus can be subdivided into distal and proximal.

The whole length of the isthmus from the uterotubal to the ampulla is about 2 to 3 cm, while the ampulla is up to 8 cm long. There is a progressive increase in the lumen diameter from the isthmus (1 mm) to ampulla (1 cm). The musculature is well developed in the isthmus, while the ampullar wall is very thin. In the mouse, the ampullar wall is so thin that the presence of a cumulus of eggs can be seen under a dissecting microscope when the intact oviduct is placed in the culture dish.

In contrast to the distal isthmus, the lumen of the proximal isthmus can be as small as 0.4 mm in humans. Together with the strong, thick layer of smooth muscle, the proximal isthmus may act as a sphincter in controlling gamete transport. The uterotubal junction is also involved in this process, though it does not have specialized structures.

The fimbriae is the distal end of the female reproductive tract. It is commonly called the oviductal funnel, which opens to the peritoneal cavity. Although there is no direct connection between the ovary and the oviduct, the funnel is closely associated with the ovarian surface. Together with its highly folded structure and numerous ciliated cells, the funnel is extremely efficient in retrieving oocytes as soon as they are ovulated. It is, however, not guaranteed 100% because even a fertilized egg can be left in the peritoneal cavity, resulting in an ectopic pregnancy that must be terminated as soon as possible. Moreover, sperms have been consistently found in the peritoneal cavity after sexual intercourse.[6]

E.   OVARIES

The ovary is located in the peritoneal cavity in all vertebrate species. In most mammals, it is usually paired with bilateral symmetry. In most reptiles, birds, platypus, and some bats, only one side is developed. The bulk of the ovary is the ovarian cortex or the stroma in which developing, mature, and atretic follicles, as well as corpora lutea, are found. This ovarian cortex is surrounded by a tough layer of connective tissues called tunica albuginea. The outermost layer is the germinal epithelium made up of squamous and low columnar cells on a thin acellular basement membrane.

The ovarian epithelium is called the germinal epithelium because it is considered to be different from the coelomic epithelium.[7] In 1961, there was still considerable speculation about whether adult germinal epithelium contained or developed into germ cells, though it had been known by that time that the proliferative activity of oogonia are completed before birth.[8] As discussed in Chapter 2, germ cells are extragonadal in origin. The germinal epithelium is derived from the coelomic epithelium. Primordial germ cells (PGCs) migrate from the hindgut to the genital ridge and pass through the epithelial layer. At this time, PGCs may be found among the epithelial cells. The germinal epithelium of the ovary, we know now, is not germinal.[9]

The ovary is enveloped by the mesovarium attached to the dorsal body wall. The junction between the peritoneum and mesovarium is called hilus where blood

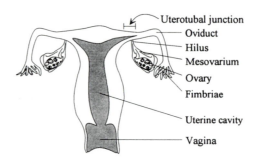

Uterotubal junction
Oviduct
Hilus
Mesovarium
Ovary
Fimbriae

Uterine cavity

Vagina

FIGURE 5.5.   The position of ovaries in humans.

vessels and nerves enter. The cells in the germinal epithelium at the hilus are found to be columnar, as are the embryonic coelomic epithelial cells. The hilus is located just beneath the uterotubal function on each side of the uterus, while the other end is orientated toward the fimbriae of the oviduct (see Figure 5.5).

The nerves come from spinal segments T_{10} and T_{11}, forming the aortorenal plexus and entering the ovary along with the ovarian artery. Sensory fibers are associated with the sympathetic fibers, while the parasympathetic is from the vagus. The nerve fibers distribute throughout the ovarian cortex, in and around follicles. The neurotransmitter is primarily norepinephrine (NE), though cholinergic fibers have also been identified. Adrenergic innervation to the ovary may be associated with follicular growth, ovarian cyclicity, compensatory ovarian hypertrophy, and ovulation. Nerve terminals are found lying close to smooth muscle cells in the theca externa of follicles.

As with innervation, there is an elaborated formation of blood capillaries in the ovary. The pair of ovarian arteries arise from the abdominal aorta inferior to the renal arteries. Through the hilus, each ovarian artery enters the ovary and ramifies into primary and secondary spiral arteries. A simple network of capillaries forms around a primary follicle and develops into a complicated system as the follicle grows. The system has an obvious important role of conveying steroid hormones and gonadotrophins as well as other necessary molecules.

F.   THE MAMMARY GLAND

All structures of the mammary gland, which is commonly known as the breast, are internal. The nipple is a structure where five to ten milk-collecting ducts open to the exterior. Each of these ducts is supplied by a lobe of 20 to 40 lobules. Each lobule is made up of 10 to 100 alveoli. The size and arrangement of these internal structures vary in different women. Although similar structures can be identified in normal men, they are much less developed.

The average adult breast is situated in an area bound by the sternal edge, second rib, midaxillary line, and sixth rib. The skin is thin and contains numerous nerve endings and sebaceous and sweat glands. In addition to vascular and lymphatic supplies, muscles are also an important part of the mammary gland. They include the pectoralis major and minor, serratus anterior, latissimus dorsi muscles, and external oblique and rectus abdominis muscles. With the support of

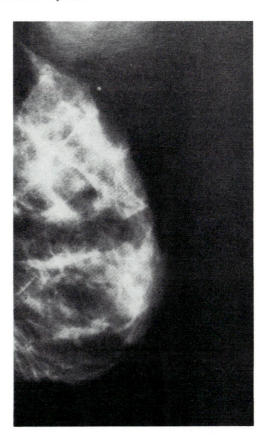

FIGURE 5.6. Mammogram of a 35-year-old woman with normal mammary glands. (From LeTreut, A. and Dilhuydy, H.M., *Mammography. A Guide to Interpretation,* C.V. Mosby, St. Louis, 1991. With permission.)

these muscles, masses of lobules with associated structures enclosed by the skin form the external shape of the breast.

The primary function of the mammary gland is lactation following pregnancy. In response to prolactin and oxytocin, milk is produced and ready for breastfeeding (details will be discussed in Chapter 9). In humans, this function becomes less important when nutritive alternatives are available, though breastfeeding is still recommended for healthy mothers. In some women, the skin of the breast is particularly sensitive, so it can be classified as a sexually responsive organ. In some extreme cases, breast stimulation alone may lead to orgasm and evokes conspicuous changes such as enlarged breast, erect nipples, and a mottled pink discoloration of the skin.[10]

Clinically, the breast poses an additional health risk for women. For example, breast cancer is the most common disease in women. Figures 5.6 and 5.7 are mammograms of normal and cancerous breasts, respectively. With the availability of improved imaging techniques of mammography, earlier diagnosis of breast

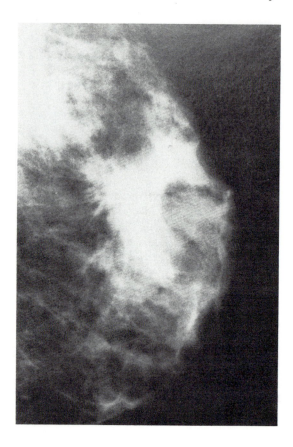

FIGURE 5.7. Mammogram of a 49-year-old woman with a 35-mm cancer of the upper and outer quadrant of the mammary gland. (From LeTreut, A. and Dilhuydy, H.M., *Mammography. A Guide to Interpretation,* C.V. Mosby, St. Louis, 1991. With permission.)

cancer is possible.[11] A recent increase in the incidence of breast cancer with frequent mammographic examinations has led to a suspicion that repetitive exposure to radiation in the routine procedure may be a causative link. Further studies are required to establish this claim.

In addition to breast cancer, there are many other diseases. Congenital abnormalities include hypoplasia (underdevelopment), amastia (completely absent), or amazia (nipple present only). Malformed muscles or dysfunctional lactation may also be found. Postnatal abnormalities are possible when pubertal breast development is inhibited.[12] Recent postsurgical complications reported in women using silicone implants are being studied.

G.   ACCESSORY SEXUAL STRUCTURES

In humans, accessory sex glands are mostly related to lubrication of the vaginal canal and the external genitalia. Cervical glands are the major source of lubricating fluid for the vagina. Bartholin's and Skene's glands are the two vestibular glands associated with the vulva. Recent studies have demonstrated the presence of endocrine cells in the human Bartholin's gland.[13] They are distributed throughout the epithelium of the duct, and some are dispersed among acinar lobules. Different cell types include serotonin-, calcitonin-, katacalcin-, bombesin-, and α-hCG-immunoreactive cells. These cells are richly granulated and show typical neuroendocrine features.

In addition, some small proteins found in human skin gland secretions have been claimed to be a possible candidate for a mammalian pheromone. However, Singer commented that, in general, many mammalian social odors do not elicit an observable specific response in the recipient and therefore strictly cannot be considered to be pheromones. Most mammalian pheromones are transferred by contact and detected by accessory olfaction.[14] Recent studies have also shown that steroids are metabolized by human epidermal keratinocytes.[15]

Amazingly, nonhuman mammalian pheromones are commonly used as perfumery ingredients that are very often marketed as having the ability to enhance sexual attractiveness. In fact, the attractive effect of perfumes is principally related to the effect of the pleasant scent. A more logical approach would be to use human pheromones that, for humans, are both more natural and more effective as true sensual attractants.[16] Androstenol and androstenone, two known sex pheromones in pigs, have also been identified in human urine, plasma, sweat, and saliva. It has been hypothesized that these two steroids are synthesized in tissues rich in 5α-reductase, such as skin, axillary sweat glands, and probably also the salivary glands.[17]

In any case, the sensitivity of the richly innervated skin to touch has led to the suggestion that it plays an important role in human sexual response. There are many areas on the female body that may be involved in the sexual response, though with considerable individual variation. During sexual excitement, some women may experience abdominal spasms. In addition to the breast, the buttocks and inner thighs are particularly sensitive in some women. It is interesting to note that, in some nonhuman primates, there is a highly vascularized edematous dermal patch, which is adjacent to the external genitalia, called sexual skin. It changes color with the reproductive cycle.[18]

With a functional neuroendocrine component, a female reproductive system with normal external genitalia and internal reproductive structures is sufficient for mating and subsequent pregnancy. In order to enhance reproductive success, two more aspects are necessary in the female: appropriate sexual and maternal behavior (see Chapters 7 and 9, respectively).

V. SEXUAL RESPONSE

Female sexual response is a necessary, integral part of the reproductive process. Appropriate sexual responses during sexual intercourse contribute to the success of the sex act. In the past two decades, systematic studies on the

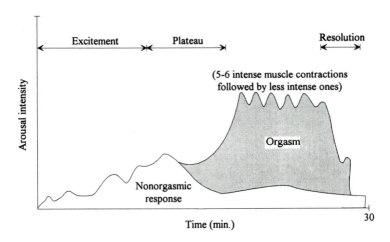

FIGURE 5.8.   The female sexual response. (After Brauer, A.P. and Brauer, D., *ESO: How You and Your Lover Can Give Each Other Hours of Extended Sexual Orgasm,* Warner Books, New York, 1983.)

human sexual response with more objective experimental designs and new instruments have provided a better understanding of human sexuality. Very often, response is considered equivalent to behavior, especially in animal studies where a certain type of activity in response to a stimulus is interpreted as behavioral reaction. In humans, the response can be divided into two parts. First are measurable changes taken by an observer. Second are the feelings described by the subject.

In the context of this chapter, sexual response is considered as a physiological response that can be measured objectively. The feelings of sexual response and their impact on human sexuality will be discussed in Chapters 7 and 12. Based on observable changes mainly in the external genitalia, the sexual response is arbitrarily divided into four sequential and continuous stages: excitement, plateau, orgasm, and resolution. Considering the high individual variation, the following is only a typical description (see also Figure 5.8).

A.   EXCITEMENT AND PLATEAU

The first phase of the female sexual response is called the excitement stage, which is likely to be induced by foreplay. Labia become darker in color, bright red or reddish purple. It is thought to be comparable to penis erection in the male. Vasocongestion leads to an increase in the size of the clitoris and the labia minora. Secretions start to be released, lubricating the vestibular area, the labia minora, and the inner surface of the labia majora. Internally, both the uterus and cervix pull away from the vagina, perhaps as a result of muscle contractions.

The plateau stage is characterized by the maximal state of all responses occurring in the excitement stage. This is the prelude to orgasm. Under normal conditions, the plateau stage is short and transient if the sexual stimulation is continuous. It is a building up of sexual excitement without release.

B. ORGASM AND RESOLUTION

Recent reports have suggested a possible homologous female prostate gland that is potentially involved in a sudden spurt of fluid being released at the moment of orgasm. A survey of female ejaculation during orgasm was performed by sending questionnaires to 2350 professional women in the U.S. and Canada with a subsequent 55% return rate.[19] Of these respondents, 40% reported having a fluid release (ejaculation) at the moment of orgasm. Furthermore, 82% of the women who reported the presence of the G-spot had also reported ejaculation with their orgasms.

Another interesting phenomenon is the simultaneous orgasm. Although orgasm can be experienced in many ways with or without a partner, partner involvement continues to be a noted preference for many women. A survey research design, which utilized the responses of 709 adult women, indicated that those women who usually experienced orgasm after their male partners perceived less physiological and psychological sexual satisfaction.[20]

In a recent comparison between 24 orgasmic and 10 anorgasmic women of age 21 to 40,[21] some psychological factors have been suggested based on self-report measures of sexual arousal while viewing explicit videotape segments depicting a variety of sexual activities. The authors reported four major points from the anorgasmic women: (1) greater discomfort in communicating with a partner regarding only those sexual activities involving direct clitoral stimulation, (2) more negative attitudes toward masturbation, (3) greater endorsement of sex myths, and (4) greater sex guilt.

Using a mathematical taxonomic method called hierarchical cluster analysis on 76 anorgasmic women, there are four distinct subtypes found based on psychosexual and psychological symptoms according to data from the Derogatis Sexual Functioning Inventory (DSFI) and the Brief Symptom Inventory (BSI).[22] Comparisons involving age, race, marital status, and social class demonstrated no significant differences among the four subtypes; however, statistical analyses of psychosexual, psychological symptom, and chart-review variables (including psychiatric diagnosis) revealed very significant distinctions among the four groups. From the resulting topology, anorgasmic subtypes were presumptively identified as "low desire" (n = 21), "histrionic/marital conflict" (n = 20), "psychiatric disorder" (n = 12), and "constitutional" (n = 16).

On the other extreme, orgasm has been reported to occur in response to imagery without any physical stimulation. Recent findings provide evidence that orgasm from self-induced imagery and genital self-stimulation can each produce significant and substantial net sympathetic activation and concomitant significant increases in pain thresholds. Orgasm from self-induced imagery or genital self-stimulation generated significant increases in systolic blood pressure, heart rate, pupil diameter, pain detection threshold, and pain tolerance threshold over resting control conditions.[23]

The length of an orgasmic episode varies greatly among different individuals and even between episodes in the same individual. The intensity also varies, and the building up of the sexual tension depends on the foreplay and the excitement

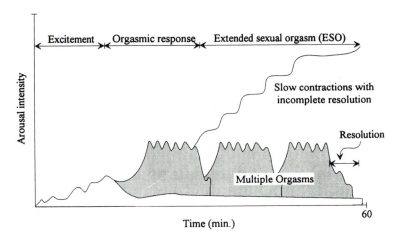

FIGURE 5.9. The female extended sexual orgasm. (After Brauer, A.P. and Brauer, D., *ESO: How You and Your Lover Can Give Each Other Hours of Extended Sexual Orgasm,* Warner Books, New York, 1983.)

stage. Orgasm is actually a rhythmic series of muscle contractions, with the last one being followed by the resolution stage. The pleasurable feeling is associated with a release of sexual tension. All the events associated with the excitement and orgasm are reversed and disappear. It should be noted that the resolution stage in some women is very short or even nonexistent, and they may sometimes have an unfinished orgasm.

C. EXTENDED OR MULTIPLE ORGASMS

The incidence of multiple orgasms among women had been reported two decades ago. A recent study based on the responses of 805 college-educated female nurses to a questionnaire indicated that 42.7% of the respondents had experienced multiple orgasms.[24] Although less than half of the women are orgasmic, while over 95% of men can easily experience orgasm, more women experience multiple orgasms than men. The biological role of multiple orgasms in human reproduction is not apparent.

The techniques leading to multiple orgasms among women have been studied, and these are collectively known as extended sexual orgasm (ESO).[25] According to Brauer and Brauer, ESO is a series of deeper vaginal muscle contractions, including the deep pelvic musculature and uterine muscles. Such contractions are longer and more pleasurable. ESO can be triggered by continual vaginal stimulation, while having the first ordinary orgasmic response. As shown in Figure 5.9, several orgasmic episodes may occur with brief resolution periods between them. As a result of incomplete resolution, the level of arousal continues to rise after each orgasmic episode. In contrast to the intermittent bursts of rapid contractions during multiple orgasms, continuous slow contractions of ESO can be sustained for over an hour. It should be noted that ESO has been claimed to occur in some women, but further physiological characterization is necessary.

The presence of such an elaborated female sexual response raises a question: What is its biological role? Since orgasmic responses associated with lordosis have been shown to be present in rats, similar sexual responses also may be experienced in animals. It is almost impossible to be certain that a rat showing physiological responses similar to orgasm is indeed "enjoying the feeling." In human introspective studies, such a conclusion about feelings is based on the verbal description of the subject. If an individual can experience these sexual pleasures during orgasm, it seems reasonable to speculate that the orgasmic response is an incentive for performing such an act.

In other species, the sex urge to copulate does provide a driving force to reproduce. In humans, the female sexual response per se is no longer relevant to the reproductive function of coitus, but rather it is part of the interaction between sexual partners. This is obvious when most coituses are nonreproductive. Being orgasmic or not is certainly not a decisive factor in the ability of the couple to reproduce, but, as shown in a recent study,[26] sexual satisfaction of both partners does contribute to marital harmony. Marital stability, at least for more than a few years, is obviously important for heterosexual partners to raise their biological children.

REFERENCES

1. **Fliegner, J.R. and Zeplin, A.J.**, Congenital absence of the vagina. Surgical treatment and perioperative care, *AORN J.*, 49, 789, 1989.
2. **DeLora, J.S., Warren, C.A.B., and Ellison, C.R.**, *Understanding Sexual Interaction*, 2nd ed., Houghton Mifflin, Boston, 1981.
3. **Davidson, J.K., Sr., Darling, C.A., and Conway-Welch, C.**, The role of the Grafenberg Spot and female ejaculation in the female orgasmic response: an empirical analysis, *J. Sex Marital Ther.*, 15, 102, 1989.
4. **Challis, J.R.G. and Olson, D.M.**, Parturition, in *The Physiology of Reproduction*, Knobil, E. and Neill, J., Eds., Raven Press, New York, 1988, 2177.
5. **Harper, M.J.K.**, Gamete and zygote transport, in *The Physiology of Reproduction*, Knobil, E. and Neill, J., Eds., Raven Press, New York, 1988, 103.
6. **Ahlgren, M.**, Sperm transport to and survival in the human Fallopian tube, *Gynecol. Invest.*, 6, 206, 1975.
7. **Mossman, H.W. and Duke, K.L.**, *Comparative Morphology of the Mammalian Ovary*, University of Wisconsin Press, Madison, 1973.
8. **Young, W.C.**, The mammalian ovary, in *Sex and Internal Secretions*, Young, W.C., Ed., Williams & Wilkins, Baltimore, 1961, 449.
9. **Byskov, A.G. and Høyer, P.E.**, Embryology of mammalian gonads and ducts, in *The Physiology of Reproduction*, Knobil, E. and Neill, J., Eds., Raven Press, New York, 1988, 265.
10. **Mastroianni, L., Jr. and Coutifaris, C.**, Reproductive physiology, in *The F.I.G.O. Manual of Human Reproduction*, Vol. 1, Fathalla, M.F., Rosenfield, A. and Indriso, C., Eds., Parthenon Publishing Group, Park Ridge, NJ, 1990.
11. **LeTreut, A. and Dilhuydy, H.M.**, *Mammography. A Guide to Interpretation*, C.V. Mosby, St. Louis, 1991.
12. **Osborne, M.P.**, Breast development and anatomy, in *Breast Disease*, Harris, J.R., Hellman, S., Henderson, I.C., and Kinne, D.W., Eds., Lippincott, New York, 1991, 1.

13. **Fetissof, F., Arbeille, B., Bellet, D., Barre, I., and Lansac, J.,** Endocrine cells in human Bartholin's glands. An immunohistochemical and ultrastructural analysis, *Virchows Archiv. B*, 57, 117, 1989.

14. **Singer, A.G.,** A chemistry of mammalian pheromones, *J. Steroid Biochem. Mol. Biol.*, 39, 627, 1991.

15. **Milewich, L., Shaw, C.B., and Sontheimer, R.D.,** Steroid metabolism by epidermal keratinocytes, *Ann. N.Y. Acad. Sci.*, 548, 66, 1988.

16. **Berliner, D.L., Jennings-White, C., and Lavker, R.M.,** The human skin: fragrances and pheromones, *J. Steroid Biochem. Mol. Biol.*, 39, 671, 1991.

17. **Smals, A.G. and Weusten, J.J.,** 16-Ene-steroids in the human testis, *J. Steroid Biochem. Mol. Biol.*, 40, 587, 1991.

18. **van Tienhoven, A.,** *Reproductive Physiology of Vertebrates,* 2nd ed., Cornell University Press, New York, 1983.

19. **Darling, C.A., Davidson, J.K., Sr., and Conway-Welch, C.,** Female ejaculation: perceived origins, the Grafenberg spot/area, and sexual responsiveness, *Arch. Sex. Behav.*, 19, 29, 1990.

20. **Darling, C.A., Davidson, J.K., Sr., and Cox, R.P.,** Female sexual response and the timing of partner orgasm, *J. Sex Marital Ther.*, 17, 3, 1991.

21. **Kelly, M.P., Strassberg, D.S., and Kircher, J.R.,** Attitudinal and experiential correlates of anorgasmia, *Arch. Sex. Behav.*, 19, 165, 1990.

22. **Derogatis, L.R., Schmidt, C.W., Fagan, P.J., and Wise, T.N.,** Subtypes of anorgasmia via mathematical taxonomy, *Psychosomatics*, 30, 166, 1989.

23. **Whipple, B., Ogden, G., and Komisaruk, B.R.,** Physiological correlates of imagery-induced orgasm in women, *Arch. Sex. Behav.*, 21, 121, 1992.

24. **Darling, C.A., Davidson, J.K., Sr., and Jennings, D.A.,** The female sexual response revisited: understanding the multiorgasmic experience in women, *Arch. Sex. Behav.*, 20, 527, 1991.

25. **Brauer, A.P. and Brauer, D.,** *ESO: How You and Your Lover Can Give Each Other Hours of Extended Sexual Orgasm,* Warner Books, New York, 1983.

26. **Greeley, A.M.,** *Faithful Attraction,* Tom Doherty Associates, New York, 1991.

27. **McLean, J.M.,** Anatomy and physiology of the vulval area, in *The Vulva,* Ridley, C.M., Ed., Churchill Livingstone, Edinburgh, 1988.

6 The Male Reproductive System

CHAPTER CONTENTS

I. INTRODUCTION

As in the female, the male reproductive system consists of the external genitalia and internal anatomical structures associated with reproduction. The neuroendocrine component involving the brain is also an important part of the system. The interactive mechanism between the testis and the brain through the "male endocrine orchestra" conducted by the pituitary gland must function well to express the necessary male characteristics. Proper use of these well-developed external and internal reproductive structures requires the neuroendocrine component and normal sexual physiology.

There are two processes unique and crucial to the male reproductive system: penile erection and ejaculation. Even with well-developed external and internal reproductive structures, the failure of these two processes will jeopardize the success of copulation and insemination (see also Chapters 7 and 8). This chapter will discuss the control of penile erection, ejaculation, and sexual responses with the involvement of neural, circulatory, and muscular systems. It will therefore emphasize the dependence of the male reproductive system on other systems.

II.   EXTERNAL GENITALIA

The male external genitalia varies greatly in structures among Eutheria, though the basic theme is identical. Two primary aims of the male genitalia are insemination and urination. Since the vas deferens is in continuation with the urethra, both semen and urine are emitted through the urethra. As described in Chapter 2, the vas deferens is derived from the Wolffian duct of the indifferent gonad. It joins with the urethra, and the pelvic portion of the urogenital sinus fuses to form the distal portion of urethra in the penis. It is interesting to compare the male genitalia with corresponding structures in the female, where most of the urogenital sinus remains open so that vaginal and urethral openings are separate.

A.   Penis

Among primates, human males have the largest penis, with a mean stretched length of a flaccid penis up to 13 cm. It consists of a long shaft with an expanded structure at the tip called the glans penis (see Figure 6.1). When flaccid, the prepuce (foreskin) usually covers most of the glans, leaving the urethral meatus exposed. In some individuals, the glans may be totally enclosed or, in contrast, totally exposed. During childhood, the prepuce may be too long so that the glans is tightly enclosed, creating a sanitary problem. Since it is believed that males with a long prepuce have a greater risk for urinary tract infection, sexually transmitted disease, phimosis, paraphimosis, and balanoposthitis, partial surgical removal of the prepuce soon after birth (neonatal circumcision) is often performed.[1] The procedure, though simple, may have complications such as infection, hemorrhage, and meatal stenosis. While the necessity of neonatal circumcision is controversial, alternatives to this surgical procedure are considered, such as foreskin retraction under local or general anesthesia. At any rate, regular foreskin hygiene is mandatory for all males, including circumcised individuals.

In Eutheria, there are different types of penises: indifferent (e.g., rodents), fibro-elastic (e.g., ruminants and whales), vascular (e.g., primates), and intermediary (e.g., elephants).[2] The indifferent penis is short, while the fibro-elastic is long and fibrous. Primate penises are long and flexible. Erection is achieved by filling the vascular tissues with blood. The elephant penis is both vascular and fibro-elastic. All types of penises can achieve erection with different erectile tissues. The human penis, as other primates, has little fibrous and no ossified tissues nor the retractor penis muscle. In all types, erection is a mechanism to

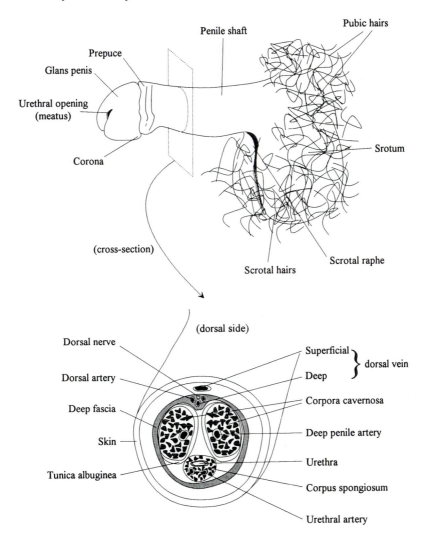

FIGURE 6.1.   Male external genital and cross-section of the penis.

enlarge the penis for insemination during coitus, but the duration of coitus varies with the type of penises. Coitus with the vascular-type penis is the longest type, whereas with the other types coitus may be as short as a few seconds.

In a normal adult human male, the glans of an erect penis is usually fully exposed (see Figure 6.1). The glans itself is enlarged and the penis shaft elongates. At the base of the glans, the rim is the corona behind which the prepuce stays during erection. Increased blood supply to the penis leads to a dramatic increase in both its length and diameter. The glans is derived from the genital tubercle, which in the female differentiates into the clitoris. Erection also leads to a change in the angle of penis relative to the body axis. All these changes are necessary for an easier penile intromission into the vaginal canal during copulation.

B.   SCROTUM

The scrotum is a sac-like structure for suspending the testes outside the body cavity. In some species with intra-abdominal testes such as elephants, armadillos, and dolphins, sperms can be produced at normal body temperature. In most mammals, spermatogenesis requires a lower temperature to operate optimally. There are additional mechanisms to enhance the cooling effect, such as the sweat glands on the scrotal skin. It is a selective advantage if the rate of spontaneous mutations in male germ cells is reduced in the lower scrotal temperature.[3]

Homologous to the labia majora of the female external genitalia, the scrotal sac is derived from the bilaterally symmetrical labioscrotal folds in the indifferent gonad. The line of fusion between the two folds becomes the scrotal raphe along the mid-ventral line of the scrotum. This median raphe of the scrotum can still be identified in adults (see Figure 6.1). In addition to these superficial structures, hairs are also found on the scrotum. Musculature can be found on the scrotal skin, and it is responsible for the movement of the scrotal sac. The scrotum can contract and relax vigorously during orgasm.

III.   INTERNAL REPRODUCTIVE STRUCTURES

A study of the male internal reproductive structures is necessary for a better understanding of penile erection, ejaculation, and semen formation. As with the male external genitalia, the arrangement of internal reproductive structures also varies greatly among vertebrates. Some have internal testes (e.g., elephant), while others may withdraw their testicles from the scrotum back to the abdominal cavity when they are frightened (e.g., rat). Human testicles remain in the scrotum at all times after fetal development.[4]

A.   PENIS

The penile erectile tissues of the human penis are the vascular type among mammals. The corpora cavernosa and corpus spongiosum are the erectile tissues richly supplied with blood vessels. This is a pair of deep arteries in the penis, each enclosed by the corpus cavernosa. As shown in the cross-section of a typical penis in Figure 6.1, the corpus spongiosum enclosing the urethra is situated at the mid-ventral position relative to the pair of corpora cavernosa. All these structures run parallel to the penile axis and are enclosed by a thick fibrous layer called Buck's fascia, which is covered by the outermost skin layer. In addition, each of the corpora is surrounded by another layer of fibrous tissue, the tunica albuginea. The corpus spongiosum extends from the base of the penile shaft to an expanded end inside the glans penis (see Figure 6.2). Two important aspects are its vasculature and innervation.

1.   Vasculature

Branches of the internal iliac or hypogastric artery become a bilateral pair of internal pudendal arteries. As shown in Figure 6.3, each pudendal artery ramifies

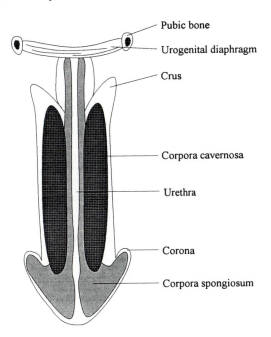

Pubic bone

Urogenital diaphragm

Crus

Corpora cavernosa

Urethra

Corona

Corpora spongiosum

FIGURE 6.2. Longitudinal section of the penis.

into the bulbar, urethral, deep penile, and dorsal arteries. The bulbar artery leads to the proximal corpus spongiosum, while the urethral artery supplies the glans penis through the whole length of corpus spongiosum. A pair of dorsal penile arteries run along the mid-dorsal line of the penis and are found between the Buck's fascia and the tunica albuginea and never enter the corpora cavernosa.

Another branch of the internal pudendal artery is the deep penile artery running inside the corpus cavernosa from the crus to the corona area. This artery divides into small helical arteries opening into the cavernous spaces separated by trabeculae. The trabeculae are made up of fibroblasts and smooth muscle cells with collagenous tissues and elastic fibers. There is a layer of endothelial cells covering the inner surface of the trabeculae. The endothelium is in continuation with the vascular endothelial layer from the small arteries and veins. In addition, there are anastomoses between the deep penile arteries of the paired corpora so that they act as a compounded unit.

For venous return, there are four major systems. First, the deep dorsal vein receives venous blood from the glans penis and the corpora cavernosa. Second, the deep vein leaves the corpus cavernosa in an area at the base of the penile shaft. Third, the bulbar and urethral veins drain the proximal corpus spongiosum. Fourth, the superficial dorsal vein running under the skin but superficial to Buck's fascia can be seen on the dorsal side of the penis. The venous drainage is very important for the degree of erection because a higher outflow resistance appears to sustain erection. Venous leakage may be a cause of erectile dysfunction leading to impotence.[5]

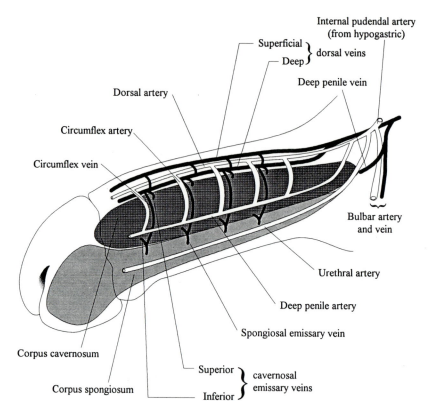

FIGURE 6.3. Vasculature of the penis.

2. Innervation

The penis is innervated by both the autonomic and somatic nervous systems (see Figure 6.4). The pelvic ganglionic plexus is located close to the rectal area and receives both sympathetic and parasympathetic nerves from thoracic (T_{10}) to upper lumbar (T_2) and the sacral (S_2 to S_4) regions of the spinal cord. Cavernosa nerves leaving the pelvic plexus run along the urethra and through the urogenital diaphragm to the dorsal medial region of the corpora cavernosa where the muscle fibers and capillaries are innervated. The pudendal nerve is the somatic innervation to the penis from sacral (S_2 to S_4) regions of the spinal cord. The nerve has a branch running parallel with the internal blood vessel, while another branch serves as the dorsal penile nerve for sensory function.

Both adrenergic and cholinergic fibers have been identified histochemically in corpora cavernosa and corpus spongiosum, but penile erection does not depend entirely on adrenergic and cholinergic systems. The involvement of vasoactive intestinal polypeptide (VIP) has been suggested.[6] In general, penile erection induced by psychogenic stimulation without physical contact with the genitalia seems to depend on the adrenergic system in some patients with spinal cord injuries. An intact sacral spinal reflex arc is required for responses to direct tactile stimuli on the genitalia.

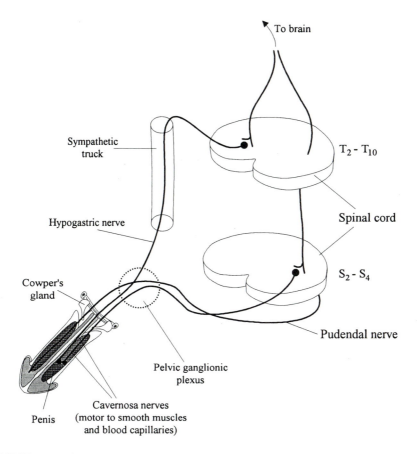

FIGURE 6.4.   Innervation of the penile structures.

B.   TESTIS, EPIDIDYMIS, AND VAS DEFERENS

The human testis and epididymis are located in the scrotum and are made up of densely packed and coiled ducts (see Figure 6.5). The connection between the testis and epididymis is the rete testis and ductuli efferentes. In 1 g of human testis, the seminiferous tubule is about 20 to 25 m long with a diameter of about 200 μm. There are about 300 lobules in a testis. Each lobule contains 1 to 4 tubules, and both ends of each tubule open into the rete testis.[7] The epididymis, in contrast, contains one single duct for sperm storage only.[8]

The rete testis is a collection of interconnecting tubules in which, unlike the seminiferous tubule, the lumen is lined by common columnar epithelial cells. As a transition zone before entering the rete testis, the lumen at the ends of each seminiferous tubule is lined by cells similar to the Sertoli cell. An aggregate of these cells forms a valvelike structure that may reduce the backflow of fluid from the rete testis to the seminiferous tubule. On the side of the rete testis joining with the transition zone of the seminiferous tubule, there is a structure called the tubulus rectus. In humans, there may be up to six seminiferous tubules connected with one tubulus rectus.[7]

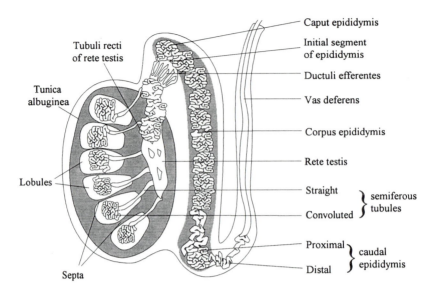

FIGURE 6.5. The human testis.

The rete testis has numerous tubuli recti on the side with seminiferous tubules and several efferent ducts on the other side with the ductus epididymis. These efferent ducts coalesce to a single epididymal duct as long as 3 to 4 m in humans. The duct is highly convoluted and is packed into a species-specific shape (see Figure 6.5). The structure is divided into four main regions: initial segment, caput, corpus, and cauda. Although some histological differences can be found among different regions of the epididymis, there are biochemical differences in the absorptive and secretory cells important for sperm maturation.[8] Other important functions of the epididymis include concentrating the semen and sperm storage.

The caudal epididymis can be subdivided further into proximal and distal regions. The distal end is connected with the vas deferens, which is a muscular duct leading to the urethra. The vas deferens enlarges at that point and becomes the ampulla where it joins with the duct of the seminal vesicle to form the ejaculatory duct. With the contralateral one, they converge to form the urethra. The whole length of the vas deferens in humans is about 25 to 35 cm. Sperm transport in both the epididymis and vas deferens is achieved by regular contractions of the wall. Ciliary action of the epithelial cells may also be helpful in the vas deferens.

Based on studies using radioactively labeled sperms, it takes 8 to 14 days for sperm to be transported from the rete testis to the vas deferens. The main sperm storage area is the caudal epididymis, and the sperms can retain their fertilizing capacity for 1 month.

C. ACCESSORY SEX GLANDS

In the semen, only about 5% are sperms, and the others are secretions mainly from the seminal vesicle and prostate gland. In addition, most of the fluid from

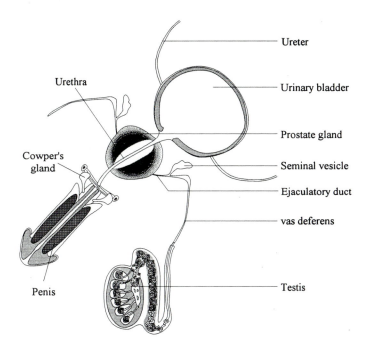

Ureter

Urethra

Urinary bladder

Prostate gland

Cowper's
gland

Seminal vesicle

Ejaculatory duct

vas deferens

Penis

Testis

FIGURE 6.6.   The male accessory sex glands.

the seminiferous tubule is reabsorbed into the epididymis where sperms are concentrated. The formation of semen mainly takes place in the vas deferens at the ampulla region. A typical sample of semen varies from 2 to 6 ml with 50 to 150×10^6/ml sperms. Figure 6.6 shows the relative positions of the accessory sex glands.

1.   Seminal Vesicle

This is a pair of glands connected to the ampulla of the vas deferens. Each gland is a collection of convoluted ducts with a secretory epithelium surrounded by a smooth muscle layer. It secretes a viscous fluid containing ascorbic acid, prostaglandins, fibrinogen, and fructose. As the major energy source for sperms, the fructose concentration can be as high as 2 to 3 mg/ml in the seminal plasma. Although sodium and potassium are the chief cations in the seminal fluid, calcium and magnesium are also high. The electrolyte usually has an alkaline pH with the presence of bicarbonate and citrate.

It should be noted that the name "seminal vesicle" was used because of a misconception. Previously, it was thought to be a receptacle for temporary storage of sperms. Seminal vesicles of lower vertebrates are for holding sperms in the female after insemination. The seminal vesicle in humans is now known to produce about half the secretions in the semen.

2.   Prostate Gland

This is a single gland larger than the seminal vesicle with more elaborated lobular structures. In humans, the prostate is densely packed and weighs about 20 g. It contains 30 to 50 tubuloalveolar glands with 15 to 30 ducts connecting to the prostatic urethra. The gland is situated at the base of the bladder where the ejaculatory ducts join. The presence of muscle fibers suggests an active secretory activity by its physical contractile property.

The prostatic fluid in humans has high calcium and potassium with abundant citrate anion (4 mg/ml seminal plasma) as an important osmotic regulator. In contrast to seminal fluid, the prostatic fluid has an acidic pH of 6.5, possibly because of high citrate. The human prostatic fluid also contains polyamines such as spermine and spermidine, which are rarely detected in other species. These polyamines can be oxidized by diamine oxidase detected in seminal plasma. This oxidation produces reactive aldehyde compounds that may be toxic to sperm and bacteria. They are also thought to give the characteristic odor of the semen. The exact function of spermine is still uncertain.[9] In a recent report, spermine and two other polyamines, putrescine and spermidine, have been shown to modulate the binding of the progesterone-receptor complex to DNA *in vitro*.[10]

Although prostaglandins were named after the prostate gland by von Euler in 1934, 25 years later it had been found out that their main source is the seminal vesicle and not the prostate gland.[11] There are many types of prostaglandins identified and detected in different tissues at lower concentrations. In the human seminal plasma, prostaglandin concentration can be up to 300 µg/ml.[12]

Another interesting component in the prostatic fluid is zinc with a mean concentration of 150 µg/ml of seminal plasma (about 350 µg/ml in prostatic fluid). As spermidine, zinc has been suggested to be antibacterial,[12] though the resistance to infection could not be shown to correlate with prostatic tissue zinc concentrations in a recent study on experimentally induced *Escherichia coli* bacterial prostatitis in dogs.[13] Zinc has also been associated with cadmium-induced prostatic cancer in a study suggesting that a higher cadmium to zinc ratio is found in populations with higher prostatic cancer rates.[14]

An immunohistochemical study demonstrated that metallothionein (MT), a binding protein for zinc or cadmium, was localized in the cytoplasm, nuclei of glandular epithelia, and secretory products in prostate glands from patients with urinary bladder cancer.[15] Most zinc ions are possibly bound to proteins as in the blood circulation. Interestingly, another protein of a smaller size (66 kDa) has been reported to form a zinc-protein complex that binds to epididymal sperms in rats.[16] When sperms with bound radiolabeled zinc-protein complexes are treated with a buffer containing 0.5% sodium deoxycholate and 40 mM EDTA, most of the labels are retained. Sansone and Abrescia suggested that the zinc proteins were kept on the plasma membrane by interactions stronger than hydrophobic bonds.[16]

3.   Cowper's (Bulbourethral) and Other Glands

This is a pair of multilobular glands connected to the urethra through ducts at a point before entering the corpus spongiosum. It is a typical glandular structure with convoluted tubules dilated into alveoli and arranged in lobules separated by septa. The whole gland is enclosed in a fibroelastic capsule. Both the capsule and septa are equipped with muscle fibers. The lumen of the secretory tubule is lined by a stratified columnar epithelium consisting of 67 cellular layers.

In the superficial layers of this epithelium, there are typical intracellular secretory granules and membrane-bound bodies with a filamentous texture that usually fuse with the mucus droplets before discharging into the lumen.[17] The mucus secretion contains a 6500-kDa mucin with a high content of sialic acid (27%).[7] Recent ultrastructural immunohistochemical studies have shown that the mucus cells of these glands have mucus droplets, which react to blood group antigens.[18] Riva et al. suggested that the glands may participate in the secretion of these antigens into the seminal plasma.

There are other glands such as the urethral glands (glands of Littré) which are small glands on the urethra in the corpus cavernosa. As other glands, they secrete mucus into the urethral lumen through small ducts. Interestingly, a recent study has demonstrated immunoreactivities of prostatic acid phosphatase (PACP) and prostate-specific antigen (PSA) in urethral glands of normal individuals by indirect immunoperoxidase staining. Kamoshida and Tsutsumi commented that the ability to express PACP and PSA is a feature common to cloacogenic glandular epithelium.[19]

IV. SPERM MATURATION AND CAPACITATION

Sperms are produced continuously in an adult testis through the processes of spermatogenesis and spermiogenesis (see Chapter 1). In the lumen of the seminiferous tubule, sperms are suspended by Sertoli cells with their tails pointing toward the center of the lumen. At different points of the seminiferous tubule, numerous differentiated sperms are released every second in a normal testis. Although a single spermatogonium takes 53 days to become a differentiated sperm, the enormous length of the seminiferous tubule is a guarantee for a continuous supply of sperms.

It should be noted that well-differentiated sperms just released into the lumen of the seminiferous tubule are immature. A maturation process occurs in the epididymis with progressive changes. Sperms recovered from caput epididymis, caudal epididymis, and ejaculated semen are different (see Figure 6.5 for different regions). Ejaculated sperms still lack the ability to fertilize oocytes. An additional process called capacitation occurring in the female reproductive tract is necessary for the sperms to acquire their fertilizing ability.

A.   EPIDIDYMAL MATURATION OF SPERMS

The major change in sperms after epididymal maturation is their increased motility. Biochemically, macromolecules attached to the sperm plasma membrane are lost, altered, or replaced by new ones from epididymal fluid. Most of these macromolecules are glycoproteins, and some are membrane lipids associated with cholesterol synthesis. There is a progressive change in osmolality and chemical composition of the fluid from the caput to the corpus to the cauda epididymis. This maturation process can be performed *in vitro* if caput sperms are demembranated and exposed to ATP, cAMP, and Mg^{2+}. Some components in the epididymal fluid may be important. Therefore, ejaculated sperms are usually in artificial insemination or *in vitro* fertilization (IVF) procedures.

B.   Sperm Capacitation

The necessity of capacitation for sperms to have their fertilizing ability was first reported by Chang in 1951.[20] By 1963, Yanagimachi and Chang[21] reported the first successful capacitation of mammalian sperms *in vitro*. According to the definition by Austin,[22] capacitation is a process through which a sperm acquires its ability to undergo the acrosome reaction. Capacitation is uniquely mammalian, while the acrosome reaction is the first mandatory step for fertilization in almost all vertebrates (see Chapter 8).

Capacitation normally occurs in the female genital tract, but the time and site are species specific.[23] It involves loss of sperm surface proteins and is dependent on the composition of the environment such as adequate free calcium, sodium, and potassium and appropriate energy substrates provided within the female reproductive tract. Biochemical changes include the alteration of membrane cholesterol to phospholipid ratios, removal of seminal plasma-coating proteins and cell-surface components, and alterations of membrane potential of the sperm head.[24] These change membrane permeability to calcium ions involving the calcium-dependent enzyme phospholipase A_2 system as well as the adenylate cyclase and cAMP-dependent protein kinase system, leading to the acrosome reaction.

The extensive modifications in the plasma membrane, such as the change in the cholesterol or phospholipid content, are not part of capacitation. Such changes would lead to premature membrane destabilization occurring later in the acrosome reaction.[25] Therefore, the beginning of the acrosome reaction indicates the end of capacitation. Although capacitation has been studied extensively *in vitro*, the process occurring *in vivo* requires shorter time and may not be the same.[26] The capacitation times *in vivo* and *in vitro* are different among several mammalian species. The capacitation time is assessed by incubating the sperms in the female reproductive tract or in a culture medium (e.g., Ham's F-10) for different times before depositing them back into recently ovulated females.

Perhaps, the requirement for capacitation may be an *in vitro* phenomenon because an exact simulation of the environment *in utero* is not possible. Very often, some heat-stable and low-molecular weight factors from the follicular fluid and blood serum are necessary. In hamsters, for example, the cumulus oophorus of the follicle is sufficient to allow capacitation. The requirements apparently vary from species to species, and there are great individual variations as well.

Another difference between capacitation *in vivo* and *in vitro* is the higher resistance of ejaculated sperms to *in vitro* capacitation than cauda epididymal sperms.[26] Both types of sperms, in contrast, are equally capacitated *in vivo*. Ejaculated sperms may have a more stable plasma membrane after exposure to seminal plasma. Epididymal sperms are similar to capacitated sperms and can fertilize a higher percentage of eggs than epididymal sperms previously exposed to seminal plasma. Therefore, ejaculated sperms are probably decapacitated by seminal plasma and need to be recapacitated in the female reproductive tract.[27,28]

C. SPERMIOPHAGY

Since sperms are continuously produced without ejaculation, there must be some ways to solve the problem of sperm accumulation. This is also a common question concerning vasectomy. Sperms were previously thought to be eliminated by "insensible ejaculation" (or nocturnal emission) and through the urine,[29] though degeneration of sperms in epididymis of the guinea pig had been reported by 1930.[30] A quantitative study on dairy bulls reported three decades later suggested that the majority of the sperms are resorbed in epididymis and vas deferens.[31] Now, we have evidence showing that the resorption is performed by phagocytic cells. Some luminal macrophages and epithelial cells in the ampullary region of vas deferens as well as the epididymis may be involved.[8]

The phagocytic process, specifically called spermiophagy, is activated by mechanical or chemical manipulation of the epididymis and vas deferens. The presence of excess or abnormal sperms is apparently a signal to initiate spermiophagy. A recent study on patients with accessory gland infections or subjects who have sperm antibodies in their semen has demonstrated the presence of macrophages with phagocytic activity on ejaculated spermatozoa.[32] With the help of the scanning electron microscopy, Blanco et al. could witness the process of spermiophagy; they wrote "... the spermatozoa were caught by the head first sometimes but by the main-piece fragment of the tail first in other instances; very rarely were they taken by the midportion, between the head and tail."

V. SEXUAL RESPONSE

Like the female sexual response, the male sexual response is divided into four continuous stages: excitement, plateau, orgasm, and resolution.[28] These stages are well defined because the responses evoked are very conspicuous; mainly indicated by penile erection and semen ejaculation (see Figure 6.7).

A. EXCITEMENT AND PENILE ERECTION

Penile erection is the excitement stage of the male sexual response. The corpus spongiosum and corpus cavernosa are endowed with abundant blood vessels and confluent spaces that become filled with blood during the excitement stage. Although the corpus spongiosum surrounding the urethra is enlarged, it remains softer than the corpus cavernosa. This allows the urethra to maintain its shape when the penis becomes rigid.

The stimulus can be either physical or psychological. Since the change in size is dramatic in a normal male, the occurrence of the sexual response toward a specific stimulus is almost indisputable. Physical touch without any psychological input can consistently produce an erection. Viewing erotic pictures or films without physical stimulation may also produce an erection in most cases. However, stress and anxiety are common causes of penile erection failure as shown in some cases of male sexual dysfunction.

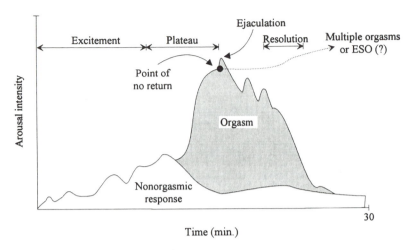

FIGURE 6.7. The male sexual response. (After Brauer, A.P. and Brauer, D., *ESO: How You and Your Lover Can Give Each Other Hours of Extended Sexual Orgasm,* Warner Books, New York, 1983.)

The degree of penile erection varies from one individual to another at different times. Penile erection may not be maintained throughout the excitement stage. Depending on the duration of the sex act, there may be recurrent penile erection. Since the major function of the penis being rigid is to facilitate insertion into the vagina, repetitive stimuli are often necessary during intromission. In some cases of male sexual dysfunction, premature ejaculation may occur prior to intromission, and penile erection is lost.

B.   ORGASM AND EJACULATION

In a normal male during a typical sexual intercourse, ejaculation occurs during orgasm. As in the female, there is a plateau stage just as all sexual responses become maximal before orgasm. At the same time, an accumulation of seminal fluid in the urethra occurs at the prostate gland. The size of the urethral bulb increases also. Under normal conditions, as compared to females, the plateau stage in males is short and transient if the sexual stimulation is continuous. At the end of the plateau, the surge toward ejaculation occurs and reaches a point where the response cannot be restrained. Ejaculation is inevitable after passing this point, and orgasm occurs.

Ejaculation or emission is usually an indication of orgasm, which consists of a series of "involuntary" muscle contractions. However, there are reports showing that orgasm can be achieved without ejaculation.[33] Experimentally, ejaculation and orgasm can be separated into two different events in animal models. There are claims that such a separation can be achieved voluntarily in humans after training.[34] This technique would be very useful for couples who employ the withdrawal method as contraception, though there is always a risk of having sperms in preejaculatory fluids.

C. Resolution and Multiple Orgasms

At the end of the series of ejaculatory muscle contractions, the resolution phase follows. The individual becomes refractory to further stimulation with a release of the sexual tension accumulated during the excitement and plateau stages. In contrast to the resolution stage in women, the "feeling of resolution" is distinct so that men often become exhausted and fall asleep. Such a gender difference is believed to be behavioral. In contrast to the refractory period of penile erection during resolution, the "feeling of exhaustion" is probably not involuntary and can be modified behaviorally.

The incidence of multiple orgasms in men has been reported and the techniques leading to multiple orgasms have been studied.[33] Ejaculation involves repetitive contractions of smooth muscle in the wall of the cauda epididymis, vas deferens, prostate, and seminal vesicles. These contractions are controlled through adrenergic fibers in the hypogastric nerves and are usually involuntary. The training technique in men to achieve multiple orgasms may be difficult, and the effectiveness varies greatly among different individuals.

D. Semen Liquefaction

Human semen is originally a liquid at the time of ejaculation. Within 5 min after ejaculation, it solidifies and becomes a coagulum. After another 5 to 10 min, the coagulum liquefies again. Recent findings indicate that the seminal vesicle-specific antigen (SVSA) is the structural component of seminal coagulum, and the prostate-specific antigen (PSA) is the enzyme which digests SVSA and liquifies the semen coagulum.[35] The coagulum is composed of sialoglycoproteins bound by copper to form protein-metal complexes.[36] The initial stage of liquefaction results from the reduction of these metal ions by L-ascorbic acid present in large quantities in the seminal plasma.

Although the coagulation process resembles blood clotting, it is not inhibited by calcium-binding agents (e.g., citrate and heparin) and does not require prothrombin, fibrinogen or factor XII, which are absent in seminal plasma.[37] There are two types of seminal plasma proteolytic enzymes involved during liquefaction. First, two plasminogen activators of 70 and 74 kDa are secreted by the prostate gland. Second, a proteolytic enzyme called seminin, a 30-kDa protein with proteinase activity, also comes from the prostate gland. Therefore, factors for coagulation originate from the seminal vesicle, while those for liquefaction are prostatic.

In contrast to the female, the male sexual response plays a more important role in the success of copulation and insemination. Penile intromission requires an erect penis that can be kept at an appropriate position in the vagina to deposit the semen. The ability of the male to ejaculate is the final but crucial step for successful insemination.

REFERENCES

1. **Robson, W.L. and Leung, A.K.**, The circumcision question, *Postgrad. Med.*, 91, 237, 1992.
2. **van Tienhoven, A.**, *Reproductive Physiology of Vertebrates*, 2nd ed., Cornell University Press, New York, 1983.
3. **Ehrenberg, L., von Ehrenstein, G., and Hedgran, A.**, Gonadal temperatures and spontaneous mutation rates in man, *Nature (London)*, 180, 1433, 1957.
4. **Williams-Ashman, H.G.**, Perspectives in the male sexual physiology of Eutherian mammals, in *The Physiology of Reproduction*, Knobil, E. and Neill, J., Eds., Raven Press, New York, 1988, 727.
5. **Wespes, E. and Shulman, C.C.**, Venous leakage: surgical treatment of a curable cause of impotence, *J. Urol.*, 133, 796, 1985.
6. **Benson, G.S.**, Male sexual function, erection, emission, and ejaculation, in *The Physiology of Reproduction*, Knobil, E. and Neill, J., Eds., Raven Press, New York, 1988, 1121.
7. **Setchell, B.P. and Brooks, D.E.**, Anatomy, vasculature, innervation, and fluids of the male reproductive tract, in *The Physiology of Reproduction*, Knobil, E. and Neill, J., Eds., Raven Press, New York, 1988, 753.
8. **Robaire, B. and Hermo, L.**, Efferent ducts, epididymis, and vas deferens: structure, functions, and their regulation, in *The Physiology of Reproduction*, Knobil, E. and Neill, J., Eds., Raven Press, New York, 1988, 999.
9. **Janne, J., Alhonen, L., and Leinonen, P.**, Polyamines: from molecular biology to clinical applications, *Ann. Med.* (Hagerstown, MD), 23, 241, 1991.
10. **Thomas, T. and Kiang, D.T.**, Modulation of the binding of progesterone receptor to DNA by polyamines, *Cancer Res.*, 48, 1217, 1988.
11. **Eliasson, R.**, Studies on prostaglandins. Occurrence, formation, and biological actions, *Acta Physiol. Scand.*, 158(Suppl. 46), 1, 1959.
12. **Coffey, D.S.**, Androgen action and the sex accessory tissues, in *The Physiology of Reproduction*, Knobil, E. and Neill, J., Eds., Raven Press, New York, 1988, 999.
13. **Cowan, L.A., Barsanti, J.A., Brown, J., and Jain, A.**, Effects of bacterial infection and castration on prostatic tissue zinc concentration in dogs, *Am. J. Vet. Res.*, 52, 1262, 1991.
14. **Ogunlewe, J.O. and Osegbe, D.N.**, Zinc and cadmium concentrations in indigenous blacks with normal, hypertrophic, and malignant prostate, *Cancer*, 63, 1388, 1989.
15. **Suzuki, T., Umeyama, T., Ohma, C., Yamanaka, H., Suzuki, K., Nakajima, K., and Kimura, M.**, Immunohistochemical study of metallothionein in normal and benign prostatic hyperplasia of human prostate, *Prostate*, 19, 35, 1991.
16. **Sansone, G. and Abrescia, P.**, Zinc-protein from rat prostate fluid binds epididymal spermatozoa, *J. Exp. Zool.*, 259, 379, 1991.
17. **Riva, A., Usai, E., Cossu, M., Scarpa, R., and Testa-Riva, F.**, The human bulbo-urethral glands. A transmission electron microscopy and scanning electron microscopy study, *J. Androl.*, 9, 133, 1988.
18. **Riva, A., Usai, E., Cossu, M., Lantini, M.S., Scarpa, R., and Testa-Riva, F.**, Ultrastructure of human bulbourethral glands and of their main excretory ducts, *Arch. Androl.*, 24, 177, 1990.
19. **Kamoshida, S. and Tsutsumi, Y.**, Extraprostatic localization of prostatic acid phosphatase and prostate-specific antigen: distribution in cloacogenic glandular epithelium and sex-dependent expression in human anal gland, *Hum. Pathol.*, 21, 1108, 1990.
20. **Chang, M.C.**, Fertilizing capacity of spermatozoa deposited in Fallopian tubes, *Nature (London)*, 168, 997, 1951.
21. **Yanagimachi, R. and Chang, M.C.**, Fertilization of hamster eggs *in vitro, Nature (London)*, 200, 281, 1963.
22. **Austin, C.R.**, Capacitation of spermatozoa, *Int. J. Fertil.*, 12, 25, 1967.

23. **Fraser, L.R.,** Requirements for successful mammalian sperm capacitation and fertilization, *Arch. Pathol. Lab. Med.,* 116, 345, 1992.

24. **Bird, J.M. and Houghton, J.A.,** The activation of mammalian sperm, *Sci. Prog. (London),* 75(297 Pt 1–2), 107, 1991.

25. **Zaneveld, L.J., De Jonge, C.J., Anderson, R.A., and Mack, S.R.,** Human sperm capacitation and the acrosome reaction, *Hum. Reprod.,* 6, 1265, 1991.

26. **Yanagimachi, R.,** Mammalian fertilization, in *The Physiology of Reproduction,* Knobil, E. and Neill, J., Eds., Raven Press, New York, 1988, 1081.

27. **Ahlgren, M.,** Sperm transport to and survival in the human Fallopian tube, *Gynecol. Invest.,* 6, 206, 1975.

28. **Mastroianni, L., Jr. and Coutifaris, C.,** Reproductive physiology, in *The F.I.G.O. Manual of Human Reproduction,* Vol. 1, Fathalla, M.F., Rosenfield, A. and Indriso, C., Eds., Parthenon Publishing Group, Park Ridge, NJ, 1990.

29. **Wilhelm, S.F. and Seligmann, A.W.,** Spermatozoa in urine, *Am. J. Surg.,* 35, 572, 1937.

30. **Young, W.C. and Simeone, F.A.,** Development and fate of spermatozoa in the epididymis and vas deferens in the guinea pig, *Proc. Soc. Exp. Biol. Med.,* 27, 838, 1930.

31. **Amann, R.P. and Almquist, J.O.,** Reproductive capacity of dairy bulls. VI. Effect of unilateral vasectomy and ejaculation frequency on sperm reserves; aspects of epididymal physiology, *J. Reprod. Fertil.,* 3, 260, 1962.

32. **Blanco, A.M., Palaoro, L., Ahedo, M.I., Palamas, M., and Zanchetti, F.,** Phagocytosis of ejaculated spermatozoa, *Acta Cytol.,* 36, 251, 1992.

33. **Dunn, M.E. and Trost, J.E.,** Male multiple orgasms: a descriptive study, *Arch. Sex. Behav.,* 18, 377, 1989.

34. **Brauer, A.P. and Brauer, D.,** *ESO: How You and Your Lover Can Give Each Other Hours of Extended Sexual Orgasm,* Warner Books, New York, 1983.

35. **Lee, C., Keefer, M., Zhao, Z.W., Kroes, R., Berg, L., Liu, X.X., and Sensibar, J.,** Demonstration of the role of prostate-specific antigen in semen liquefaction by two-dimensional electrophoresis, *J. Androl.,* 10, 432, 1989.

36. **Polak, B. and Daunter, B.,** Seminal plasma biochemistry. III: characterization of coagulum components, *Eur. J. Obstet. Gynecol. Reprod. Biol.,* 35, 223, 1990.

37. **Polak, B. and Daunter, B.,** Seminal plasma biochemistry. IV: enzymes involved in the liquefaction of human seminal plasma, *Int. J. Androl.,* 12, 187, 1989.

7 Sexual Behavior and Copulation

CHAPTER CONTENTS

I. INTRODUCTION

Sexual behavior plays an important role in the reproductive process. To achieve sexual union, an appropriate pattern of sexual behavior specific to a particular species is necessary. This statement also applies to different races, cultures, or even among different individuals in human society. Some people may find others' sexual behavior unacceptable, while others insist on performing a unique ritual before copulation. The compatibility of sexual behavior between two heterosexual partners is crucial to the success of sexual union and their joint reproductive life. The distinction between normal and deviant sexual behavior is often controversial and varies from time to time in different cultures. From an evolutionary viewpoint, any behavior leading to a loss of reproductive potentials can be classified as deviant sexual behavior. Contraception to achieve childlessness throughout one's lifetime is apparently against the Darwinian principle of reproductive fitness for species survival.

The practice of contraception has become an integral part of human sexual behavior. It provides a mechanism comparable to the reproductive cycle. For example, seasonal breeders cannot reproduce when the dark period is long because of gonadal regression and low sex drive. These animals are endowed with a natural mechanism of contraception under unfavorable conditions and have well-defined endocrine changes and observable anatomical adjustments to achieve contraception. Without these neuroendocrine mechanisms, how can we regulate our reproductive process? Although some neuroendocrine mechanisms remain operative in humans, we are not truly seasonal (see also Chapter 11). The human species may be evolving toward a greater dependence on neural or cognitive control of reproduction.

The human brain is endowed with a natural mechanism to regulate its own reproductive process: creativity. Humans have indeed done a brilliant job in the past several decades to create contraceptive means for reproductive control (see also Chapter 10). Unlike seasonal animals with restrictive reproductive cycles, humans prefer having freedom of choice. The act of not having a reproductive control is a choice itself. With the advancement of reproductive technology, the list of choices lengthens from time to time. We have a more precise timing control of conception and have safer ways to cope with infertility diseases. A couple can now choose to have a child at any time during the fertile period. All these inventions of our brain shape human sexuality and thus our reproductive pattern (see Chapter 12).

Diversified contraceptive methods are available in a human society advocating freedom of choice, such as the U.S. Some can effectively regulate their conception rates by saying yes or no, while others must rely on drugs or contraceptive devices. Physicians may help others to achieve or terminate pregnancy, while some activists insist on forbidding others' sexual behavior and reproductive choices. In more restrictive societies, couples have to obey laws limiting the number of children they should have and even how they should perform their sex acts. All these are part of the natural mechanism to regulate our reproductive process. This is human sexual behavior.

As a focus in this chapter, the main purpose of sexual behavior is to achieve copulation. The process involves development of appropriate behaviors, courtship for bringing females and males in close proximity, and final physical contact leading to copulation. In addition to normal female and male reproductive structures, well-defined female and male sexual behaviors are necessary for courtship and the drive to copulate. Since more objective experimental data on the control of sexual behavior are available for laboratory animals, our understanding of human sexual behavior is mostly derived from animal studies. With cautious interpretations of animal data extrapolated to humans and of often subjective human studies, this chapter will emphasize the role of sexual behavior and gender differences in human reproduction.

II.   SEXUALLY DIMORPHIC BEHAVIOR

Sexual dimorphism in anatomical structures is so conspicuous that two individuals of opposite sexes of the same species can be mistaken as two different species. Based on casual examination of the external genitalia, a novice can find no resemblance at all between a penis and a vulva, even in humans. These subtle structural differences lead one to speculate that sexual dimorphism in the brain exists and that sexual behavior is also sexually dimorphic. There are many studies searching for sexually dimorphic behaviors correlated with anatomical differences between male and female brains in humans. Sexually dimorphic behavior provides initial clues for gender recognition, a crucial step to initiate the interaction between two sexes. Sexual attraction and courtship allow screening of competent partners before copulation. Figure 7.1 is an overview of sexual attraction leading to courtship in humans. Several theories have been proposed to explain the complex set of factors in mate selection. In the Process Theory, a series of selection filters was conceived by Klimek as a screening mechanism from sexual attraction to courtship.[1] We will discuss more about these theories later in this chapter. Sexually dimorphic behavior is not limited to mate selection. Aggression, maternal behavior, and cognitive behavior may also be sexually specific.

A.   REPRODUCTIVE BEHAVIOR

Reproductive behavior includes, in addition to sexual behavior, other behaviors related to reproduction, such as migration and maternal behavior. Some migratory species travel from tropical areas to arctic breeding sites. As a common example, the migratory salmon spends a long time with great efforts to swim upstream to spawn once in a lifetime and die. Some males fight with other males or their own intended mates for several hours. If the courtship is successful, they have a brief copulation of only a few seconds.

In humans, the institution of marriage may be viewed as a mechanism to achieve copulation for reproductive purposes. About 50% of married couples in the U.S. spend their lives in monogamous relationships. Americans typically start courtship in their twenties and get married. During their fertile married life, they copulate and produce several children until menopause. Many couples then choose to stay together until the end of their lives. Since only about 30 to 40% of married individuals admit having extramarital copulations, we can assume that most of these lifelong monogamous couples have only intramarital copulations. Predominant reproductive behaviors in civilized human societies such as the U.S. are lifelong monogamy and serial monogamy, though polygamy also exists in some minor human societies with diversified courtship behaviors (see Chapter 12).

In most species including humans, mating partners have to perform the following three steps, which are sexually dimorphic, in order to achieve copulation: courtship, intromission, and insemination. The initial step is identification and

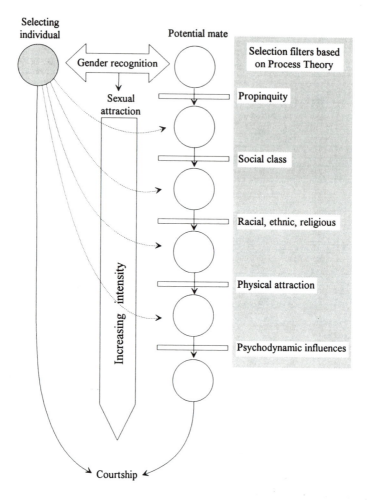

FIGURE 7.1. Sexual attraction leading to courtship. (After Klimek, D., *Beneath Mate Selection and Marriage*, Van Nostrand Reinhold, New York, 1979.)

courtship, followed by physical contact and intromission. The final step is insemination accompanied by genital reflexes (see Chapter 8). Identification is obviously an important prelude to courtship. There are two levels of identification: species and gender.

1.   Species Identification

The first level of identification is species recognition that is necessary to avoid futile copulations. Even for humans, the ability to identify our own species may fail in some mentally abnormal individuals. The identification process indeed requires complex brain functions. Species identification involves the display of species-specific features and the ability to identify them by different senses including visual, auditory, and olfactory. Interspecies mating does occur, and the process in which the oocyte is activated by a sperm from another species is called hybridogenesis. With a few exceptions, the outcome is usually lethal or the interspecies hybrids are at least sterile.

In some freshwater viviparous fishes of the genus *Poeciliopsis*, interspecies reproduction results in viable and fertile offspring. For example, hybrids of *P. monacha* oocytes activated by *P. lucida* sperms are all females with only the *P. monacha* genome intact. It is a result of segregation failure in the hybrid zygote, so that paternal genome is eliminated in the polar body, while the oocyte carrying the maternal genome develops into an embryo.[2] In a recent study, the incidence of liver tumors was compared in these fishes exposed to diethylnitrosamine. The incidence was significantly higher in *P. lucida* (89.0%) than in *P. monacha* (18.9 to 36.8%), while the nine hybrid clones of *P. monacha-lucida* had a graded occurrence ranging from 3.8 to 52.9%.

In *Drosophila*, interspecies hybrids usually cannot survive, but a mutation, Hmr, has recently been found to rescue hybrid males from the cross of *D. melanogaster* females to males of its three sibling species, *D. simulans, D. mauritiana*, and *D. sechellia*. Although this rescue is recessive, the hybrid males survive. There are also other mutations found to rescue hybrid females.[3]

Interspecies pregnancies in laboratory mammalian species have been created: a murine model using *Mus musculus* and *M. caroli*, an equine model involving horse and donkey, and a bovine model between sheep and goat. An immunological barrier appears to restrict interspecies pregnancy, probably involving interactions between trophoblast and endometrium.[4] Under natural conditions, the famous example is the sterile mule, a hybrid between a donkey and a mare. Interestingly, a recent report has shown that, by chromosomal analysis, some female mules (jack donkey × mare) and hinnies (stallion × jenny donkey) are fertile.[5]

2. Gender Recognition

The second level of identification is gender recognition, a more difficult task. The identification requires distinct differences in body sex and/or secretions. It is very easy to observe in laboratory mice that a male or female is mounting on another of the same sex. In a study on homosexual mounting in a bisexual one-male troop of free-ranging Hanuman langurs in northwestern India over a period of 6 years, female-female mounts (n = 524) occurred during all months. The function of homosexual female mounting is uncertain, though it appears to be stimulated by sexual arousal as in heterosexual mounting. Srivastava et al. suggested that, as a form of intrasexual competition, "pseudocopulations" may satisfy the mountees so that the number of their solicitations addressed to the male is reduced.[6]

The mechanism of gender recognition is highly complex. As discussed in Chapter 1, there are different levels of sex determination. The gender identity of an individual is established based on some physical attributes that must be developed during sexual differentiation. Figure 7.2 shows the expression of genetic sex through proper genital and gonadal sex. Under an appropriate

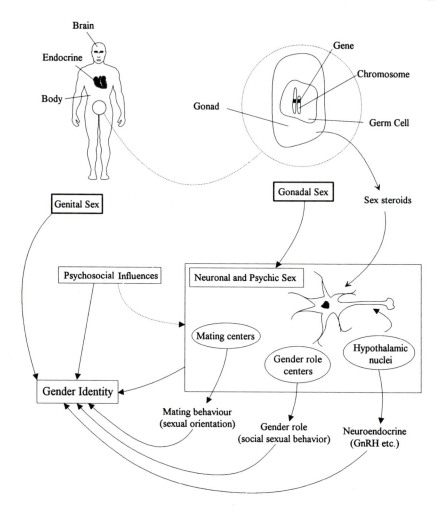

FIGURE 7.2. The roles of genital and gonadal sex in gender identity and recognition.

neuroendocrine environment, neuronal or brain sex is differentiated, leading to a set of gender-specific behaviors. All these physical and behavioral attributes must also be interpreted correctly by possible mates. The recognition is initially performed by visual cues. Courtship will then allow intimate physical contact during which body sex can be identified by examining external genitalia and other sexual features. All these steps rely heavily on cognition. Both mates have to recognize structures with correct interpretations in the context of sexual interactions. In humans, one can easily infer that a person can be attracted to another of the opposite sex. Attraction and gender recognition are so innate that we overlook the complexity of the neuronal mechanism generating the consciousness of being a female or male. One must successfully identify the sex of prospective mates and play the proper gender role according to this self-concept of gender identity.

The next step is copulation, which involves mounting and penile intromission. The urge of mounting is possibly related to pheromones. Recent evidence showed that the mucus of the female bovine genital tract contains low molecular weight mount-inducing pheromones. This mucus induces physiological and behavioral responses in other animals.[7] In mice, genital sniffing and mounting by the male was stimulated by ovarian-dependent chemosignals such as estradiol, vaginal fluids, and preputial extract from estrous females.[8] Data showing chemical stimulation of mounting behavior are available, but may not be related to gender recognition. A simple component of gender recognition may be explained by a stimulus-response model. Sex-specific stimuli can possibly evoke responses from the opposite sex.

In females, lordosis is the complimentary response to mounting by a male. It is a reflex arching of the back. Again, such a reflex can also be observed in males. It should be noted that the medial preoptic area (MPOA) in the female rat responds to intracerebroventricular administration of oxytocin that enhances sexual receptivity.[9] Treatment with 500 ng oxytocin significantly elevated lordosis. Mounting by males significantly increased levels of immunoreactive oxytocin and decreased the number of oxytocin-immunostaining cells in the MPOA of sexually receptive rats pretreated with estrogen, which suppresses lordosis.[10] The stimulus-response system is possibly linked with the neuroendocrine systems involved in the reproductive process. The MPOA may be a primary site of oxytocin facilitation of sexual receptivity where oxytocin may be released during mating.

B. AGGRESSIVE BEHAVIOR

The gender difference in aggressiveness can easily be demonstrated by putting two sexually mature male mice in one cage. If the cage is small, they soon start to fight for their territory. In a recent study on adult males, higher testosterone levels are found in groups selected for high levels of aggressiveness.[11] Despite a clear causal link between testosterone and aggression in animal studies, data on psychiatric and behavioral effects related to libido in human studies are often inconsistent.[12] The possible effects of androgens during prenatal and prepubertal development in humans is also inconclusive.

As for female mice, ten of them can share a small cage without any signs of fighting. However, a female mouse becomes extremely aggressive if she is a mother feeding her litter of pups. It has been found that removal of pups from the cage for more than 5 h depresses the maternal aggression, while it has no effect if the time of removal is only 1 h. The suppressed aggression is reversed if the pups are returned to the cage only a few minutes before the aggression test.[13] Suckling stimulation is suggested to be essential for postpartum aggression, and additional work has shown that surgical excision of nipples (thelectomy) on day 5 postpartum in mice accelerates the decline in aggression.[14] On the other hand, the postpartum aggression in mice is also suppressed by the removal of the vomeronasal organ, suggesting an involvement of a chemical signal.[15] Further experiments in rats have demonstrated that electrolytic lesions of the medial hypothalamus or parasagittal knife cuts along the lateral border of the ventromedial hypothalamic nucleus decreased maternal aggression.[16]

In humans, an increased emotional instability occurs during the early postpartum period in some women. The symptoms include higher anxiety, depression, irritability, and hostility, but the phenomenon should not be considered to be the same as the maternal aggression in rats and mice. It is often compared to premenstrual syndrome (PMS), showing similar symptoms. Interestingly, higher plasma prolactin levels are found in women showing PMS and postpartum depression. Treatment lowering prolactin levels also reduced their symptoms.[13] This does not indicate a direct causal relationship of prolactin with PMS and postpartum depression. The mechanism is more complex with possible genetic involvement.

C. COGNITIVE BEHAVIOR

Sexually dimorphic cognitive behavior is the most controversial part of the debate over gender differences, especially in humans. In rhesus monkeys, the frontal lobe of the brain is sexually dimorphic, but the difference disappears by puberty. Human data are inconsistent. The assessment methods may vary and be invalid in different studies. There may be a difference before or during puberty, but training may eliminate or reverse the difference. This raises questions on the validity of interpretation of these gender differences in cognitive behavior. They may be caused by different preferences instead of limitations imposed by biological differences.

According to Jacklin et al.,[17] the generalized sex differences were females are better at verbal expression and males are good at quantitative and spatial abilities. Such a difference seems to disappear in recent studies. For example, among the SAT math scores for precocious 12-year-old children, boys predominate at the top, but this trend is disappearing in recent years. In a later study on 6-year-old children by the same group in 1988, there were no significant differences between boys and girls in cognitive ability assessment based on reading, numbers, listening, and spatial ability. In the same study, they also assayed testosterone, androstenedione, estradiol, estrone, and progesterone in the umbilical cord blood at birth and 6 years later. Among children at age 6, higher levels of perinatal testosterone and androstenedione were significantly associated with low spatial ability in girls, while no significant correlation could be found for boys.

Figure 7.3 is a two-dimensional map for an interesting cognitive exercise involving mental imagery. Suppose you want to travel by car from point A to point B along the route indicated by the dotted line. Your task is to memorize the map and then reconstruct three-dimensional images as if you were driving the car slowly. At the end, you stop at point B and see the tower. While you are creating these mental images, describe verbally your directions and buildings to your colleagues. Some may find this task difficult, while others enjoy it. You will see a considerable variation among different individuals and probably discover a gender difference in the preference of ways to deal with these mental exercises.

This mental game can be modified in different ways such as changing the height and color of the buildings. More women may not like the game. The continuity of three-dimensional images may be disrupted if they communicate with others verbally simultaneously. Some women may overcome this interference

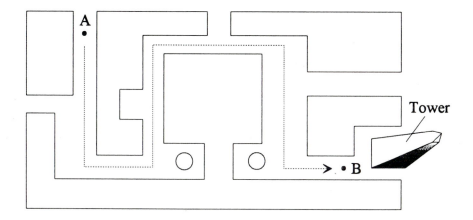

FIGURE 7.3. A cognitive exercise of mental imagery: three-dimensional reconstruction of a two-dimensional map.

by training if they want to. Many women prefer to describe directions sequentially with words instead of mental pictures, while many men memorize directions by images. This is associated with a possible gender difference in spatial ability suggested by earlier studies. If the spatial ability can be acquired by training in both sexes, these gender differences are caused by preferences rather than limitations.

Undoubtedly, females and males are different in many ways ranging from reproductive structures to brain activities. These differences may not lead to gender differences in the limitation of cognitive power. Instead, they make a difference in personality such as preferences, sexual orientation, and the way of thinking. In other words, the possible gender difference observed in the above mental game is subjective. The spatial ability is irrelevant. If they prefer to learn the skill well, both sexes can excel in the performance. As Hare-Mustin and Marecek[18] wrote, "A difference that makes no difference is no difference." Some may just prefer having such differences as flavors of human sexuality.

D. BRAIN SEXUALITY

One indisputable gender difference in the human brain is that all neurons in the female brain are XX, while those in the male brain are XY. The controversy lies not on the genetic sex of the brain, but on whether such a genetic difference contributes to a gender difference in the brain activity and, subsequently, the behavior. It is important to establish correlative gender differences in structures and activities of the brain associated with sexual behavior.

According to Kelley,[19] there are two kinds of mechanisms leading to sexually dimorphic behavior. First, one sex possesses a certain type of behavior, while the other sex does not because of differences in external stimuli or endocrine environment (e.g., maternal behavior in rodents). Second, the brain or CNS areas responsible for the behavior are different in males and females (e.g., courtship and copulatory behavior). Kelley suggested that cellular mechanisms leading to these

TABLE 7.1.
Anatomical Differences Between the Human
Female and Male Brains

Brain region	Difference	Comments
Hypothalamus		Strongest data,
• SDN	2.5 times in ♂	5 times in male rats,
• Other nuclei	2 of 4 larger	related to sexual
		behavior
Thalamus		
• Massa Intermedia	More often absent in ♂	Difficult to quantify differences
Corpus callosum		Conflicting data
• Splenium	More bulbous in ♀	entire callosum
• Isthmus	Larger in ♀	shrinks with age in men; related to brain lateralization
Anterior commissure	Larger in ♀	Little data
Onuf's nucleus	More motoneurons in ♂	Related to copulation

Note: Most data from Forger, N.G. and Breedlove, S.M., *Proc. Natl. Acad. Sci. U.S.A.,* 84, 8026, 1986 and Gibbons, A., *Science,* 253, 957, 1991.

differences in the effector neurons responsible for sexually dimorphic behavior, including sensitivity to hormones, cell number, and synaptic connectivity, may depend on generating a different degree of developmental arrest. For example, sexually dimorphic hormone-sensitive neurons or muscles are immature at stages when other cells have completed differentiation.

If this notion is correct, it would not be surprising to find anatomical differences between the male and female brains. Some examples are shown in Table 7.1. Some problems have been suggested in these findings. First, the results are often not reproducible. Results from human studies are difficult to interpret since postmortem specimens are usually obtained from patients with fatal diseases. For example, a previous study on 14 postmortem brains demonstrated gender differences in the splenium of the human corpus callosum. The larger splenium in females reflects less hemispheric lateralization, or "specialization," than the male brain for visual-spatial functions. In a later study, measurements of the human corpus callosum using magnetic resonance images of 37 living subjects failed to confirm reported gender differences in the splenium.[20] Existing knowledge of the functions of the corpus callosum does not permit correlations between variations in callosal size and shape and variations in cognitive functions.

In addition, intrahemispheric language organization was examined by determining the location of lesions causing aphasia using computerized tomography.

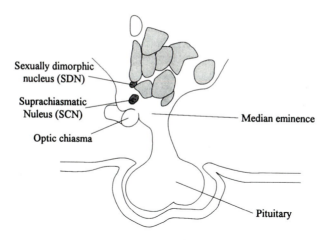

Sexually dimorphic
nucleus (SDN)

Suprachiasmatic
Nuleus (SCN)

Optic chiasma

Median eminence

Pituitary

FIGURE 7.4. Location of the sexually dimorphic nuclei in humans.

No gender difference in the incidence of anterior, posterior, or central lesions was found. The distribution of left-hemisphere lesions in stroke patients, with or without aphasia, was also equal among the sexes. This study does not support the postulated gender difference in intrahemispheric cerebral organization.[21]

Some of these anatomical differences really exist, such as the sexually dimorphic nucleus (SDN) identified in the preoptic area (see Figure 7.4). SDN is extremely sensitive to testosterone and estrogen. In a study, male rat pups were castrated, and half of the neurons in SDN died. This effect could be reversed if testosterone was injected between days 1 and 5 after birth. It became irreversible afterward. In female neonatal rats, androgen treatment induces SDN enlargement until it is similar to the one in male. SDN is five times larger in males. In addition, the Onuf's nucleus, located in the sacral spinal cord, has also been found to be sexually dimorphic in humans and dogs.[22] This nucleus innervates perineal muscles involved in copulatory behavior and has significantly more motoneurons in males.

Many neuroanatomical gender differences have been identified in the human brain.[23] For example, the shape of the suprachiasmatic nucleus (SCN), which is involved in the regulation of circadian rhythms and reproductive cycles, is elongated in females and more spherical in males. In addition, an extremely large SCN was observed in the brains of homosexual men who died from AIDS. Both the volume of the SCN and the number of vasopressin neurons were about twice as large as in a male reference group. In contrast to the SCN, in which only shape differences were found in relation to gender, the volume and cell number of the SDN of the preoptic area (SDN-POA) showed a marked sexual dimorphism. The mean volume of the SDN-POA was 2.2 times larger in males than in females and contained about twice as many cells. The function of this sexually dimorphic area in humans is not known, but presumably it is involved in the control of male sexual behavior. No difference in either volume or cell number was observed between the SDN-POAs of homosexual and heterosexual men. This finding shows a selectivity of the SCN in this respect and contradicts the view that male homosexuals have a "female" hypothalamus.

More recently, LeVay reported a difference in part of the anterior hypothalamus which governs sexual behavior.[24] The third interstitial nucleus of the anterior hypothalamus (INAH3) in homosexual males was similar to that in females. Actually, such a difference between homosexuals and heterosexuals is a second finding. In 1990, Hofman and Swaab reported an enlarged SCN in homosexual males.[23] However, SCN is not involved in controlling sexual behavior, but it does regulate circadian rhythms. As LeVay has pointed out, these differences are just anatomical. The results need to be repeated and have no direct evidence that this difference causes homosexuality. There are several problems in the study pointed out by others. First, all 19 homosexuals died of AIDS, while only 6 of the 16 heterosexuals died this way. Second, sexual information of 14 of the heterosexuals is uncertain (i.e., they were presumed to be exclusively heterosexuals). Third, there was no homosexual woman for comparison.

If LeVay's findings are correct, the dimorphic INAH3 area is associated with sexual orientation. If confirmed, these findings provide further support for sexual dimorphism in brain anatomy and possibly in human sexual behavior. Recent clinical evidence shows that these anatomical sex differences correlate with behaviors in some prevailing mental disorders and responses to psychotrophic medications. Gonadal hormones might be involved in these differences and in differential cognitive functions.[25] Even if both anatomical and behavioral differences can be found consistently, one must be cautious to correlate them with behavioral differences. It is a typical problem of "cause and effect." Anatomical differences may be a result of postnatal changes induced by behavioral differences or vice versa.

III. SEXUAL ATTRACTION

Sexual attraction is a general term describing the phenomenon of two individuals being brought closer to each other as a result of olfactory, auditory, or visual responses. In birds, auditory and visual displays are mainly used as a means of sexual attraction, while pheromones and olfactory senses are usual among mammals, especially in nocturnal rodents. In humans, powerful sexual attraction does exist, but the process is compounded by the cognitive power governing the sexual response. Human sexual attraction is a complex behavioral phenomenon involving all senses with an orchestrated coordination of the brain. Despite the lack of conclusive evidence of human pheromones, their possible presence in humans still cannot be eliminated.

A. PHEROMONES

The word "pheromone" was originally coined by Karlson and Butenandt in 1959 for a chemical signal released to the exterior by insects.[26] The concept of pheromone signaling has now been extended to fish,[27] amphibians and reptiles,[28] mammals,[29] and even yeast.[30] Pheromone signaling is mainly associated with the reproductive process and more specifically with sexual behavior. So far, birds have been thought to rely on visual and auditory cues for mate attraction and selection rather than pheromones.[31] Despite the addition of nonhuman mammalian pheromones to perfumes, the evidence for the effects of pheromones on humans is inconclusive.[32]

The mechanism of pheromone signaling consists of two components: production and reception of the chemosignal. The process requires structures or tissues for synthesis, secretion, and detection of the chemosignal. Since the responses to the chemosignal in mammals are mostly behavioral, higher centers of the brain must be involved. Besides, most of our understanding is based on animal data.

1.   Pheromone Production

Pheromones are thought to be produced in subcutaneous glands, though the internal glandular secretions of the reproductive systems are also a significant source. Some excretory products or other factors in the urine may be involved. It is known that all body odors are chemosignals, and the effects are very much dependent on the reception of the partner. The regulation of pheromone production in these tissues is likely to be associated with sex steroids.

The skin is known to metabolize steroids that regulate the size and secretory activity of glands in the skin. Similarly, the preputial gland is also dependent on steroids. In a study on the preference of female mice for castrated, castrated-preputialectomized, and preputialectomized males, no significant difference was noted. The females, however, preferred a mixture of urine from preputialectomized males and castrated males rather than from preputialectomized males and castrated-preputialectomized males. The urinary factor is suggested to be androgen dependent, and the preputial factor is possibly not.[33]

2.   Pheromone Receptors

There are four chemoreceptor systems possibly involved: the nervus terminalis, the trigeminal system, the septal organ and the vomeronasal organ.

The nervus terminalis is present in almost all vertebrates including humans.[34] The nervus terminalis is a cranial nerve that is a part of the accessory olfactory system, which projects directly from the nose to the septal-preoptic nuclei in the brain. During development, LHRH-immunoreactivity is detected in the peripheral parts of the nervus terminalis before it is found in the brain. By LHRH immunocytochemistry and ^{3}H-thymidine autoradiography, a recent study has shown that LHRH neurons originate in the medial olfactory placode of the developing nose in fetal mice, migrate across the nasal septum, and enter the forebrain with the nervus terminalis, arching into the septal-preoptic area and hypothalamus. This intimate relationship between the olfactory organ and the septal-preoptic nuclei could be used to explain the link of gonadotrophin deficiency with anosmia in Kallmann's syndrome.[35] In adult, the nervus terminalis still contains high levels of LHRH, but the function is uncertain.

The trigeminal system may play a role in modulating the olfactory bulb in response to irritating odors. The nerve begins with sensory nerves innervating the upper and lower mandibles and buccal cavity and ends with nerves projecting to jaw muscles.

The septal organ is located at the nasal septum anterior to the main olfactory epithelium, but its function is also uncertain.

The vomeronasal or Jacobson's organ and accessory olfactory system are present in most terrestrial vertebrates except birds and higher primates. The system is important in many behavioral and physiological responses to pheromones. The sensory neurons in the organ respond to both volatile and nonvolatile chemosignals as social and reproductive cues. The stimulation may elicit an intracerebral release of LHRH, leading to changes associated with reproductive physiology.[36]

Vomeromodulin, a 60-kDa glycoprotein, is localized immunocytochemically in the lateral nasal glands and the posterior septal and vomeronasal glands, but it is not detected in many other tissues including the mucus of the main olfactory neuroepithelium. Khew-Goodall et al. suggested that vomeromodulin may play a role in the process by which pheromones of low volatility bind with their receptors in the vomeronasal organ.[37] Although this organ is confirmed to have receptors for pheromones and to play a significant role in sexual responses in many mammalian species, it is absent in humans.

3.   Signal Interpretation and Responses

In yeast, it is known that peptide pheromones are capable of inducing mating, which involves mitotic arrest and transcription initiation. As shown in Figure 7.5, the mating process in yeast is evoked by an exchange of factors between an α-cell and an a-cell. The α-factor secreted by the α-cell is a short peptide of 13 amino acids, while the a-factor has only 12 amino acids. Various gene products are involved in the signal transduction of the receptor for these factors. A group of mutant genes designated as "ste" is known to cause sterility in yeast. The wild type genes are called STE. Their gene products are members of the signal transduction pathway.

α-Factor binds to the pheromone receptor STE2 on the membrane of the a-cell and initiates the signal transduction. The pathway begins with the pheromone receptor bound by the G-protein. Protein kinases and DNA-binding proteins also participate in the process; genes involved have also been sequenced.[30] The final protein in the pathway is STE12, which binds with the pheromone response element (PRE) of the gene sequence and triggers transcription. The gene products are used for generating the mating response, such as the change in cell shape (see Figure 7.5), forming the so-called shmoos. Eventually, the two cells fuse to become a zygote, and the mating process is completed.

The involvement of pheromones has also been demonstrated in bacterial conjugation, such as in *Enterococcus (Streptococcus) faecalis*. A small hydrophobic peptide induces a complex mating response, resulting in plasmid transfer from

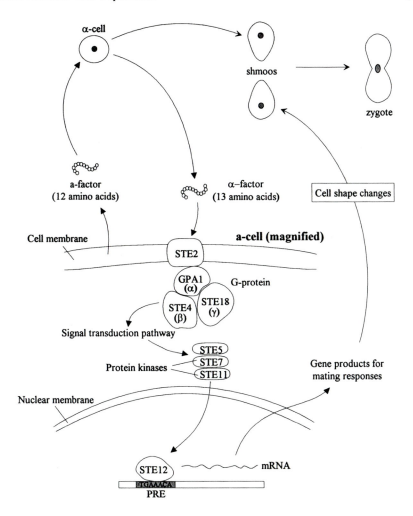

FIGURE 7.5. Signal transduction pathway in an a-cell of *Saccharomyces cerevisiae* (yeast) in response to pheromone secreted by an α-cell during mating. (PRE) pheromone response element; (STEn) wild types of sterile mutant genes, ste; and (GPA1) a protein with homology to G-protein α-subunit. (After Fields, S., *Trends Biochem. Sci.*, 15, 270, 1990.)

the donor cell. The effective concentration of the pheromone can be as low as 1 to 5 molecules per responder cell. The pheromone response includes cell-cell aggregation for promoting close contact between mating cells and surface exclusion for preventing plasmid transfer between aggregated donor cells.[38]

Although these prokaryotic models provide an excellent approach to elucidate the molecular mechanism of pheromone signaling, the signal interpretation and responses in mammals are substantially different. It is a series of complex signals conveyed from the receptor cells to the effector cells via the nervous system. The simplistic model of yeast may be equivalent to the receptor cell in, say, the vomeronasal organ. The stimulated receptor cell sends signals to the brain via the vomeronasal nerves, resulting in an increase in copulatory behavior. In the golden hamster *(Mesocricetus auratus)*, the vaginal discharge elicits several sexual responses from the male. They include approaching and sniffing the external genitalia, licking and ingestion of the secretion, reduced aggressiveness, and increased sexual arousal and urge to copulate. Physiologically, a rise in plasma testosterone can also be detected.[31]

In rhesus monkeys, the vaginal secretion from estrogen-stimulated females contains a complex mixture of fatty acids producing an odor and is attractive to males. In some mammalian species, the onset of puberty can be accelerated or inhibited by pheromones. Since their presence at the time of the response is not required, they are called priming pheromones. In females, the accelerated onset of puberty occurs in response to a stimulatory signal in the male urine, while delayed puberty occurs in groups of females without a male. In addition, there is a synchronization of ovarian cycles in these grouped females. When female mice are exposed to males, there is a rapid decrease in serum prolactin, which is possibly an effect of hypothalamic dopamine release. Therefore, neuroendocrine modulation of prolactin secretion is probably the signaling mechanism mediated by priming hormones.[31]

B.   SEX ATTRACTANTS

Since the discussion is mainly on human sexual behavior, the term "sex attractants" is used in a broader sense. Both fragrances and pheromones are included. In other words, all types of chemical compounds capable of enhancing sexual attraction are called sex attractants. As discussed earlier, pheromones found mostly in nonhuman mammals are sex attractants. These compounds are commonly added to perfumes for a primary purpose as a fixative or odor carrier rather than for their pheromonal effects. Perfumes are often advertised as having the ability to enhance sexual attractiveness. The attractive effect of perfumes is not related to the pheromonal effects, but to the effect of the pleasant scent.[32] Although the compounds producing the pleasant scent should not be taken as human pheromones, they are sex attractants because they do enhance sexual attraction in humans.

It should be added that some 16-ene-steroids synthesized in the human testis are found identical to the boar sex pheromone precursor androsta-5, 16-diene-3β-ol (ADL). In contrast to boars, the human testis has no 5α-reductase activity and no 5α-reduced 16-androstenes, but two known boar sex pheromones, androstenone and androstenol (see Figure 7.6 for their chemical structures), have been identified in the urine, plasma, sweat, and saliva of men and women. It was hypothesized that the two sex pheromones are synthesized in humans from ADL peripherally in tissues rich in 5α-reductase, such as skin, axillary sweat glands, and probably also the salivary glands.[39] Perhaps, these types of pheromones with higher effectiveness may be used in fragrances as a real pheromonal sex attractant.

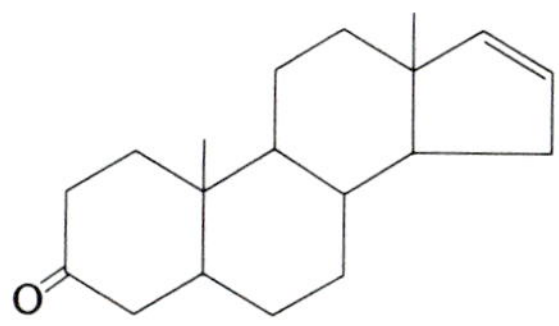

Androst-16-en-3-one

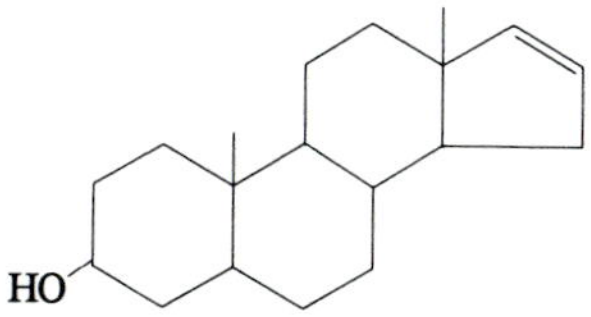

Androst-16-en-3-ol

FIGURE 7.6. Chemical structures of steroidal sex pheromones androstenone and androstenol from the boar.

C. GENDER IDENTIFICATION AND MATE SELECTION

The major purpose of sexual attraction is mate selection and, more specifically, the recognition of individuals of the proper gender. In hamsters, based on olfactory cues, males can discriminate odors of females and prefer those not recently mated. Female rats, however, prefer to approach a previous mating partner instead of a new one. These types of recognition may involve a holistic interpretation of all chemosignals and may be found in many mammalian species including primates.[31] Similar mechanisms are employed in the identification of gender, species, or even subspecies. Sex steroids, and possibly the endocrine system, may play a role in mediating behavior during mate selection.[40]

During sexual selection, according to Darwin,[41] individuals compete with members of their own sex for reproductively relevant resources held by members of the opposite sex. This may possibly happen in humans.[42] Mate selection is a complex process involving species, gender, and individual identification. Besides hormonal involvement, other modalities such as olfactory, auditory, and visual functions are employed. In humans, the mechanism of sexual attraction should be considered much more complicated than these basic instincts. Although the involvement of chemical attraction cannot be ruled out, the highly developed cognitive power seems to be the superseding control over physiological responses among average individuals.

Therefore, mate selection in humans does not depend entirely on sexual attraction. It is generalized as "attraction and love." According to Murstein,[43] human attraction is a three-stage process: stimulus, value comparison, and compatible expectations. The first stage depends on physical attributes, while the second is a period of mutual testing for values. The final stage is the fulfillment

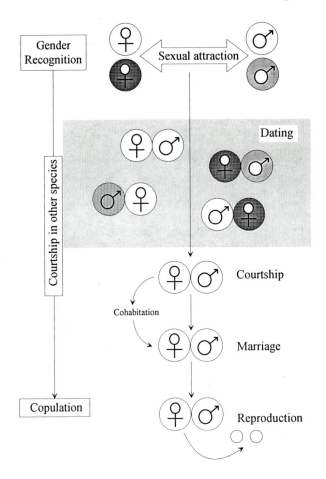

FIGURE 7.7.   Courtship in humans and other species.

of expectations upon each other based on ideal self and ideal other images. This is the social exchange theory based on the consideration of rewards and costs during the process of mate selection. A uniquely human term, "dating," is used to describe the activities during this process (see Figure 7.7).

According to Lasswell and Lasswell,[44] dating is an interaction between two persons, presumably to enjoy mutual recreational activities. Although there is no commitment, one or both of them may have a desire to initiate courtship or to engage in sexual activities. Dating partners often have sexual involvement including copulation, though such acts are prohibited by some. As suggested by Cupach and Metts,[45] sexual involvement is interpreted as a turning point from a friendship to a dating relationship. In other words, friendship is considered to be platonic, while a dating relationship implies sexual involvement. If these copulations are nonreproductive, they can be viewed as activities during courtship as in other species.

IV. COURTSHIP AND COPULATION

After successful sexual attraction, courtship is initiated as a prelude to copulation (see Figures 7.1 and 7.7). The duration varies from brief seconds to hours or days in different species. In animals, courtship is normally considered to follow sexual attraction brought about by pheromones and is part of the mate selection. After successful courtship, sexual partners will copulate, reproduce, and rear the young. For example, ringdoves usually spend 1 week or so for courtship and nesting, followed by 2 weeks of egg incubation and 3 weeks of parental care. Mostly, courtship consists of display or fighting activities, leading to the final physical contact between potential sexual partners. The style, timing, and events vary greatly even within the same species. The basic theme of courtship, however, remains the same; it is advertisement and selection prior to copulation.[1] The biological significance of courtship and copulation in humans is compared to that in other species.

A. COURTSHIP

In humans, courtship is a protracted series of interactions between two people in which one is attempting to persuade the other to marry him or her or sometimes to engage in some specific social behavior.[44] Despite exceptions to the norm, legal marriage is still the formal way adopted by the majority to establish a heterosexual relationship for reproduction. In this sense, the basic theme of courtship still holds, and nonmarital copulations resulting in pregnancy are unacceptable. A typical heterosexual interaction begins with the initial attraction and platonic friendship followed by dating and courtship, leading to marriage and subsequent establishment of a family (see also Chapter 12).

The distinction between dating and courtship in humans is often vague because commitment may also be transient during courtship. The degree of sexual involvement is often used as an indicator of commitment, but, realistically, the relationship may cease any time during courtship. Normally, courtship represents a period of strong commitment before marriage. According to a recent survey,[46] about half of unmarried couples between ages 18 and 24 are engaged in premarital sexual intercourse, while 40% of married couples have cohabited before marriage. Although the actual figures may vary among different studies, they provide an idea about commitment and sexual involvement during courtship in humans. There are still some couples who prefer to abstain from sexual intercourse until the wedding day, though they may have other forms of sexual interactions.

There has been no conclusive evidence showing an impact of cohabitation on the success of subsequent marriage. Although cohabitation is not as formal as marriage, there are laws governing cohabiting couples, but they vary greatly from state to state; it may be illegal in some states. There are still pressures from parents or relatives for these cohabiting couples to marry or terminate living together.[44] Some lawyers like Paul Ashley[47] recommend that cohabiting couples establish legal contracts. Cohabitation may evolve into a legal relationship as complicated as marriage. If one can have children legally without marriage, cohabitation and marriage are essentially the same except for some details of legality. In some rural communities of other countries, there is no restriction for couples to be married without official certification.

In comparison to other species, all the stages in humans from initial attraction, dating, courtship, cohabitation, and/or an early marital period before having children can be considered as a period of mate selection or courtship for reproduction (see Figure 7.7). Although the couples are said to be committed to lifelong monogamous relationships at the time of courtship, such a promise is not kept in almost 50% of the cases. A divorced individual may prefer to remarry and initiate another sequence of courtship behavior as if entering a second reproductive cycle. If this individual copulates again to reproduce with the new spouse, the biological result is identical to that of a seasonal breeder who mates with multiple sexual partners in successive reproductive cycles (see Figure 7.8).

B.   COPULATION

True intromittent organs are found in most vertebrates from sharks to birds and mammals for copulation. The major purpose is to deposit sperms into the female reproductive tract. This is valid for humans except in cases of artificial insemination. However, the word "copulation" is seldom used to describe sexual intercourse in humans; it usually refers to coitus for reproduction. "Sexual intercourse" is a more general term for the human sex act. Specifically, coitus is an act of inserting the penis into the vagina, excluding other forms of sexual intercourse such as oral or anal intercourse.[44]

In a biased way, we assume that all animals copulate instinctively for reproduction only. Since castrated animals continue to perform copulation, they have the sexual urge and can possibly experience the pleasurable feeling associated with coitus. Although the exact mechanism leading to erotic sensation is still uncertain, the sexual experience associated with orgasm is known to involve the interaction of psychological and somatic processes (see Figure 7.9). As suggested by Bancroft, this interactive system can be represented by the psychosomatic circle of sex.[48] Disruption of a component of this circle would cause a failure in the sexual response. For example, the lack of awareness of sexual response can be a cause of impotence, even though other components in the system are functional.

If the limbic system and cognitive power are involved in the sexual experience, the orgasmic response has a strong subjective element in humans. There are individual preferences of areas for tactile stimuli and the type of sexual foreplay. Another example is the coital position, which is irrelevant to reproductive outcomes. In most animals, copulation is usually performed with the male behind the female, comparable to the "rear entry position" in humans. The most popular position for Americans reportedly is the "missionary position," with the man on top.[49] (The name is thought to have been given by Pacific islanders who observed such a common coital position among Western missionaries.) The preference of coital positions is primarily associated with sexual pleasure and has no known biological significance. Some positions, however, may be more appropriate under certain health conditions such as pregnancy, arthritis, and heart problems.

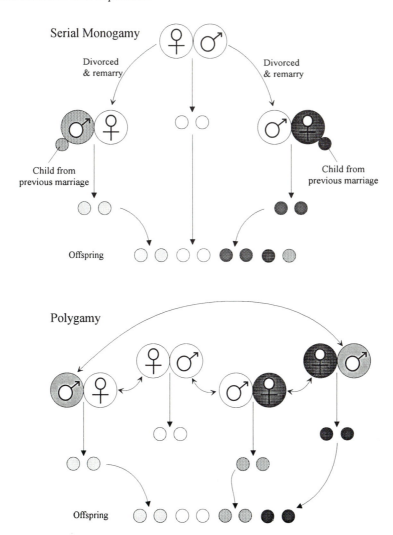

FIGURE 7.8. Comparison of serial monogamy and polygamy.

More than 4 million coituses occur every hour among humans worldwide.[50] Based on a fecundity ratio of 1:100 in humans, 99% of these copulations are nonreproductive. This apparently futile practice is the most important characteristic of human sexuality. Undoubtedly, these futile acts of copulation in humans provide sexual satisfaction, which may contribute to the stability of mating partners. The ultimate purpose of copulation in humans is still for reproduction. Its role remains crucial in determining the pattern of human reproduction. Despite the institution of marriage or the practice of cohabitation, the primary purpose of courtship is to bring two heterosexual individuals together so that they can copulate and reproduce. This way leading to sexual union is uniquely human.

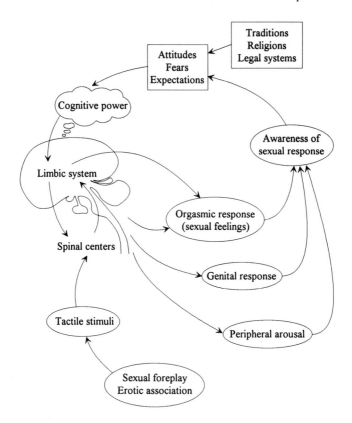

FIGURE 7.9.   The psychosomatic circle of sex. (After Bancroft, J., *Human Sexuality and Its Problems,* Churchill Livingstone, New York, 1989.)

REFERENCES

1. **Klimek, D.,** *Beneath Mate Selection and Marriage,* Van Nostrand Reinhold, New York, 1979.
2. **Schultz, M.E. and Schultz, R.J.,** Differences in response to a chemical carcinogen within species and clones of the livebearing fish, *Poeciliopsis, Carcinogenesis,* 9, 1029, 1988.
3. **Hutter, P., Roote, J., and Ashburner, M.,** A genetic basis for the inviability of hybrids between sibling species of *Drosophila, Genetics,* 124, 909, 1990.
4. **Anderson, G.B.,** Interspecific pregnancy: barriers and prospects, *Biol. Reprod.,* 38, 1, 1988.
5. **Rong, R., Chandley, A.C., Song, J., McBeath, S., Tan, P.P., Bai, Q., and Speed, R.M.,** A fertile mule and hinny in China, *Cytogenet. Cell Genet.,* 47, 134, 1988.
6. **Srivastava, A., Borries, C., and Sommer, V.,** Homosexual mounting in free-ranging female Hanuman langurs *(Presbytis entellus), Arch. Sex. Behav.,* 20, 487, 1991.
7. **Nishimura, K., Utsumi, K., Okano, T., and Iritani, A.,** Separation of mounting-inducing pheromones of vaginal mucus from estrual heifers, *J. Anim. Sci.,* 69, 3343, 1991.
8. **Weinhold, L.L. and Ingersoll, D.W.,** Modulation of male mouse genital sniff, attack, and mount behaviors by urogenital substances from estrous females, *Behav. Neural Biol.,* 50, 207, 1988.

9. **Caldwell, J.D., Jirikowski, G.F., Greer, E.R., and Pedersen, C.A.,** Medial preoptic area oxytocin and female sexual receptivity, *Behav. Neurosci.,* 103, 655, 1989.
10. **Hasegawa, N., Takeo, T., and Sakuma, Y.,** Differential regulation of estrogen-dependent sexual development of rat brain by growth factors, *Neurosci. Lett.,* 123, 183, 1991.
11. **Archer, J.,** The influence of testosterone on human aggression, *Br. J. Psychol.,* 82, 1, 1991.
12. **Uzych, L.,** Anabolic-androgenic steroids and psychiatric-related effects: a review, *Can. J. Psychol.,* 37, 23, 1992.
13. **Numan, M.,** Maternal behavior, in *The Physiology of Reproduction,* Knobil, E. and Neill, J., Eds., Raven Press, New York, 1988, 1569.
14. **Garland, M. and Svare, B.,** Suckling stimulation modulates the maintenance of postpartum aggression in mice, *Physiol. Behav.,* 44, 301, 1988.
15. **Bean, N.J. and Wysocki, C.J.,** Vomeronasal organ removal and female mouse aggression: the role of experience, *Physiol. Behav.,* 45, 875, 1989.
16. **Hansen, S.,** Medial hypothalamic involvement in maternal aggression of rats, *Behav. Neurosci.,* 103, 1035, 1989.
17. **Jacklin, C.N., Wilcox, K.T., and Maccoby, E.E.,** Neonatal sex-steroid hormones and cognitive abilities at six years, *Dev. Psychobiol.,* 21, 567, 1988.
18. **Hare-Mustin, R.T. and Marecek, J.,** On making a difference, in *Making a Difference,* Hare-Mustin, R.J. and Marecek, J., Eds., Yale University Press, New Haven, 1990, 1.
19. **Kelley, D.B.,** Sexually dimorphic behaviors, *Annu. Rev. Neurosci.,* 11, 225, 1988.
20. **Byne, W., Bleier, R., and Houston, L.,** Variations in human corpus callosum do not predict gender: a study using magnetic resonance imaging, *Behav. Neurosci.,* 102, 222, 1988.
21. **Kertesz, A. and Benke, T.,** Sex equality in intrahemispheric language organization, *Brain Language,* 37, 401, 1989.
22. **Forger, N.G. and Breedlove, S.M.,** Sexual dimorphism in human and canine spinal cord: role of early androgen, *Proc. Natl. Acad. Sci. U.S.A.,* 84, 8026, 1986.
23. **Hofman, M.A. and Swaab, D.F.,** Sexual dimorphism of the human brain: myth and reality, *Exp. Clin. Endocrinol.,* 98, 161, 1991.
24. **LeVay, S.,** A difference in hypothalamic structure between heterosexual and homosexual men, *Science,* 253, 1034, 1991.
25. **Halbreich, U., Lemus, C.Z., Lieberman, J.A., Parry, B., and Schiavi, R.C.,** Gonadal hormones, sex and behavior, *Psychopharmacol. Bull.,* 26, 297, 1990.
26. **Karlson, P. and Butenandt, A.,** Pheromones (ectohormones) in insects, *Annu. Rev. Entomol.,* 4, 39, 1959.
27. **Tavolga, W.N.,** Chemical stimuli in the reproductive behavior of fish: communication, *Experientia,* 32, 1093, 1976.
28. **Madison, D.M.,** Chemical communication in amphibians and reptiles, in *Chemical Signals in Vertebrates,* Müller-Schwarze, D. and Mozell, M.M., Eds., Plenum Press, New York, 1976, 135.
29. **Singer, A.G.,** A chemistry of mammalian pheromones, *J. Steroid Biochem. Mol. Biol.,* 39, 627, 1991.
30. **Fields, S.,** Pheromone response in yeast, *Trends Biochem. Sci.,* 15, 270, 1990.
31. **Vandenbergh, J.G.,** Pheromones and mammalian reproduction, in *The Physiology of Reproduction,* Knobil, E. and Neill, J., Eds., Raven Press, New York, 1988, 1679.
32. **Berliner, D.L., Jennings-White, C., and Lavker, R.M.,** The human skin: fragrances and pheromones, *J. Steroid Biochem. Mol. Biol.,* 39, 671, 1991.
33. **Ninomiya, K. and Kimura, T.,** Male odors that influence the preference of female mice: roles of urinary and preputial factors, *Physiol. Behav.,* 44, 791, 1988.
34. **Fuller, G.N. and Burger, P.C.,** Nervus terminalis (cranial nerve zero) in the adult human, *Clin. Neuropathol.,* 9, 279, 1990.
35. **Schwanzel-Fukuda, M. and Pfaff, D.W.,** Origin of luteinizing hormone-releasing hormone neurons, *Nature (London),* 338, 161, 1989.
36. **Meredith, M.,** Sensory processing in the main and accessory olfactory systems: comparisons and contrasts, *J. Steroid Biochem. Mol. Biol.,* 39, 601, 1991.

37. **Khew-Goodall, Y., Grillo, M., Getchell, M.L., Danho, W., Getchell, T.V., and Margolis, F.L.,** Vomeromodulin, a putative pheromone transporter: cloning, characterization, and cellular localization of a novel glycoprotein of lateral nasal gland, *FASEB J.,* 5, 2976, 1991.

38. **Dunny, G.M.,** Genetic functions and cell-cell interactions in the pheromone-inducible plasmid transfer system of *Enterococcus faecalis, Mol. Microbiol.,* 4, 689, 1990.

39. **Smals, A. and Weusten, J.J.,** 16-Ene-steroids in the human testis, *J. Steroid Biochem. Mol. Biol.,* 40, 587, 1991.

40. **Wingfield, J.C. and Marler, P.,** Endocrine basis of communication in reproduction and aggression, in *The Physiology of Reproduction,* Knobil, E. and Neill, J., Eds., Raven Press, New York, 1988, 1647.

41. **Darwin, C.,** *The Descent of Man, and Selection in Relation to Sex,* John Murray Ltd., London, 1871.

42. **Buss, D.M.,** The evolution of human intrasexual competition: tactics of mate attraction, *J. Pers. Soc. Psychol.,* 54, 616, 1988.

43. **Murstein, B.I.,** Mate selection in the 1970s, *J. Marriage Fam.,* 42, 777, 1980.

44. **Lasswell, M. and Lasswell, T.,** *Marriage and the Family,* 3rd ed., Wadsworth Publishing Co., Belmont, CA, 1991.

45. **Cupach, W.R. and Metts, S.,** Sexuality and communication in close relationships, in *Sexuality and Close Relationships,* McKinney, K. and Sprecher, S., Eds., Lawrence Erlbaum Associates, Hillsdale, NJ, 1991, 93.

46. **Greeley, A.M.,** *Faithful Attraction,* Tom Doherty Associates, New York, 1991.

47. **Ashley, P. P.,** *Oh Promise Me, But Put It in Writing: Living-Together Agreements Without, Before, During and After Marriage,* McGraw-Hill, New York, 1978.

48. **Bancroft, J.,** *Human Sexuality and Its Problems,* Churchill Livingstone, New York, 1989.

49. **Reinisch, J.M. and Beasley, R.,** *The Kinsey Institute New Report on Sex. What You Must Know To Be Sexually Literate,* Kent, D., Ed., St. Martin's Press, New York, 1990.

50. **Chronicle Wire Services,** The world has sex 100 million times daily, *San Francisco Chronicle,* June 25, 1992, A1.

8 Insemination and Fertilization

CHAPTER CONTENTS

I. INTRODUCTION

Insemination is the deposition of semen into the female reproductive tract. The main purpose of insemination is to achieve fertilization. As in most other vertebrates, insemination in humans is achieved by copulation, though internal fertilization is not necessarily brought about by copulation. For example, some lizards may deposit their semen as spermatophores that are picked up by cloacal labia in the female.[1] Artificial insemination in humans is an interesting case of fertilization without copulation analogous to the reptilian way of mating.

There are three possible sites of insemination: vagina, cervix, and uterus. Uterine insemination is rare among vertebrates, while cervical insemination is common among horses, cattle, and swine. As in rabbits and rats, the site of insemination in humans is vaginal. Despite the site of semen deposition, sperms have to be transported to the oviducal ampulla where they fertilize the oocytes. During the sperm transport in the female reproductive tract, they undergo capacitation through which the sperms acquire the fertilizing capacity.

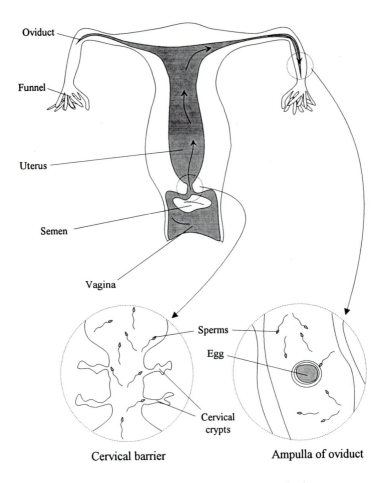

FIGURE 8.1.   The route of sperm transport in the female reproductive tract.

II.   SPERM TRANSPORT

In humans, sperms in the semen deposited in the vagina have to be transported through several barriers: cervix, uterus, uterotubal junction, and oviduct. Although normal sperms are actively motile, their locomotory ability does not contribute significantly to sperm transport in the female reproductive tract. The route of sperm transport is summarized in Figure 8.1.

A.   SPERMS IN THE VAGINA

An average ejaculate contains 200 to 500 million sperms. The semen in humans coagulates immediately following ejaculation and liquefies about 10 min later. Semen coagulation in rodents such as mice leads to the formation of vaginal plugs that do not liquefy. An enzyme vesiculase from the anterior lobe of the prostate gland (coagulating gland) is present in the coagulation. The plugs are thought to reduce the loss of semen after copulation. In humans, the role of coagulation and liquefaction is unclear, though the changes do not affect the transport. Sperms are normally found in the cervical barrier within 1 to 2 min after ejaculation.

Since the acidic environment in the human vagina is hostile to sperms, prolonged storage in the vagina for up to 6 hours is detrimental to sperms. They become nonmotile with reduced fertilizing capacity. This is thought to be a selective mechanism to eliminate abnormal or nonmotile sperms left in the vagina. If the sperms are normal, they should reach the uterine cavity within minutes.

B.   SPERMS AND CERVICAL MUCUS

The cervix is the first barrier to sperm ascent. It is rich in secretions which are collectively known as cervical mucus. The secretory activity varies with the menstrual cycle. During the proliferative phase, a high level of estrogen enhances the secretion, leading to a decrease in mucus viscosity and an increase in pH. Just prior to ovulation, the amount of mucus produced reaches 700 mg/day as compared to about 30 mg/day during the early proliferative phase. At the same time, the lumen of the cervix enlarges, reaching a diameter of up to 3 mm just before ovulation. As progesterone level increases after ovulation, the secretion of cervical mucus ceases, while the cervical opening reduces in size.

Inside the cervical canal, sperms are temporarily stored in cervical crypts (see Figure 8.1). In contrast to the vaginal canal, the environment in these structures with cervical mucus is optimal for sperms. Although their fertilizing capability may not be retained, motile sperms can still be found in cervical crypts more than 1 week after insemination.

C.   SPERMS IN THE UTERINE CAVITY

Myometrial contraction of the uterus is the main driving force of sperm transport in the uterine cavity. The presence of prostaglandins in semen has been suggested to be a crucial factor in uterine contractility. Oxytocin may also be another candidate and has been detected in the blood circulation of women after orgasm. Although sperms in the uterine cavity are actively motile, their movement is random and nondirectional. The passive nature of sperm transport has further been shown by the movement of inert particles from the cervix to the oviduct. With a mechanism in the uterine cavity to remove dead, nonmotile, damaged, or extra sperms, only a few sperms enter the oviduct. Leukocytes are found to play an important role in the phagocytosis of these sperms.[2]

D.   SPERMS IN THE UTEROTUBAL JUNCTION

The second barrier to sperm ascent is the uterotubal junction. Interestingly, there is no structural barrier such as a sphincter or valve regulating the passage of sperms. The lumenal diameter of the oviduct adjacent to the uterotubal junction is about 0.1 to 1 mm. In humans, inert particles are found to pass through the uterotubal junction. Apparently, there is a mechanism operating to screen and select motile sperms. Normally, only about 0.5% of the sperms in the ejaculate are found in the oviduct.

E.   SPERM TRANSPORT IN THE OVIDUCT

In the oviduct, there are two phases of sperm transport to the ampullar region where fertilization occurs. The first phase is fast; a few sperms are rapidly transported to the ampullar region, but they are not the ones fertilizing the oocytes. The second phase occurs later and is a slower transport of sperms; they remain less motile in the proximal isthmus until the time of ovulation. This is a compensation for the time difference between ovulation and sexual intercourse.[2]

Although about 1000 sperms can successfully reach the oviduct, about 100 can be brought in close vicinity with the oocytes in the ampullar region. There are some, however, that manage to pass through the oviduct and progress out of the oviducal funnel into the peritoneal cavity. These "escaped sperms" are eventually reabsorbed. Despite the high sperm motility, the major transport force is still the oviducal muscular activity and fluid flow.

III.   FERTILIZATION

Fertilization occurs in the oviducal ampulla that is a diluted portion of the tube close to the oviducal funnel. Sperms transported from the vaginal canal to this region are capacitated and ready to fertilize oocytes. Although sperms and oocytes are brought together in the small ampulla of the oviduct, there is still a vast distance between a sperm and its prospective partner. The final journey of the sperm is to find the oocyte, to penetrate through the cumulus oophorus and corona radiata, and to bind with the specific sperm receptor on the zona pellucida. At this time, fertilization is said to have occurred, accompanied by a signal to block attachment by other sperms. The process of fertilization is completed when the female and male nuclei come together in the egg cytoplasm. The union of the nuclei indicates the formation of a zygote.[3]

A.   SPERM-EGG ATTRACTION AND SPERM HYPERACTIVATION

As shown in rabbits, sperms in the ampullar are much more motile than those in the isthmus. Such an increase in motility is called hyperactivation, allowing the sperm to have a stronger thrusting power. It plays an important role in sperm penetration through the cumulus oophorus of the oocyte. This phenomenon has also been demonstrated in humans.[4] Both intracellular Ca^{2+} and cAMP are crucial for sperm tail movement; an increased level of Ca^{2+} in the ampullar fluid and intracellular cAMP may be the cause of the sperm hyperactivation.

B.   SPERM PENETRATION THROUGH THE CUMULUS OOPHORUS

There are two possible mechanisms by which sperms penetrate the cumulus oophorus: physical and enzymatic. It is tempting to conclude that highly motile

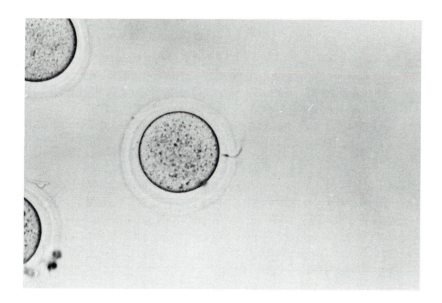

FIGURE 8.2. Mouse oocyte penetrated by a sperm.

capacitated sperms can actively disperse the cumulus oophorus. Under *in vitro* conditions, the dispersion of the cumulus oophorus by sperms is evident when the oocytes are inseminated with a large number of sperms. The cumulus oophorus is dispersed by the sperms or artificially by an enzyme hyaluronidase before *in vitro* fertilization, but the presence of cumulus cells in the same culture dish enhances the fertilization rate.

Under *in vivo* conditions, only a few sperms can successfully reach the ampulla in the vicinity of the oocytes. Physical dispersion of the cumulus oophorus does not seem feasible. In contrast to *in vitro* fertilization, the oocyte is fertilized before the cumulus oophorus is dispersed. The sperm, in fact, can penetrate the cumulus oophorus. If the sperm can reach the zona pellucida, the dispersion of the cumulus oophorus is unnecessary and may be disadvantageous for blocking polyspermy. Figure 8.2 shows a mouse oocyte penetrated by a sperm *in vitro*. Note that the cumulus oophorus has been dispersed. In contrast to fertilization *in vivo*, a large number of sperms (at least 10^5 sperms per milliliter culture medium) are placed in the culture dish containing the oocytes. The dispersion of cumulus oophorus by active sperms can easily be observed under a microscope.

Although the enzyme hyaluronidase has been shown to be bound on the acrosome surface of the sperm, its role in penetrating the cumulus oophorus is controversial. Nevertheless, antihyaluronidase antibodies and hyaluronidase inhibitor (e.g., myocrisin or sodium aurothiomalate) have been shown to inhibit fertilization. Suggested functions of hyaluronidase include depolymerizing hyaluronic acid in the cumulus matrix and serving as a lubricant. It may also play a role in penetrating the zona pellucida.

C. SPERM ATTACHMENT TO THE ZONA PELLUCIDA

Prior to penetrating the zona pellucida, sperms are attached to specific sperm receptors. The zona pellucida is a translucent acellular layer. The major component is glycoproteins. The outer surface of the zona pellucida is lattice-like ultrastructurally with fenestrated regions where hyaluronic acid molecules of the cumulus oophorus are anchored.

The zona pellucida contains three fractions of sulfated glycoproteins: ZP1, ZP2, and ZP3. These protein fractions are about 200, 120, and 83 kDa, respectively, in the mouse. Sperm receptors are mainly found in ZP3, the primary sperm receptor. ZP2 is the secondary sperm receptor, while ZP1 seems to have no contribution to sperm binding to the zona pellucida. After the initial binding to the primary sperm receptor (ZP3), the sperm proceeds to zona penetration, which requires a series of biochemical changes in the acrosome known as acrosome reaction. At the conclusion of the acrosome reaction, the sperm becomes bound to the secondary sperm receptor (ZP2).

Complimentary to the sperm receptors on the zona pellucida, there are zona receptors on the sperm. The zona receptor for ZP3 is located on the plasma membrane of the acrosome in capacitated sperms. At this stage, the zona receptor for ZP2 is not detectable until the acrosome reaction is completed and it resides on the plasma membrane over the equatorial segment and inner acrosomal membrane.

D. ACROSOME AND CORTICAL REACTIONS

During the penetration of a sperm through the zona pellucida, a drastic reaction occurs in its acrosome. The acrosome is a membrane-bound structure analogous to the lysosome and contains a battery of hydrolytic enzymes. The two major enzymes are hyaluronidase and acrosin present in the acrosomal matrix, though some others are in or on the acrosomal membrane. Acrosome reaction involves multiple fusions of the acrosomal membrane and outermost plasma membrane. Since these membranes are thin and delicate, they may also be damaged in dead sperms; this phenomenon is called false acrosome reaction.

In true acrosome reaction during zona penetration in humans, the fusion between the outer acrosomal and the plasma membranes starts to occur at the equatorial segment of the acrosome. The whole acrosome reaction takes about several minutes. Some physical and chemical agents can trigger acrosome reaction. The natural inducers found in the zona pellucida are possibly proteins in the ZP3 fraction. The cumulus oophorus also has to ability to induce the acrosome reaction, but this is controversial.

The mechanism of acrosome reaction has been studied extensively in sea urchin sperms, but it is less studied in mammalian sperms. According to Yanagimachi,[3] a massive influx of Ca^{2+} is necessary to inactivate Na^+-K^+ ATPase. This leads to an increase in intracellular Na^+ and an efflux of H^+, resulting in a rise of intracellular pH. At the same time, Ca^{2+} activates membrane phospholipases, which then convert phospholipids to arachidonic acid and lysophospholipids. As

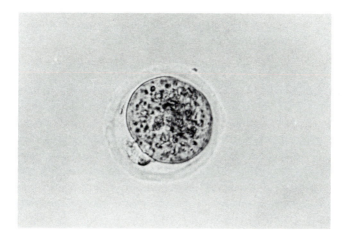

FIGURE 8.3. Fertilized mouse oocyte with female and male pronuclei near the center. Note also the shrunken oocyte cytoplasm and wide perivitelline space with polar bodies.

membrane fusion occurs, proacrosin is converted to acrosin, which is responsible for dispersing the acrosomal matrix.

The passage of the sperm through the zona pellucida may be both mechanical and enzymatic. The strong thrusting power of the sperm's tail is necessary, while the repetitive binding and release processes between proteins are crucial for the specificity of sperm-zona interaction. The zona reaction is an integral part of the whole process and is an important mechanism which prevents further binding of other sperms.

After passing the zona, the sperm head reaches the perivitelline space, which is a minute gap between the inner surface of the zona and the oocyte plasma membrane. Interestingly, the sperm head does not collide with its bald area onto the oocyte surface. It actually lands sideways with its postacrosomal area touching the oocyte surface where numerous villi are found. Sperm-oocyte fusion occurs as their plasma membranes integrate with each other.

At the time of sperm-oocyte fusion, the oocyte is activated metabolically, causing a rise in intracellular Ca^{2+}. It resumes its meiotic division. The exact mechanism is uncertain; the primary cause is probably the membrane fusion and the injection of Ca^{2+} carried by the sperm. Accompanying the flow of ions, there is an electrical change across the oocyte membrane. The first noticeable change is the cortical granule reaction, which is the release of small cortical granules underlying the plasma membrane. These granules contain hydrolytic enzymes and are present in unfertilized eggs. They disappear after fertilization and are thought to be released by exocytosis at that time.

The oocyte becomes a fertilized egg. The whole oocyte cytoplasm appears to shrink, leaving a wider perivitelline space as observed during *in vitro* fertilization (see Figure 8.3). As the sperm head proceeds with its integration with the oocyte, the whole sperm tail is pulled into the perivitelline space and eventually incorporated with the cytoplasm of the oocyte. These changes provide a further block to the entry of other sperms, reducing the chance of polyspermy.

E. FUSION OF PRONUCLEI AND ZYGOTE FORMATION

Once the sperm head is inside the egg cytoplasm, the nuclear envelope disintegrates and the chromatin materials are liberated. At the same time, decondensation of the nucleus occurs while the whole mass of materials moves centripetally. On the other hand, the egg nucleus completes its second meiotic division, liberating the second polar body. The newly formed egg nucleus, now known as female pronucleus, also moves centripetally to meet the sperm nucleus. A new nuclear envelope is developed from endoplasmic reticulum and probably old nuclear membrane materials around the male chromatin materials, forming the male pronucleus.

With the help of a network of microfilaments or microtubules, the female and male pronuclei are brought together at the center of the egg (see Figure 8.3). The pronuclei contain a haploid set of chromosomes with large characteristic nucleoli, but the DNA content is doubled. The nuclear envelopes of both start to disintegrate, and the chromosomes begin to align as if they are in mitotic metaphase. At this time, the egg becomes diploid and is called a zygote or conceptus. Pregnancy is considered to begin on this day, which is designated as day 1.

IV. PREIMPLANTATION ZYGOTE

A description of the early rabbit zygote by van Benenden in 1875 is probably the first accurate account of the early development of a mammalian conceptus.[5] Following this work, other careful structural studies on zygotes of other species such as the mouse[6] had supported van Benenden's observations. A fertilized mammalian egg cleaves into a mass of cells and becomes a morula at the eight-cell stage. It then undergoes compaction, the first morphologically discernible differentiation, during which intercellular boundaries become indistinct.[7] The zygote continues to develop into a blastocyst consisting of an outer cell layer called the trophectoderm or trophoblast. An inner cell mass is attached to the trophectoderm asymmetrically and is suspended in the blastocyst cavity.

In the inner cell mass, the primitive ectoderm is separated from the blastocyst cavity by a cell monolayer, the primitive endoderm, which extends to cover the whole inner surface of the trophoblast.[6] In all of these stages, the size of the zygote does not change and is enclosed in the zona pellucida. Later, the zygote "hatches" from this clear envelope and attaches to the endometrial epithelium of the uterus. The attachment process is called implantation, a crucial event in the establishment of pregnancy. In humans, only about 40% of the preimplantation zygotes can implant successfully under optimal conditions.[8]

Implantation is an important event which marks the division lines between preimplantation and postimplantation zygotes. The preimplantation zygote is also called a "preembryo."[9] In a postimplantation zygote, part of the inner cell mass differentiates into an embryo with embryonic cell layers enclosing the fetus. For some reasons, the word "embryo" has been used loosely as conceptus or even the fetus. In order to avoid confusion, these terms have to be defined rigorously here, though some other authors may not agree completely.

As the smallest part of a zygote, the fetus is a complete set of cells that will develop into an individual. A human fetus comes to existence a few days after implantation when a part of an embryo differentiates into recognizable fetal structures. An embryo consists of the fetus surrounded by embryonic membranes or a set of cells that will develop into these structures. Therefore, the embryo exists before the emergence of the fetus and is part of the egg cylinder in an early postimplantation conceptus. The embryo proper is enclosed by extraembryonic membranes developed from the outer layer of the egg cylinder. Since these membranes are called "extraembryonic," they are not part of the embryo.

Strictly speaking, an embryo does not exist before the differentiation of the extraembryonic membranes. The entire mass of structures should be called the egg cylinder, which is a differentiated inner cell mass after implantation. At the time of implantation, there is only the inner cell mass enclosed by a trophoblast. The inner cell mass develops into the egg cylinder, while the trophoblast will form part of the placenta. The entire structure is the zygote or conceptus, which has differentiated from the fertilized egg with the zona pellucida removed. Hence, an embryo does not exist before implantation, and the entity should be called a preimplantation zygote or preembryo. Although zygote and conceptus can be used interchangeably, conceptus is often used for the zygote after implantation.

The fusion of the female and male pronuclei turns the haploid gametes into a single diploid cell. This event signifies the end of fertilization, and the mother is said to have conceived. In humans, it takes about 12 h from sperm penetration to this stage, and it will require 1 day more for this fertilized egg to finish its first mitotic division. In total, it takes about 36 h to become a two-cell zygote after fertilization (see Figure 8.4). All these events occur in the ampullar region of the oviduct. When the two-cell zygote is formed, its journey from the ampulla to the uterine cavity begins as it continues to cleave. It takes 1 to 2 days more to complete the journey.

A. COMPACTION

A two-cell zygote takes about 12 h to become a four-cell zygote (see Figure 8.5) and another 12 h to form a morula (see Figure 8.6a). The individual cells in the zygotes are called blastomeres. At this stage, compaction occurs as the first event showing cell commitment. This process can be described in terms of four types of cell reorganization, one of which is intracellular reorganization, while the others are intercellular reorganization. The intracellular reorganization is the polarization of blastomeres on which surface microvilli become localized apically.[10] The three intercellular changes are cell flattening against each other,[7] development of tight junctions,[11] and formation of low-resistance channels between basolateral membranes in gap junctional complexes.[12]

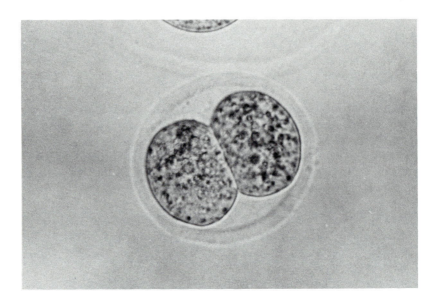

FIGURE 8.4.   Two-cell mouse zygote.

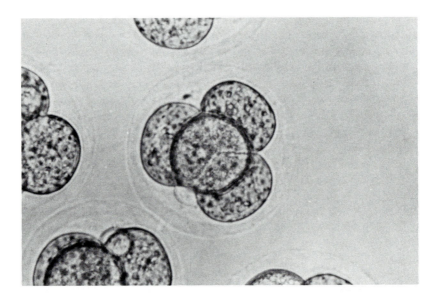

FIGURE 8.5.   Four-cell mouse zygote.

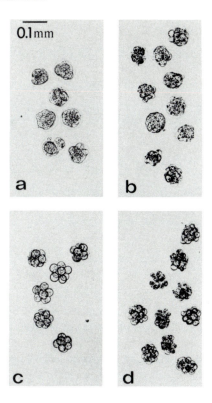

FIGURE 8.6. Mouse morulae, compacted 8- to 16-cell zygotes, cultured in (a) normal medium, (b) medium containing 10 μg/ml cadmium chloride, (c) calcium-free medium, and (d) calcium-free medium containing 10 μg/ml cadmium chloride.

The polarization of blastomeres in a morula is possibly initiated by some positional signals generated as a result of the arrangement of cells exposed to different microenvironments.[13] Some blastomeres are enclosed by the peripheral ones whose apical ends are in contact with the zona pellucida and the basolateral surfaces with adjacent cells, while the inside cells are only in contact with adjacent cells. This is the "inside-outside" hypothesis, which was proposed in the 1960s to explain how differences in cell-cell interaction can provide positional clues.[14,15]

The blastomeres in an eight-cell zygote can be disaggregated experimentally. Polarized blastomeres can divide and generate both polar and apolar daughter cells. Apolar daughter cells are still able to polarize when exposed to asymmetrical contact among cells. During normal development, the apolar blastomeres are enclosed at the center of the zygote in symmetrical contact with outside cells. These blastomeres do not polarize and are destined to form the inner cell mass.[16]

Cell flattening is likely to be mediated via a homotypic Ca^{2+}-dependent cell-cell adhesion system (CDS), which contributes to the synchronization of blastomere polarization and orientation of polarization axis.[16] This notion is supported

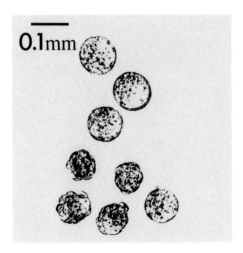

FIGURE 8.7.   Mouse blastocysts.

by reports showing that the formation of the inner cell mass is impaired by a monoclonal antibody which specifically binds the CDS. The treated blastomeres appear to lose their ability to recognize the presence of an adjacent cell. The CDS may lead to a local depolymerization of microtubules, and the process is regulated by CDS activation at a posttranslational level.[13]

Since compaction is an energy-requiring process, it can be disrupted if the zygote is exposed to cytotoxic substances. As shown in Figure 8.6b, decompaction occurs in mouse zygotes treated with cadmium, which interferes with mitochondrial functions and general energy metabolism. Subsequent developmental failure of these treated zygotes is caused by cadmium cytotoxicity rather than decompaction. Transient failure of compaction has no observable effect on development if the delay is insignificant.

In a Ca^{2+}-free culture medium, compaction is inhibited.[17] Individual blastomeres are still distinctly separated at the 16-cell stage (see Figure 8.6c), though blastomere polarization persists.[18] Despite the failure of compaction, blastomeres are still healthy. They are distinctly different from degenerate blastomeres in cadmium-treated zygotes (see Figure 8.6d). If normal culture medium is replaced within several hours, compaction can resume in those zygotes in Figure 8.6c. Most of them can resume their normal development.

B.   CAVITATION

On day 4 after fertilization, a 16- to 32-cell morula develops into a blastocyst when a fluid-filled blastocoel or blastocyst cavity is formed (see Figure 8.7). The appearance of this cavity is called cavitation. The blastocoel is enclosed by the mural trophectoderm in which the cells are assembled by tight junctional complexes.[19] Trophectoderm is the first epithelium to develop during mammalian embryogenesis, and cavitation is considered to be the first functional expression of the trophectoderm phenotype.[20] Nascent trophectoderm cells are morphologically polarized with asymmetrical distribution of organelles.

Mitochondrial and lipid droplets are localized in apposed borders of blastomeres, and K^+-sensitive transport Na^+K^+-ATPase are also found on the surface of these apposed cells. Ouabain and extracellular K^+ and Na^+ affect the activity of Na^+K^+-ATPase and the polarization of these nascent trophectoderm cells. Following a marked increase in lipid metabolism,[21] excess fluid enters the intercellular spaces when the influx is greater than efflux. Small vesicles are formed and coalesce to become the blastocoel. The blastocyst does not increase in size at this stage as a result of a compensatory decrease in lipid volume.[20]

It should be noted that a cavitation-like process is induced in two-cell zygotes by wheat germ agglutinin (WGA) with a high lectin-binding affinity for *N*-acetylglucosamine and sialic acid residues.[22] WGA binds the zona pellucida and vitelline membrane, blocking fertilization.[23] As ouabain, WGA inhibits ATPase activity, but it fails to cross the plasma membrane. It has selective inhibition on externally located ATPase only and may lead to a compensatory increase in internal ATPase activity in response to ionic and osmotic changes. This is a possible explanation for its induction of cavitation.[22]

At mid to late blastocyst stages, the apical junctions in the trophectoderm become tight, and transcellular fluid movement increases, resulting in blastocyst expansion. There are about 50 cells in a blastocyst at about 12 h after the onset of cavitation, but the cells in the inner cell mass are still capable of regenerating the trophectoderm.[24] Mitosis still occurs during blastocyst expansion. Figure 8.8 shows a flat histological preparation of a blastocyst for determining the number of blastomeres by counting the nuclei. A late blastocyst of 100 cells can be recovered on day 5 of pregnancy, that is about 100 to 140 h after fertilization in humans. The size and cell number of blastocysts, however, vary from one to another without significant differences in their developmental potentials.[25]

C. HATCHING

The zona pellucida has to be removed before implantation to allow direct cell-cell interactions between the trophoblast and uterine epithelial cells. Under *in vitro* conditions, mouse blastocysts undergo hatching or herniation following a series of alternating contraction and relaxation.[26] This process may be an *in vitro* phenomenon only and can be seen readily under an inverted microscope (see Figure 8.9). There are conspicuous differences between hatching *in vitro* and *in vivo*. No strong evidence is available to show that hatching *in vitro* is equivalent to the dissolution of zona pellucida *in utero*.[27]

Hatching *in vitro* appears to be a more pronounced splitting of the zona pellucida than that *in vivo*.[28] Figure 8.10 shows a hatched mouse blastocyst and its shed zona pellucida. In the rabbit blastocyst, the zona pellucida appeared to be digested enzymatically *in utero*.[29] A similar zonalytic protease has also been found in the uterine fluid of mice.[30] In addition, hatching *in vitro* is a more prolonged process, and the blastocyst has to attain a greater size before hatching,

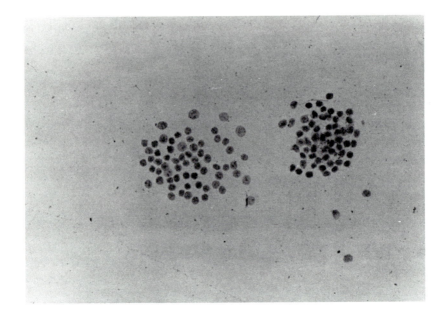

FIGURE 8.8.   Blastomere nuclei of two mouse blastocysts on a flat, dried histological preparation stained in Giemsa.

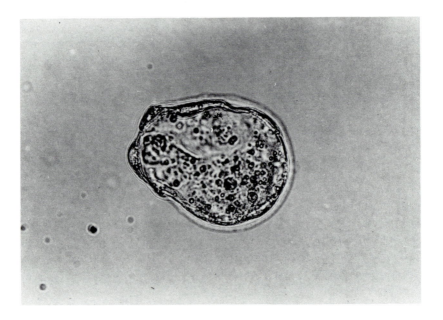

FIGURE 8.9.   A hatching mouse blastocyst.

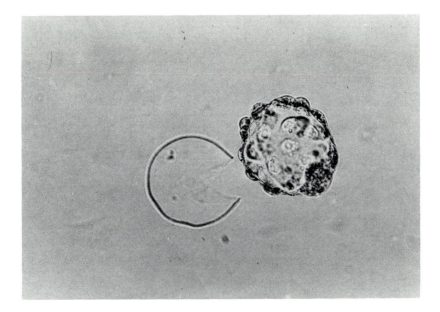

FIGURE 8.10.   A hatched mouse blastocyst and its shed zona pellucida.

whereas the removal of zona pellucida *in utero* occurs rapidly in smaller blasto-cysts.[28,29] A similar hatching process is observed in human blastocysts, and recent studies have shown that assisted hatching enhances the success rate of pregnancy after fertilization *in vitro*.[31]

A hatched blastocyst is ready for implantation. From the time of cavitation to this stage, the blastocyst floats freely in the uterine cavity for about 3 days. At optimal conditions, implantation occurs on days 6 to 7 of pregnancy in humans. The success depends on the preparation of endometrium and the normality of the zygote. Some fertilized eggs may not cleave at all, while other developing ones may be abnormal and die. Less than 40% of the zygotes can actually implant in a normal healthy woman. For an average woman, a fecundity ratio of 1:100 is generally agreed; in other words, there is one successful pregnancy out of 100 sexual intercourses.[32]

Although the preimplantation period is designated as the first week of pregnancy in humans, an actual contact of the zygote with maternal tissues occurs at, and embryogenesis begins after, implantation. The preimplantation zygote is virtually a collection of living cells floating in the uterine fluid. This raises an ethical question about whether this is human life or not. Scientifically, of course, life exists whenever there are living cells of either plants or animals.

It should be reiterated that reproduction is the continuation of life. Life never ends in the reproductive process, but in modern society "ownership" of the collection of new cells generated has become an issue. An individual has no problem claiming the ownership of the cells in his or her arm. Likewise, sperms and unfertilized eggs are unequivocally agreed to be the property of those who produce them. However, once an egg is fertilized and develops into a collection of cells, the ownership of these cells becomes problematic. Even if these cells are considered autonomous with a consciousness of their own, biological priority should be given to the one carrying them. If maternal health is in jeopardy, then from a biological viewpoint, abortion of a particular pregnancy may be necessary to preserve a woman's potential for reproduction and the continuation of human life.

REFERENCES

1. **van Tienhoven, A.,** *Reproductive Physiology of Veı tebrates,* 2nd ed., Cornell University Press, Ithaca, NY, 1983.
2. **Harper, M.J.K.,** Gamete and zygote transport, in *The Physiology of Reproduction,* Knobil, E. and Neill, J., Eds., Raven Press, New York, 1988, 103.
3. **Yanagimachi, R.,** Mammalian fertilization, in *The Physiology of Reproduction,* Knobil, E. and Neill, J., Eds., Raven Press, New York, 1988, 135.
4. **Burkman, L.J.,** Characterization of hyperactivated motility by human spermatozoa during capacitation: comparison of fertile and oligospermic sperm populations, *Arch. Androl.,* 13, 153.
5. **van Benenden, E.,** De la maturation d'oeuf, de la fecondation, et des premiers phenomenes embryonnaires chez les mammiferes, d'apres les observations faites chez le lapin, *Bull. Acad. R. Sci. Belg.,* 1875.
6. **Jenkinson, J.W.,** A reinvestigation of the early stages of the development of the mouse, *Q. J. Microsc. Sci.,* 43, 61, 1900.
7. **Lewis, W.H. and Wright, E.S.,** On the early development of the mouse egg, *Contrib. Embryol.,* 24, 133, 1935.
8. **Glasser, S.R.,** Laboratory models of implantation, in *Reproductive Toxicology,* Dixon, R.L., Ed., Raven Press, New York, 1985, 219.
9. **Clarke, M.,** IVF: another bill bites the dust, *Science,* 319, 349, 1986.
10. **Reeve, W.J.D. and Ziomek, C.A.,** Distribution of microvilli on dissociated blastomeres from mouse embryos: evidence for surface polarization at compaction, *J. Embryol. Exp. Morphol.,* 62, 339, 1981.
11. **Magnuson, T., Demsey, A., and Stackpole, C.W.,** Characterization of intercellular junctions in the preimplantation mouse embryo by freeze fracture and thin section electron microscopy, *Dev. Biol.,* 61, 252, 1977.
12. **Lo, C.W. and Gilula, N.B.,** Gap junctional communication in the preimplantation mouse embryo, *Cell,* 18, 399, 1979.
13. **Levy, J.B., Johnson, M.H., Goodall, H., and Maro, B.,** The timing of compaction: control of a major development transition in mouse early embryogenesis, *J. Embryol. Exp. Morphol.,* 95, 213, 1986.
14. **Mintz, B.,** Formation of genetically mosaic mouse embryos, and early development of "lethal (t12/t12)-normal" mosaics, *J. Exp. Zool.,* 157, 273, 1964.
15. **Tarkowski, A.K. and Wroblewska, J.,** Development of blastomeres of mouse eggs isolated at the four- and eight-cell stage, *J. Embryol. Exp. Morphol.,* 18, 155, 1967.
16. **Johnson, M.H., Maro, B., and Takeichi, M.,** The role of cell adhesion in the synchronization and orientation of polarization in 8-cell mouse blastomeres, *J. Embryol. Exp. Morphol.,* 93, 239, 1986.
17. **Whitten, W.K.,** Nutrient requirements for the culture of preimplantation embryos *in vitro,* *Adv. Biosci.,* 6, 129, 1971.
18. **Pratt, H.P.M., Ziomek, C.A., Reeve, W.J.D., and Johnson, M.H.,** Compaction of the mouse embryo: an analysis of its components, *J. Embryol. Exp. Morphol.,* 70, 113, 1982.

19. **Enders, A.C. and Schlafke, S.J.,** The fine structure of the blastocyst: some comparative studies, in *Preimplantation Stages of Pregnancy: A Ciba Foundation Symposium,* Wolstenholme, G.E.W. and O'Connor, M., Eds., Churchill, London, 1965, 29.

20. **Wiley, L.M.,** Trophectoderm: the first epithelium to develop in the mammalian embryo, *Scanning Electron Microsc.,* 2, 417, 1988.

21. **Flynn, T.J. and Hillman, N.,** The metabolism of exogenous fatty acids by preimplantation mouse embryos developing *in vitro, J. Embryol. Exp. Morphol.,* 56, 257, 1980.

22. **Johnson, L.V.,** Wheat germ agglutinin induces compaction- and cavitation-like events in two-cell mouse embryo, *Dev. Biol.,* 113, 1, 1986.

23. **Parkening, T.A. and Chang, M.C.,** Effects of wheat germ agglutinin on fertilization of mouse ova *in vivo* and *in vitro, J. Exp. Zool.,* 195, 215, 1976.

24. **Fleming, T.P., Warren, P.D., Chisholm, J.C., and Johnson, M.H.,** Trophectodermal processes regulate the expression of totipotency within the inner cell mass of the expanding mouse blastocyst, *J. Embryol. Exp. Morphol.,* 84, 63, 1984.

25. **Chisholm, J.C., Johnson, M.H., Warren, P.D., Fleming, T.P., and Pickering, S.J.,** Developmental variability within and between mouse expanding blastocysts and their ICMs, *J. Embryol. Exp. Morphol.,* 86, 311, 1985.

26. **Hsu, Y.,** Time-lapse cinematography of mouse embryo development from blastocysts to early somite stage, in *Cellular and Molecular Aspects of Implantation,* Glasser, S.R. and Bullock, D.W., Eds., Plenum Press, New York, 1981, 383.

27. **Ebert, K.M. and Black, D.L.,** Effects of immunoglobulins on *in vitro* hatching of preimplantation rabbit embryos, *J. Reprod. Immunol.,* 4, 39, 1982.

28. **Enders, A.C., Chavez, D.J., and Schlafke, S.,** Comparison of implantation *in utero* and *in vitro,* in *Cellular and Molecular Aspects of Implantation,* Glasser, S.R. and Bullock, D.W., Eds., Plenum Press, New York, 1981, 365.

29. **Denker, H.W.,** Trophoblastic factors involved in lysis of the blastocyst coverings and in implantation in the rabbit: observation on inversely oriented blastocysts, *J. Embryol. Exp. Morphol.,* 32, 739, 1974.

30. **Pinsker, M.C., Sacco, A.G., and Mintz, B.M.,** Implantation associated protease in mouse uterine fluid, *Dev. Biol.,* 38, 285, 1974.

31. **Alikani, M. and Cohen, J.,** Advances in clinical micromanipulation of gametes and embryos. Assisted fertilization and hatching, *Arch. Pathol. Lab. Med.,* 116, 373, 1992.

32. **Chronicle Wire Services,** The world has sex 100 million times daily, *San Francisco Chronicle,* June 25, 1992, A1.

9 Pregnancy and Reproductive Immunology

CHAPTER CONTENTS

I. INTRODUCTION

Pregnancy is established after successful fertilization. The two major processes are implantation and organogenesis. In humans, implantation occurs at the end of the first week and marks the dividing point between the preimplantation and postimplantation periods. An embryo forms after implantation, and organogenesis begins by the fourth week. Most organs are developed by the 8th to 12th weeks, including the gonads and external genitalia. After this time, there is only fetal enlargement until parturition by the 38th week from the time of fertilization. In clinical terms, human pregnancy is divided into three trimesters. Differentiation occurs in the first trimester, fetal growth in the second and third trimesters.

Since a typical conceptus contains only 50% of genetic materials from the maternal genome, the other 50% from the paternal genome creates an immunological problem. In a successful pregnancy, paternal antigens do not elicit a classical immune response to an allogenic organ graft. Despite the immunosuppressive mechanism, there are still antibodies detected with cellular and morphological responses to these antigens. The frequency and magnitude of responses actually increase with the number of pregnancies, but remain steady after the fifth pregnancy.[1]

The key lies in placental trophoblast cells that constitute a cellular barrier between maternal blood and fetal tissues. The highly regulated expression of the human leukocyte antigen (HLA) is thought to play an important role in suppressing the immune response. These cells express HLA-G, a nonpolymorphic gene, but not the highly polymorphic class I HLA-A, -B, and -C genes responsible for stimulating graft rejection. In addition, they do not express class II genes for HLA-D antigens nor respond to factors enhancing HLA expression such as interferons.[2]

Some factors from the preimplantation zygote have been found to function as regulatory signals for the uterus.[3] These factors may be necessary to prevent maternal rejection of the fertilized egg carrying paternal genes during oviducal transport. On the other hand, the partially suppressed immune responses may serve as signals for maternal recognition. Pregnancy may be recognized at very early stages, even before fertilization. Transfer of preimplantation zygotes developed from ova fertilized *in vitro* to the uterus of the biological or surrogate mothers results in live births. It appears that preimplantation zygotes can provide sufficient clues for maternal recognition of pregnancy.

II. IMPLANTATION

Implantation is a process universal to mammalian reproduction involving a series of complex interactions between the blastocyst and epithelial cells of the endometrium. It occurs at the beginning of the second week of pregnancy in humans. The steps include attachment, penetration of the uterine epithelium, and decidualization of the endometrium. The trophoblast of the blastocyst first touches the endometrial epithelium and penetrates deeper into the cell layer to form the syncytiotrophoblast and cytotrophoblast. The inner cell mass differentiates into a bilaminar germ disc consisting of the endodermal germ layer separating the ectodermal germ layer from the blastocyst layer.

In humans, an interstitial type of implantation occurs during the second week of pregnancy. A day-9 human blastocyst is firmly embedded beneath the uterine mucosa, and the hole left on the epithelium is plugged by a fibrin coagulum. While the inner cell mass is at the egg cylinder stage, lacunae develop in the syncytiotrophoblast and maternal sinusoids form around the conceptus. The lacunae and maternal sinusoids will later join to establish the uteroplacental circulation. As the conceptus continues to grow, dramatic cytological changes in the endometrial stroma occur, leading to a gross increase in uterine size and weight. This decidualization of the endometrium closely resembles an immune response to trophoblast-associated antigens of the allogenic intrauterine conceptus.[4] The process of implantation is completed by day 14.

A.   ATTACHMENT

Before attachment, a hatched blastocyst aligns itself correctly in the uterine lumen in a nonrandom fashion with an unknown mechanism.[5] It involves a complex interaction between the blastocyst and uterine epithelium.[6] The initiation of attachment *in utero* may involve changes in cell surface properties of both the trophoblast and uterine epithelial cells[7] and two-way cell-cell interactions between the two cell types.[2] This entails the synchrony between zygotic and uterine development.[8] As shown in mice, late blastocysts fail to implant in an asynchronous uterus 2 days in advance, and there is a "nonreceptive" state developed in the uterus after the appropriate time of implantation. A uterine blastotoxic factor may be present after the implantation time, and it inhibits the development of blastocysts *in vitro* in both rats and mice.[9]

The implantation process can be divided into two phases: apposition and adhesion. The zygote does not require the presence of endometrial epithelium in these two initial processes. Under *in vitro* conditions, the zygote can adhere to a nonliving substratum and continue to differentiate. Figure 9.1a shows an early postimplantation mouse zygote attached to a plastic culture dish. Note the well-formed inner cell mass surrounded by a sheet of trophoblast cells. Its cross-section is shown in Figure 9.1e. The trophoblast is a monolayer of multinucleated giant cells attached firmly to the flat surface. In contrast to implantation *in vivo*, the inner cell mass is above the trophoblast instead of being enclosed inside (see Figure 9.2 for an implanted human zygote *in vivo*).

The trophoblastic invasiveness is a necessary quality of the zygote for successful implantation. The trophoblastic area of a cultured zygote is a quantitative measure of this characteristic. In addition to morphological assessment, this characteristic has been used for sensitive *in vitro* embryotoxicity testings.[10] Attached zygotes exposed to embryotoxic substances at different doses show various degrees of degenerative responses. The attached zygotes in Figures 9.1b, 9.1c, and 9.1d were cultured for 72 h in culture media containing cadmium chloride at 0.5, 1.0, and 5.0 µg/ml, respectively. Note that the inner cell masses of all three zygotes degenerated, while the size of their trophoblasts became smaller with increasing dosages. The degenerated zygote eventually detached from the substratum, suggesting that trophoblast attachment is an active process.

B.   PENETRATION OF ENDOMETRIAL EPITHELIUM

In all mammalian species except those with epitheliochorial type of placentation, the conceptus penetrates the endometrial epithelium to implant. There are three major types of endometrial penetration by the conceptus: intrusive,

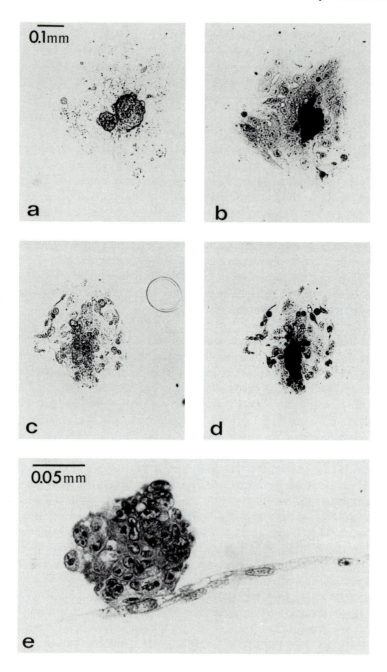

FIGURE 9.1. Mouse early postimplantation zygotes cultured in normal medium (a) or in media containing cadmium chloride at different concentrations: (b) 0.5, (c) 1.0, and (d) 5.0 μg/ml. Part (e) is a histological section of the zygote in part (a).

displacement, and fusion. As in guinea pigs, ferrets, and rhesus monkeys, the penetration is intrusive in humans.[11] In rodents, displacement penetration is found in rats and mice, while fusion penetration occurs in rabbits.[12]

In the fusion type of penetration, syncytial knobs of the abembryonic trophoblast are fused with the apical membrane of the endometrial epithelial cells to form cytoplasmic connections during attachment. In displacement penetration, these epithelial cells are replaced with the trophoblast penetrates. There is cell death and detachment of the epithelium. These trophoblastic cells phagocytize the dead cells and contact the basal lamina.

Although intrusive penetration, as the displacement type, may also involve cell death and phagocytosis, a healthy epithelium is still crucial for anchorage of the trophoblast. Since the conceptus is highly invasive, the cellular changes are more dramatic. Endometrial basal lamina penetration and stroma invasion may be due to the presence of proteolytic enzymes such as collagenase and the urokinase-like plasminogen activator in the human trophoblast.[13]

The mechanism of trophoblast invasion of basement membrane and stroma is possibly similar to that of invasive tumor cells.[14] First, the cell attaches to the basement membrane by binding to basement membrane components such as laminin. Second, the cell has to detach from the basement membrane component prior to its penetration involving some oligosaccharides on the cell surface. Third, the basement membrane components are broken down by trophoblast-derived metalloproteases (type IV and interstitial collagenase) and serine proteases (plasminogen activator). Trophoblast-derived metalloproteases may be activated by plasmin derived from plasminogen, binding to laminin, or decidua-derived transforming growth factor-β (TGF-β).

C. ENDOMETRIAL DECIDUALIZATION

In response to the attachment of an invasive zygote, the endometrial epithelium reacts with an inflammation-like process called decidualization (see Figure 9.2). The decidual reaction is the major morphological response to the implanting conceptus and is crucial to the success of implantation. The process involves decidualization of the endometrial fibroblasts accompanied by an accumulation of large numbers of large granular lymphocytes.[15] The maintenance of pregnancy depends on the trophoblast which can prevent significant entry of maternal lymphocytes across the trophoblast and protect the conceptus from maternal immune rejection by features of its cell surface molecular structure and/or its synthesis of factors that render it insusceptible to antibody- or cell-mediated immune lysis *in vivo*. Alternatively, maternal recognition and immunoregulatory processes which are different from expected rejection reactions may also operate.[4]

Prolactin synthesis in human endometrium and decidua has recently been demonstrated, and expression of the prolactin gene has been confirmed by the successful isolation of prolactin mRNA from the human endometrium.[16] Endometrial prolactin is predominately glycosylated and begins to be secreted in the late luteal phase of the menstrual cycle with increasing amounts of nonglycosylated

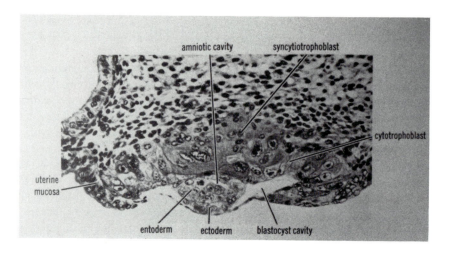

FIGURE 9.2. Decidualization of human endometrium. (From Langman, J., *Medical Embryology. Human Development — Normal and Abnormal,* 3rd ed., Williams & Wilkins, Baltimore, 1975. With permission.)

prolactin after implantation. Prolactin may be necessary for the normal production of macrophage-activating factors, including interferon, which may reduce human endometrial prolactin secretion. Thus, it may have a possible local immunomodulatory role in human implantation. The exact function of prolactin in decidualization is unknown.

III. POSTIMPLANTATION DEVELOPMENT

In humans, implantation takes the entire second week of pregnancy to complete. The conceptus around this time is called a periimplantation zygote. Inside the trophoblast, the inner cell mass continues to differentiate into the egg cylinder. The region of trophoblast where the egg cylinder is attached is the polar trophectoderm. Cells in this region later form the ectoplacental cone and secondary trophoblastic giant cells. Generally, most postblastocyst culture media fail to nourish the conceptus from preimplantation stages to the early primitive-streak stage on days 15 to 16. This stage also marks the termination of the preembryo stage, followed by the formation of a true embryo that will develop into a fetus.[17] In contrast to most mammals, the gestation period in humans is much longer. A typical human gestation period is 266 days (38 weeks) from the time of fertilization. For convenience, it is often estimated as 280 days (40 weeks) from the first day of the last menstrual bleeding. It is divided into three periods: first, second, and third trimesters. All drastic development changes occur during the first trimester, while the increase in fetal size occurs in the second and third trimesters.

The first trimester is the first 3 months from the time of fertilization to the eighth week, including the first week of preimplantation development, the second week of implantation followed by embryogenesis, and the period of organogenesis (or embryonic period) from the fourth to eighth week. At the beginning of the second trimester, the fetus is still as small as 10 to 45 g in weight, though most organs are well formed. At this stage, the morphology appears to be similar across different mammalian species.

During the first month of the second trimester, the initially lateral eyes become ventral as the head enlarges. With the general increase in size and weight, the limbs become more proportional to the body. The face develops into a recognizable human form. By the 12th week, the external genitalia become visible, and the sex can be determined by external examination of the fetus. From the 12th to 24th week, there is a considerable increase in the crown-rump length (about 5 to 15 cm), though the weight is still less than 500 g at the end of this trimester. At this time, the movement of the fetus can be felt by the mother.

The third trimester is the final 3-month period of intrauterine life, which is from the 25th week to term. Tremendous growth occurs during this time, especially during the last 2 to 3 months during which half the neonatal weight is gained. Under intensive care, some fetuses after the sixth month may still survive. The respiratory and nervous systems are last to develop, and their coordination is crucial in fetal survival for early labor. The mean length and weight at birth are 36 cm and 3200 g, respectively.

A. EMBRYOGENESIS

In a day-7 human implanting blastocyst, a cavity called the amniotic cavity starts to develop between the ectoderm of the inner cell mass and trophoblast. The cell layer of trophoblast lining the amniotic cavity is the amnioblast. The central area of the ectoderm facing the amniotic cavity is the region that will become the embryo. The formation of the embryo is called embryogenesis.

Around day 9, the blastocyst cavity can be named as the exocoelomic cavity or the primitive yolk sac. On the other hand, cavities are found in the extraembryonic mesoderm of the trophoblast, and they coalesce to form the extraembryonic coelom or the future chorionic cavity. The inner exocoelomic cavity is separated from the outer concentric extraembryonic coelom by a cellular layer known as Heuser's membrane, in continuation with the entoderm underlying the ectoderm.

By day 9, the internal side of the Heuser's membrane is invaded by proliferating endodermal cells, which form the lining of the new but smaller secondary yolk sac. Part of the original exocoelomic cavity remains as a exocoelomic cyst without the internal lining by endodermal cells. At the same time, the chorionic cavity expands considerably and is enclosed by the chorionic plate derived also from the extraembryonic mesoderm. The resultant conceptus on day 13 is a central mass of tissues suspended in the chorionic cavity. The central mass of tissues consists of two cavities, the amniotic cavity and yolk sac, separated by the germ disc where embryogenesis begins 1 day later.

The germ disc is originally a bilayer: ectoderm and entoderm. By day 14, another layer is formed between these two layers with actively migrating mesodermal cells. As the first sign of a developing embryo, the primitive streak appears on the ectoderm in the amniotic cavity. Two prominent formations during the third week of development are the notochord and allantois. The notochord develops from the notochordal process that is part of the mesoderm. The allantois forms as a small diverticulum from the yolk sac, but unlike lower vertebrates, it does not have a functional role in embryonic development.

During the same week, the trophoblast differentiates further into a more complex tissue surrounding the chorionic cavity. It consists of primary, seconding, and tertiary villi well dispersed with maternal blood sinuses in the intervillous space. At the end of the third week, the embryo is clearly suspended in the chorionic cavity by a stalk derived from extraembryonic mesoderm. This stalk is the future umbilical cord acting as the major connection between the placenta and embryo.

B. ORGANOGENESIS

From the fourth to eighth weeks, there is a change from a presomite embryo to a somite embryo. Most of the organs are developed from the three germ layers of the embryos: ectoderm, mesoderm, and endoderm.

1. The ectoderm consists of cells that form the nervous system, skin and external sensory epithelia, mammary gland, pituitary gland, and the enamel of teeth.
2. The mesoderm layer contributes to the formation of somites or segments. The first somite is formed at the end of the third week, and the number of somites comes up to 34 to 35 on day 30. Each somite is a primitive segmental unit of structures including muscle, skeletal elements, and connective tissues. These somites are combined later in development. The future tissues are connective tissue, muscle, cartilage, bone, circulatory and lymphatic systems, urinogenital system, spleen, and adrenal cortex.
3. The endoderm develops into the alimentary canal, the epithelial lining of urinary bladder, urethra, and respiratory tracts, as well as parenchymal tissues of glands such as thyroid, thymus, liver, and pancreas.

During this period of organogenesis, discernible external features include limb buds, face, ear, nose, and eyes. Another important change is the folding of the embryo. The amniotic cavity folds bilaterally around the yolk sac with the formation of intraembryonic coelom where the gut is suspended. As a result, the amniotic cavity is enclosed by an inner fetal membrane called the amnion that is, in turn, surrounded by the chorionic cavity. The outer fetal membrane is known as the chorion.

C. FETAL DEVELOPMENT

At the end of the eighth week, the period of organogenesis ends. Although the fetal period begins at this time, the fetus and accompanying fetal membranes

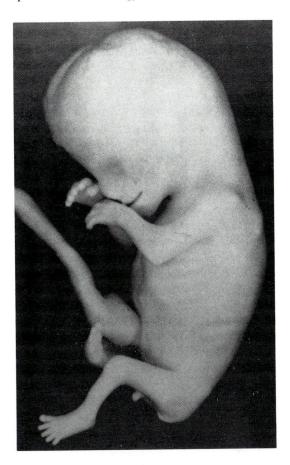

FIGURE 9.3. A 3-month human fetus. (From Langman, J., *Medical Embryology. Human Development — Normal and Abnormal,* 3rd ed., Williams & Wilkins, Baltimore, 1975. With permission.)

(amnion and chorion) are formed during the second month. There are important changes in the placental development and the differentiation into a recognizable human form. Figure 9.3 is a 3-month human fetus. All internal organs are well formed at this stage, but the fetus will not survive if removed from the mother. Figure 9.4 shows a sagittal section of a mouse fetus on day 15. This is equivalent to a fully developed human fetus during the early second semester. Note that all the organs are well differentiated, including the brain and spinal cord. In contrast to mouse fetuses, a human fetus takes 8 months to grow in size before parturition.

IV. PARTURITION AND LACTATION

Parturition is the birth of the infant at the end of the pregnancy period. The timing varies from 37 to 43 weeks after conception and is considered normal

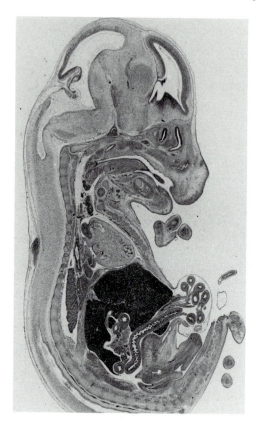

FIGURE 9.4.   Sagittal section of a day 15 mouse fetus.

within this range. If the delivery occurs earlier (i.e., before week 37), as in 5 to 9% of all deliveries in the U.S., the baby is classified as premature or preterm.[18] After the 43rd week, the parturition is postmature. Despite the advent of sophisticated methods of postnatal care, preterm labor is still the major problem in obstetrics and gynecology.

As a preparation for parturition, there are hormonal changes which induce appropriate alterations to facilitate the expulsion of the fetus. The process involves a complex interaction between the maternal physiology and the maturing endocrine system of the fetus. Relaxin, for example, is a 6-kDa polypeptide hormone produced in increasing amounts before parturition by the placenta and the corpus luteum in the ovary. This hormone causes the relaxation of the connective tissue between the pelvic bones and inhibits uterine contraction. The cervix softens because of the dissociation of collagen fibers.

Oxytocin is another agent secreted at a much higher level during the last month of pregnancy, while the uterine tissues become more sensitive to oxytocin. Oxytocin is synthesized and secreted by oxytocin neurons originated from both paraventricular and supraoptic nuclei (PVN and SON) (see Chapter 3). Oxytocin

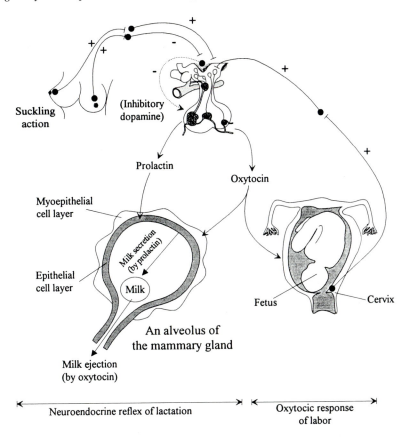

FIGURE 9.5.   Roles of oxytocin and prolactin in lactation and parturition.

produces a series of uterine contractions to expel the fetus. This effect is known as oxytocic response of labor. Oxytocin is also involved in the induction of lactation, which is another important event for postnatal care after parturition. Milk ejection induced by oxytocin is called galactogogic effect. Therefore, there is a series of steps from parturition initiation to fetal expulsion, recovery, and lactation (see Figure 9.5).

A.   INDUCTION OF LABOR

In addition to relaxin and oxytocin, steroids and possibly prostaglandins are also involved. Oxytocin, estrogens, PGE, and PGF can induce uterine contraction. As relaxin, progesterone suppresses uterine contraction, but it has no effect on pelvic relaxation. Since progesterone is mainly produced by the placenta, there is a steady increase in progesterone level since the late first trimester in humans. This steroid does not decrease in level prior to parturition.

The initiation of labor may be related to the decrease in the ratio of progesterone to estrogens as estrogen level increases before parturition. Such a decrease in this ratio may be interpreted as a decrease in progesterone level. It is evident that estrogen concentration is increased prior to parturition. It is found both in maternal peripheral plasma and amniotic fluid during the last 2 weeks of gestation. In addition, estrogens may also inhibit progesterone production and promote stimulatory effects of other agents.

PGE$_2$ and PGF$_{2\alpha}$ have been suggested to be responsible for inducing labor based on their potent stimulatory actions on human myometrial tissues. The mechanism may possibly involve prostaglandin-induced increase in free intracellular Ca^{2+}. Besides, there is an increase in their levels during labor. The production of PGE$_2$ and PGF$_{2\alpha}$ in human decidua is stimulated by oxytocin. Therefore, oxytocin may have both direct and indirect promoting effects on uterine contractility.

B.   LABOR

The induction of uterine contractions by oxytocin plays a crucial role in labor. At the onset of labor, the intensity, duration, and frequency of uterine contractions increase considerably. The frequency is about two contractions per minute with a duration of about 30 s. This increases to 20 to 30 contractions per minute with a duration of about 1 min. The contraction starts at the uterine fundus and propagates downward to the cervix, forcing the fetus toward the cervical opening. The amplification of this effect involves a neuroendocrine positive feedback loop of oxytocin.

As a result of uterine contraction, the cervix is stretched, and a signal is sent to the hypothalamus to enhance oxytocin release. This neurohypophyseal hormone further induces uterine contractions. The sensitivity of the myometrium to oxytocin also increases as the level of oxytocin in the circulation is elevated. This positive feedback mechanism amplifies the rhythmic contractions. They become much more intense in comparison to the tonic weak contractions, or Braxton-Hicks contractions, occurring throughout gestation. Sometimes, just prior to labor, there are episodes of false labor as these contractions become too strong.

There are three stages in true normal labor: cervical dilatation, delivery of the fetus, and expulsion of the placenta. As a result of the positive feedback effect of oxytocin, the cervix dilates 2 to 10 cm in diameter. This first stage of labor may take several hours to 1 day and is a prelude to the delivery of the fetus. When the cervix is fully dilated, the fetus is pushed through the cervical opening by the powerful rhythmic uterine contractions. Once the fetus is in the vaginal canal, there is a reflex action from the abdominal muscles, causing abdominal contractions. At the end of this stage, the infant is pushed through the vagina, but the placenta is still retained inside the uterus. The second stage takes about 30 min to 1 h.

The final stage of labor is the separation of the placenta from the myometrium. This is an important step contributing to the success of a normal labor. Improper position of the placenta or erroneous handling may lead to excessive bleeding. In a normal delivery, it takes less than 30 min with the assistance of continued myometrial contractions. Maternal blood loss is minimized by constriction of capillaries in the placental area of the myometrium. Oxytocin is very often used clinically to induce more uterine concentrations to reduce hemorrhage.

C.   RECOVERY

Since the original size of the uterus is much smaller, the recovery requires 1 to 2 months. Involution of the uterus starts immediately after the expulsion of the placenta, which is the major source of estrogens and progesterone. With the increased oxytocin, the fall of the steroid levels contributes to the process of uterine involution. The tissue remains in the uterus become necrotic and are shed within 1 month after labor. The vaginal discharge is often called "lochia," and its removal is assisted by the uterine contractions induced by oxytocin.

D.   LACTATION

The primary function of oxytocin is thought to be an inducer of milk ejection. Lactation is a crucial process in mammals after the birth of the infant. It can be considered as the final step of the mammalian reproductive process. In humans, however, maternal milk can be replaced by animal milk, though recent evidence suggests that the former is more advantageous to the infant.

1.   Milk

Milk is a highly complex secretion from the epithelial cells of alveoli of a lobule of the mammary gland. Its composition varies from time to time and is dependent on the maternal physiology. During the first 5 days postpartum, the milk produced contains high salt concentration and proteins, but a low lactose level and fat content. This type of milk is called colostrum, which is known to have high concentrations of antibodies contributing to the passive immunity of the neonate.

From days 5 to 10 postpartum, the milk composition continues to change, and it is called transitional milk. It later becomes mature milk with a more stable composition. It has high concentrations of lactose, fat, calcium, phosphate, casein, α-lactalbumin, vitamins, and other ingredients such as minerals and hormones. The composition varies from species to species, so that human milk is unique and may be very specific on an individual basis.

2.   Lactogenesis

Lactogenesis is the initiation of lactation involving a cascade of events occurring before labor. First, the alveolar cells in the lobule of the mammary gland have to become fully differentiated at the time of parturition. Second, an intense secretion of milk must occur immediately after parturition. There is an array of hormones involved such as prolactin, oxytocin, estrogens, progesterone, placental lactogen, cortisol, insulin, thyroid and parathyroid hormones, growth hormone (GH), prostaglandins, and epidermal growth factor, though only prolactin and oxytocin are responsible for the actual secretion and ejection of milk. The other hormones are essential for cytodifferentiation during lactogenesis and preparation for lactation.[19]

Estradiol promotes the growth of the ducts, and progesterone enhances the alveolar-lobular differentiation during puberty. As their concentrations increase during pregnancy, there is extensive hypertrophy and hyperplasia of the alveoli. Alveolar development during pregnancy is further enhanced by the increasing secretion of prolactin and hCS. The mammary glands are fully developed by the second trimester, with a drastic increase in the enzymes necessary for milk production. Progesterone, however, inhibits lactogenesis and counteracts the effects of estrogens.

Cortisol induces differentiation of rough ER and Golgi apparatus necessary for milk production. Its effects are mediated by prostaglandins and are necessary for the action of prolactin. Insulin, thyroid and parathyroid hormones, GH, and epidermal growth factors may also be involved in the development of alveolar cells and the stimulated proliferation of the epithelial cells. Suppression of these hormones leads to a reduction in milk secretion. These hormones are thought to regulate the process at the level of gene expression and at a cellular level.

3.   Milk Secretion

After labor, the production and secretion of milk are stimulated by an increase in prolactin release from adenohypophysis (see Figure 9.5). The suckling action has a suppressive effect on the dopaminergic neuron that produces the prolactin-inhibiting factor (PIF or dopamine). The lowering of this inhibitory effect leads to an increased prolactin secretion. Prolactin acts on the alveolar epithelial cells of the mammary gland responsible for milk production. More milk is secreted into the lumen of the alveolus for ejection.

Myoepithelial cells surrounding the epithelial cell layer are responsive to oxytocin. The suckling action also stimulates oxytocin release and induces con-traction of these myoepithelial cells. As the alveolar lumen contracts, milk is ejected to the exterior through the alveolar duct. The maintenance of milk production also depends on this suckling stimulation, so that continual breastfeeding is necessary to induce uninterrupted lactation.[20]

It should be noted that breastfeeding in women delays the resumption of ovarian cyclicity and menstruation; this is called lactational amenorrhea, with a duration ranging from months to years. Ovulation may occur in some women, but the luteal phase is often deficient. This is suggested to be the reason for reduced fertility of breastfeeding women with resumed menstrual cycles. In those with lactational amenorrhea, LH secretion is suppressed, and estradiol fails to induce a positive feedback response of either LH or FSH. The pulsatile LH secretion fails to resume, and the preovulatory LH surge is absent. Continual breastfeeding at night further suppresses the resumption of normal LH secretion, leading to a longer lactational amenorrhea. All these may be attributed to the high levels of prolactin, which acts directly on the ovary and indirectly on other neuroendocrine systems.[21]

When there is no suckling action at weaning of the infant, prolactin secretion is reduced so that the signal for milk synthesis and secretion is lost. The produc-tion process still continues, though the milk ejection reflex ceases as oxytocin release is reduced. This causes an accumulation of milk and enlargement of the breast. The increased pressure in the alveoli also acts as a signal to suppress milk production and secretion. In some women, the engorgement of the breast becomes so uncomfortable that artificial removal of the milk is needed.

V.   REPRODUCTIVE IMMUNOLOGY

In a broader sense, reproductive immunology is the study of immune responses relevant to the reproductive process. It includes both the male and female. There are immunological techniques such as radioimmunoassay for quantitation of sex steroids and passive and active immunization against sex hormones. The use of these techniques for contraception will be discussed in Chapter 10. Reproductive immunology also includes studies on H-Y antigens (see Chapter 1) and antispermic antibodies as a result of a vasectomy (see Chapter 10). The fertilization process involves the response of the oocyte to a sperm carrying sperm surface antigens foreign to the maternal system (see Chapter 8). Therefore, some topics are discussed elsewhere in other chapters, but also will be discussed below from an immunological point of view.

The most interesting immunological problem in the reproductive process is pregnancy. The first problem is insemination, during which a large batch of antigens is introduced into the female reproductive canal. Since the genetic makeup of the male is often very different from that of the female, the materials in the semen are foreign and analogous to an "allograft." The immunological problem becomes more obvious when fertilization is successful, followed by the establishment of the placenta. Placentation is not unique to mammals nor even to vertebrates. It is defined as any intimate apposition or fusion of the fetal organs to the maternal or paternal tissues for physiological exchange. This condition occurs in many phyla of invertebrates and vertebrates exhibiting viviparity.[22]

The conceptus carrying paternally derived antigens is often called an allograft transplanted on the uterine wall. Medawar[23] was the first to raise these problems and suggested this analogy. Although the analogy is a convenient comparison for educational purposes, it should not be considered as an immune response equivalent to that of an organ graft. In most species studied, including humans, it is now known that the immune response of the maternal system to the paternal component of the fetal placental unit appears to direct against broadly shared class I antigens and not against the classical class I transplantation antigens responsible for common tissue rejection. So far, there is no consistent evidence for a physiological role of immunoregulatory substances in the implantation process, though some immunological factors are associated with gestational abnormalities.[24]

A.   Fertilization and Preimplantation Development

In a recent review,[25] it has been shown that 1 to 30% of infertility in couples is associated with antispermic antibodies. Infertility may be attributed to decreased acrosome reaction and/or suppressed sperm binding to the zona pellucida. There is a rare but serious allergic reaction reported in some young women who have hypersensitivity to human seminal plasma and require immunotherapy.[26] In both men and women, antispermic antibodies are developed, but serious allergic reactions are not observed. Immunosuppressive therapy and IVF have been suggested to be possible treatment methods.[27]

Since only 5% of sperms finally reach the oviduct, a stringent selection process is thought to occur in the uterus. It is possible that the selection process has an immunological basis.[22] The immunity would become hazardous if it were abnormally enhanced. Autoimmunization of the male and isoimmunization of the female with spermatozoal or testicular material leading to infertility have been proposed to be contraceptive methods. However, immunity to sperms is possibly a relative phenomenon. The efficiency varies from time to time in different individuals.[28]

Fertilization presents another immunological barrier to the sperm. This is the well-known recognition mechanism of sperms from different species. The specific sperm receptor on the zona pellucida governs the ability of sperm binding. Therefore, antibodies specific or nonspecific to the sperm receptor which are capable of binding to the zona pellucida are inhibitory to sperm binding. In some women with autoimmune diseases, they can be infertile if antibodies against the zona pellucida are developed. There is a disease entity called autoimmune oophoritis with which patients are often presented with symptoms of premature ovarian failure.[29] In these cases, the patients have a general immunological problem with autoimmune reactions to ovarian tissues.

The zona pellucida is another source of antigens. It contains three fractions of sulfated glycoproteins: ZP1, ZP2, and ZP3. These protein fractions are about 200, 120, and 83 kDa, respectively, in the mouse. Sperm receptors are mainly found in ZP3, which is called the primary sperm receptor, while ZP2 is the secondary sperm receptor. In a recent report, a peptide (amino acid sequence: CSNSSSSQFQIHGPR) isolated from the sperm-binding component (ZP3) of the mouse zona pellucida had been used to induce autoimmune disease of the ovary in the murine model.[30] ZP3 is a potential contraceptive vaccine for immunization against fertilization.[31]

After fertilization, the conceptus carries paternal genetic materials and is transported along the oviduct to the uterine cavity for implantation. This period of time represents a high level of wastage; more than half of the fertilized ova are eventually lost. The primary cause of embryonic wastage is genetic abnormalities of the zygote, including improper maternal-fetal histocompatibility. This serves as an early screening process before committing subsequent physiological investment for postimplantation development. Increased concentrations of immunosuppressive factors such as α-fetoprotein, α_2-globulin, and β_1-globulin in maternal blood of pregnant women apparently suggest a possible but controversial physiological role of the immune response. Cytotoxic T lymphocytes against paternal antigens have also been detected by the time of implantation. In humans, the frequency and amplitude of the antibody titer increases to a plateau after the fifth pregnancy.[1]

So far, there is no clear evidence showing maternal immune reaction to preimplantation zygotes until the time when implantation is initiated.[32] The implanting conceptus evokes the appearance of some immunoregulatory factors involved in the decidual reaction. The central issue is whether such a reaction has a physiological role or is merely a residual response of the suppressed immunity to paternal antigens. It seems reasonable to speculate that the evolution of viviparity might have to overcome the severe maternal immunity of the conceptus carrying paternal genes. Successful pregnancy in humans today may represent a suppressed version of such an immune response. This evolutionary legacy is inherited to maintain a certain degree of selectivity in the recognition process during implantation.

Recently, it has been proposed by Daunter[33] that a normal allogeneic immune response is initiated at the time of blastocyst implantation. The immune response regulates the invasiveness of the trophoblast based on an interplay between maternal and paternal HLA and trophoblast antigens. Daunter also suggests that the immune response involving lymphocytes and leukocytes in the peripheral blood is not important. The local uterine immune response suppressing the expression of allogeneic HLA may play a pivotal role. This unifying hypothesis remains to be evaluated.

B. POSTIMPLANTATION AND POSTNATAL INTERACTIONS

Despite the embryonic wastage incurred by implantation, the implanted conceptus is still not guaranteed to full term and is presented with another immunological problem during placentation. In contrast to ovoviviparity in lower vertebrates where the mother only provides shelter for the developing young, the placenta is mandatory for fetal nourishment in viviparous species. In addition, the placenta also provides a protective filter against microorganisms that are terminated by antibodies in maternal blood. Despite different varieties of placentas among mammals, the immunological problem is overcome by separating the maternal and fetal vascular systems in all types. Physical damages or parturition causing the mixing of maternal and fetal blood can create an immune reaction associated with some antigenic factors such as blood groups (see Section V.C.2).

In the hemochorial placenta of humans, being well integrated with the poorly antigenic placenta, the fetal trophoblast without conventional class I and class II HLA molecules is insusceptible to immune attack.[32] As a way to circumvent the lack of immunity in early conceptus, transplacental immunization has been shown to occur in humans.[1] Maternal IgG antibodies are transmitted across the placental trophoblast by receptor-dependent mechanisms for this purpose. Maternally acquired IgG is available for up to 9 months of gestation. This capability, however, can become pathological when fetal erythrocytes, leukocytes, and platelets are somehow transferred into the maternal circulation. IgG isoantibodies thus produced can gain access to the fetus through similar mechanisms. Autoantibodies associated with various diseases may similarly pass into the fetus, though the effects are usually mild and transient. The fetal immune system starts to express and develop early; it can react to intrauterine infections as early as the 12th week of gestation.[32]

Despite the immunological barrier provided by the placenta, there are still occasional transfers of fetal red blood cells and platelets to the maternal circulation or the escape of maternal stem cells to the fetus. Maternal sensitization to red blood cell antigens may lead to anemia, hydrops, and death in the fetus.[34] Other entities that have access to the fetal blood are viruses. It has been observed in the recent AIDS epidemic in which maternal HIV virus infections have become a leading cause of immunodeficiency in children; the risk of HIV transmission from an infected mother to the fetus is 13 to 39%.[35] Diagnosis of HIV infection in the newborn is complicated by transplacental transfer of the HIV antibody. In addition to standard serologic tests, a positive p24 core antigen test, a positive viral culture or AIDS-defining criteria with immune abnormalities are also required for diagnosis in children younger than 15 months.

α-Fetoprotein (αFP) is a product of fetal guts and liver. A similar protein can also be detected in neoplastic cells of hepatocyte or of germ cell origin in adults. This protein belongs to a gene family phylogenetically related to serum albumin which has structural similarity to αFP. The difference between the two proteins occurs in the first 135 amino acid residues, with about 42% of the remaining 590 residues of the human proteins being identical.[36] As αFP is transferred to maternal circulation, the measurement of its concentration in maternal serum has been used as a marker of fetal abnormality since the 1970s.[37] αFP may play a role in fetal immune function or in maintaining osmotic pressure. In infants with congenital deficiency of serum αFP, it is a benign genetic trait comparable to analbuminemia, a congenital deficiency in albumin.[38]

The passive antibody-mediated immunity in the fetus provided by the mother continues even beyond pregnancy; immunoglobins are transferred to breast-fed infants through milk.[39] Clinical data suggest that human milk provides not only antimicrobial factors, but also anti-inflammatory agents. A complex host defense system exists in human milk to fight against common microbial pathogens possible in the alimentary or respiratory tracts of the infant. In addition, there are major anti-inflammatory agents such as anti-proteases, lysozyme, lactoferrin, and IgA with some antioxidants such as cysteine, ascorbate, α-tocopherol, and β-carotene.[40] The presence of antioxidants may be beneficial to the infant's developing immune system, which is susceptible to oxidant damage.

Although breastfeeding is apparently an important type of postnatal interaction with the mother immunologically, a recent comparative study between breast-fed and formula-fed infants cannot demonstrate drastic differences in secretory antibodies.[41] In this study, salivary IgA, anti-*Escherichia coli,* anti-β-lactoglobulin, and antipoliovirus type 1 IgA and IgM in serum and saliva were evaluated in two groups of infants over the first 6 months of life. The only difference found was that the salivary IgA in breast-fed infants increased more rapidly and was significantly higher than that in formula-fed infants at 6 months.

C.   IMMUNOGENETIC FACTORS AND REPRODUCTIVE FAILURE

Since the reproductive process is continuous, immunogenetic factors exert their effects throughout the whole process at different time points. When these factors are operating within normal parameters, they may have important regulatory roles in the selection process and maternal-fetal recognition. Reproductive failure is part of the stringent selective mechanism. In severe cases, the extreme response is infertility to prevent passing these defective genes to the next generation.

1. Autoimmune Responses

An association exists between abnormal autoimmune response and reproductive failure, especially in patients with autoimmune reactions in reproductive organs.[42] Despite the lack of definitive evidence of autoimmune diseases of the gonads in humans, immunologic factors of human infertility are implicated in both clinical cases and experimental animal models involving ovarian and testicular dysfunction.[43]

The presence of antispermic antibody is one of the causes of male-factor infertility (see also Chapter 10). This is a type of autoimmune disease in the male. Other male factors are poor sperm quality, oligozoospermia, or even azoospermia, though they may not be immunologically related.[44] These deficiencies ultimately lead to a low rate of fertilization. Similar antispermic antibodies produced in the female would also jeopardize the chance of fertilization.

One interesting clinical disorder in pregnant women is the antiphospholipid syndrome.[45] For some unknown reasons, autoantibodies against several types of negatively charged phospholipids are developed in these patients. For example, there are anticardiolipin antibodies and the lupus anticoagulant. The measurement of these factors is employed in current diagnostic methods. Fortunately, under careful clinical management, these patients can usually carry a baby to full term.

2. Blood Groups

The Rhesus (Rh) and ABO blood group antigens are the two major antigenic systems involved in the immunological interaction between maternal and fetal blood. There are rare cases in which maternal sensitization is elicited when some minor serological factors are involved. For example, there is a reported case of hemolytic disease of the newborn due to anti-K (Cellano) during a fifth pregnancy.[46] This is a rare pregnancy disorder in Caucasians. The newborn requires an exchange transfusion immediately after delivery.

The Rh incompatibility is a result of an immune response in an Rh– mother to an Rh+ fetus who inherits the Rh+ factor from an Rh+ father. The Rh factor, which was first found in the Rhesus monkey, consists of six antigens located on the red blood cell (RBC). Only three of them, C, D, and E, are responsible for the Rh antigenicity and are present in Rh+ individuals. When Rh+ red blood cells are injected into Rh– individuals without these three antigens, anti-Rh agglutinins (IgG antibodies) develop slowly. The severity of the reaction depends on the combination of dominant and recessive components; CDe appears to be less severe than cDE (lower-case letters for recessive). Fortunately, over 85% of all people are Rh+, so these types of incompatibility problems are not too common.

Since IgG antibodies can pass through the placenta into fetal circulation, an Rh+ fetus dies in an Rh– mother before birth in some cases. In other cases, the newborn is extremely anemic; this is caused by progressive destruction of RBCs by antibodies, a condition called erythroblastosis fetalis. Since the macrophage system converts hemoglobin released from destroyed RBCs into bilirubin, the baby's skin becomes yellow and is said to be jaundiced. Currently, some physicians recommend performing amniocentesis to measure the bilirubin level in amniotic fluid in cases of severe Rh incompatibility.[47] An intrauterine transfusion of blood without anti-Rh agglutinins may be performed, but usually the transfusion should be done immediately after birth.

The common ABO blood group system can also create incompatibility problems during pregnancy. With two types of antigens, A and B, on the plasma membrane of the RBC, there are four possible types of RBCs: A, B, both, or none. They are designated as AO, BO, AB, and O, respectively. Since antigens A and B are lacking in individuals with blood group O, anti-A and anti-B agglutinins are developed if they are injected with blood from AB individuals. Therefore, an O mother carrying an A, B, or AB fetus would have ABO incompatibility and produce IgG against A and/or B antigens, leading to erythroblastosis fetalis.

A or B mothers may produce anti-B and anti-A, respectively, but the antibodies are mainly IgM, unlike IgG, which does not pass through the placenta significantly. In the case of O mothers, IgG crosses the placenta but, in contrast to Rh incompatibility, the hemolytic disease of the newborn is only mild. The low incidence of ABO incompatibility problems has been explained by the finding that a large amount of soluble blood-group glycoproteins are produced by the fetus, so that most of the maternal antibodies are bound.[1] A recent study on 1944 pregnant women, however, suggests that the incidence may increase with maternal serum immune antibody titer. The author recommended that pregnant women with a titer higher than 1:64 should be followed up regularly and those above 1:128 should be treated immediately.[48]

It is interesting to note that ABO incompatibility has a protective effect against Rh incompatibility. It is suggested that ABO incompatibility causes an increased removal of fetal RBCs from maternal circulation, reducing the chance of further maternal immunization against Rh antigens from the fetus. In addition, a recent report linked sex ratio with blood-group incompatibility.[49] The highest sex ratio with more males was found in Rh(D)⁻ newborns of Rh(D)⁺ mothers (172.7), while the lowest is among Rh(D)⁺ newborns of Rh(D)⁺ mothers (113.5). Rex-Kiss offered an explanation that the incompatibility exerts a negative effect on the X chromosome, resulting in a higher elimination rate of the zygotes carrying two X chromosomes.

3.   Major Histocompatibility Complex (MHC)

MHC in humans is called HLA (H-2 in mouse) and is a DNA region of 4×10^6 bp containing over 70 known genes on chromosome 6. There are three regions: the telomeric region of class I, the centromeric region of class II, and the class III in the region between the former two.[50] There is a high degree of polymorphism at all MHC gene loci with considerable ethnic differences.[51] Figure 9.6 shows the

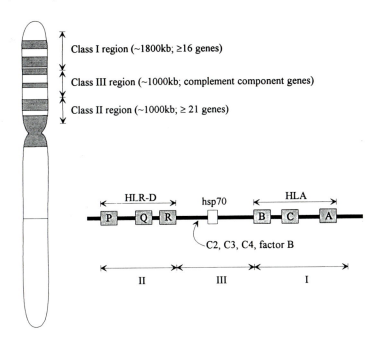

Homo sapiens Chromosome 6 (HSA6)

FIGURE 9.6. Location and structure of the MHC on human chromosome 6 (see text for abbreviations). (After Srivastava, R., Ram, B.P., and Tyle, P., *Immunogenetics of the Major Histocompatibility Complex,* Srivastava, R., Ram, B.P., and Tyle, P., Eds., VCH Publishers, New York, 1991.)

location of MHC loci on chromosome 6 and the gene structure of the MHC. In humans, there are four loci called A, B, C, and D in the HLA region. HLA molecules, on the surface of antigen-presenting cells, bind foreign peptides. This antigen complex is then recognized by T lymphocytes and triggers the alloresponse against the peptide.

The class I region contains major genes HLA-A, -B, and -C. These types of antigens can be found in almost all tissues. In the class II region, there are at least 21 genes encoded; three major genes are DP, DQ, and DR (see Figure 9.6). DR encodes heterodimers expressed on the surface of B lymphocytes, while DP and DQ genes play a role in binding antigens stimulatory to T-cell proliferation. There are also allelic variants of DP, DQ, and DR genes linked with some autoimmunity cases. These variants are possibly more capable of directing the T-cell response against self-antigens.[52] In the 100-kb segment of DNA for class III, there are two clusters of genes encoding proteins involved in the activation of C3, C2, C4, and factor B. The complement (C) system has two activation pathways: classical and alternative.

In the classical pathway, there are 9 enzyme precursors (designated as C1 through C9) responsible for the cascade reactions when an antibody binds with an antigen. Factor B is the central component of the alternative pathway. It cleaves in response to antigen activation. Fragments of factor B modulate prestimulated B lymphocytes by binding to their cell surface receptors. Class III region is thus an important part of the complement component genes of the immune system.[53] The gene of the well-known heat shock protein (hsp70) is also embedded in the subregion of this class III region.[54]

The regulatory proteins factor H, C4BP, CR1, and DAF, which are involved in the control of C3 convertase activity, are encoded by closely linked genes (termed the regulators of complement activation or RCA linkage group) that have been mapped to human chromosome 1.[53] There are also genes for minor histocompatibility (MIH) antigens scattered over the entire genome. MIH antigens are thought to be responsible for graft rejection in HLA-identical siblings and are recognized by T cells but not antibodies. The genes encoding them are found in almost all chromosomes, including the Y chromosome where the H-Y antigen gene is located.[54]

MHC products are normally not expressed during early development so that the fetus can escape recognition by maternal lymphocytes.[55] There is evidence that MHC-linked genes encoding peptide transporter molecules and possibly components of a proteolytic complex are necessary for MHC class I assembly and stability at the cell surface. The MHC class I assembly may be defective in early embryonic cells, suggesting that the tolerance of fetal allograft may in part be controlled at the level of peptide-dependent MHC class I assembly. Later in the development, only some paternal class I antigens are expressed in the trophoblast. In a normal pregnancy, the maternal immune response is not against those class I antigens responsible for the classical type of tissue rejection.

4.   Spontaneous Abortions

Maternal-fetal histocompatibility caused by sharing of MHC antigens between males and females may increase the incidence of spontaneous abortion.[56] A spontaneous abortion can be considered as a maternal selective mechanism to terminate as early as possible her investment to carry an immunologically incompatible baby of low developmental potential. Perhaps such incompatibility is a result of abnormal gene expression. There are two common types of immunogenetically related abnormalities leading to spontaneous abortion: toxemia of pregnancy and choriocarcinoma.

Toxemia of pregnancy is also known as eclampsia or preeclampsia. The characteristic clinical features of eclampsia are high blood pressure and edema. The symptoms occur mostly during the latter half of pregnancy in humans. A similar disorder cannot be found in other mammalian species. The severity also varies greatly among different women: from mild hypertension to placental ischemia and proteinuria in severe preeclampsia and further to even maternal death after a full eclamptic attack. At autopsy, cerebral hemorrhage is usually found with extensive small vessel thrombosis. A conservative estimate of all forms of preeclampsia/eclampsia is 5%.[57]

Preeclampsia is a placental disorder that is sometimes dependent on paternal genes in the conceptus. Two stages have been hypothesized in this pregnancy disease. First, there are processes leading to smaller spiral arteries or vascular obstruction and poor placentation or acute arthrosis. The conditions worsen in the second stage during which placental ischemia and eventually abortion occur.[58] The disease entity is probably genetic and is suspected to be caused by a recessive Mendelian expression. Paternal HLA antigens, which are part of the MHC system, may also be involved (see Section V.C.3). Fortunately, in most preeclamptic women, the risk of preeclampsia induced by the same partner is reduced after the first pregnancy.[57]

Choriocarcinoma is another gestational problem possibly related to HLA antigens. It is a type of benign or malignant trophoblastic tumor. There are data suggesting, not conclusively, that HLA compatibility between maternal and paternal genes favors the development of choriocarcinoma through sharing of HLA antigens.[57] In nonmetastatic cases, the disease progression may be inconspicuous and can be limited to a few villi. Unfortunately, there is no optimal treatment for metastatic cases with grossly evident involvement of the placenta. In severe cases, the prognosis is usually poor for both mother and infant.[59]

REFERENCES

1. **Gill, T.J., III.,** Immunological and genetic factors influencing pregnancy, in *The Physiology of Reproduction,* Knobil, E. and Neill, J., Eds., Raven Press, New York, 1988, 2023.
2. **Hunt, J.S. and Orr, H.T.,** HLA and maternal-fetal recognition, *FASEB J.,* 6, 2344, 1992.
3. **Hodgen, G.D. and Itskovitz, J.,** Recognition and maintenance of pregnancy, in *The Physiology of Reproduction,* Knobil, E. and Neill, J., Eds., Raven Press, New York, 1988, 1995.
4. **Billington, W.D.,** Maternal immune response to pregnancy, *Reprod. Fertil. Dev.,* 1, 183, 1989.
5. **Glasser, S.R.,** Laboratory models of implantation, in *Reproductive Toxicology,* Dixon, R.L., Ed., Raven Press, New York, 1985, 219.
6. **Heap, R.B., Flint, A.P.F., and Gadsby, J.E.,** Embryonic signals and maternal recognition, in *Cellular and Molecular Aspects of Implantation,* Glasser, S.R. and Bullock, D.W., Eds., Plenum Press, New York, 1981, 311.
7. **Sherman, M.I. and Wudl, L.R.,** The implanting mouse blastocyst, in *The Cell Surface in Animal Development,* Poste, G. and Nicholson, G.R., Eds., North-Holland, Amsterdam, 1976, 81.
8. **Hoppe, P.C. and Coman, D.R.,** Reduced survival *in utero* from transferred mouse blastocysts compared with morulae, *Gam. Res.,* 7, 161, 1983.
9. **Psychoyos, A. and Casimiri, V.,** Uterine blastotoxic factors, in *Cellular and Molecular Aspects of Implantation,* Glasser, S.R. and Bullock, D.W., Eds., Plenum Press, New York, 1981, 327.
10. **Yu, H.S. and Chan, S.T.H.,** Effects of cadmium on preimplantation and early postimplantation mouse embryos *in vitro* with special reference to their trophoblastic invasiveness, *Pharmacol. Toxicol.,* 60, 129, 1987.
11. **Lindenberg, S.,** Experimental studies on the initial trophoblast endometrial interaction, *Dan. Med. Bull.,* 38, 371, 1991.

12. **Weitlauf, H.M.,** Biology of implantation, in *The Physiology of Reproduction,* Knobil, E. and Neill, J., Eds., Raven Press, New York, 1988, 231.

13. **Flamigni, C., Bulletti, C., Polli, V., Ciotti, P.M., Prefetto, R.A., Galassi, A., and DiCosmo, E.,** Factors regulating interaction between trophoblast and human endometrium, *Ann. N.Y. Acad. Sci.,* 622, 176, 1991.

14. **Lala, P.K. and Graham, C.H.,** Mechanisms of trophoblast invasiveness and their control: the role of proteases and protease inhibitors, *Cancer Metastasis Rev.,* 9, 369, 1990.

15. **Enders, A.C.,** Current topic: structural responses of the primate endometrium to implantation, *Placenta,* 12, 309, 1991.

16. **Healy, D.L.,** Endometrial prolactin and implantation, *Baillieres Clin. Obstet. Gynaecol.,* 5, 95, 1991.

17. **McLaren, A.,** Embryo research, *Science,* 320, 570, 1986.

18. **Challis, J.R.G. and Olson, D.M.,** Parturition, in *The Physiology of Reproduction,* Knobil, E. and Neill, J., Eds., Raven Press, New York, 1988, 2177.

19. **Tucker, H.A.,** Lactation and its hormonal control, in *The Physiology of Reproduction,* Knobil, E. and Neill, J., Eds., Raven Press, New York, 1988, 2235.

20. **Wakerley, J.B., Clarke, G., and Summerlee, A.J.S.,** Milk ejection and its control, in *The Physiology of Reproduction,* Knobil, E. and Neill, J., Eds., Raven Press, New York, 1988, 2283.

21. **McNeilly, A.S.,** Suckling and the control of gonadotrophin secretion, in *The Physiology of Reproduction,* Knobil, E. and Neill, J., Eds., Raven Press, New York, 1988, 2323.

22. **Kaye, M.,** Immunological relationships between mother and fetus during pregnancy, in *Immunological Aspects of Reproduction and Fertility Control,* Hearn, J.P., Ed., MTP Press, Lancaster, 1980, 3.

23. **Medawar, P.B.,** Some immunological and endocrinological problems raised by the evolution of viviparity in vertebrates, *Symp. Soc. Exp. Biol.,* 7, 320, 1953.

24. **Cooper, D.W.,** Immunological relationships between mother and conceptus in man, in *Immunological Aspects of Reproduction and Fertility Control,* Hearn, J.P., Ed., MTP Press, Lancaster, 1980, 33.

25. **Peters, A.J. and Coulam, C.B.,** Sperm antibodies, *Am. J. Reprod. Immunol.,* 27, 156, 1992.

26. **Presti, M.E. and Druce, H.M.,** Hypersensitivity reactions to human seminal plasma, *Ann. Allergy,* 63, 477, 1989.

27. **Alexander, N.J.,** Reproductive immunology: relevance to infertility practice, *Arch. Immunol. Ther. Exp.,* 38, 23, 1990.

28. **Schumacher, G.F.,** Immunology of spermatozoa and cervical mucus, *Hum. Reprod.,* 3, 289, 1988.

29. **Bannatyne, P., Russell, P., and Shearman, R.P.,** Autoimmune oophoritis: a clinicopathologic assessment of 12 cases, *Int. J. Gynecol. Pathol.,* 9, 191, 1990.

30. **Rhim, S.H., Millar, S.E., Robey, F., Luo, A.M., Lou, Y.H., Yule, T., Allen, P., Dean, J., and Tung, K.S.,** Autoimmune disease of the ovary induced by a ZP3 peptide from the mouse zona pellucida, *J. Clin. Invest.,* 89, 28, 1992.

31. **Paterson, M., Koothan, P.T., Morris, K.D., O'Byrne, K.T., Braude, P., Williams, A., and Aitken, R.J.,** Analysis of the contraceptive potential of antibodies against native and deglycosylated porcine ZP3 *in vivo* and *in vitro,* *Biol. Reprod.,* 46, 523, 1992.

32. **Billington, W.D.,** The normal fetomaternal immune relationship, *Baillieres Clin. Obstet. Gynaecol.,* 6, 417, 1992.

33. **Daunter, B.,** Immunology of pregnancy: towards a unifying hypothesis, *Eur. J. Obstet. Gynecol. Reprod. Biol.,* 43, 81, 1992.

34. **Jackson, G.M. and Scott, J.R.,** Alloimmune conditions and pregnancy, *Baillieres Clin. Obstet. Gynaecol.,* 6, 541, 1992.

35. **Sleasman, J.W. and Scott, G.B.,** Pediatric HIV infection. An update, *J. Fl. Med. Assoc.,* 78, 673, 1991.

36. **Deutsch, H.F.,** Chemistry and biology of α-fetoprotein, *Adv. Cancer Res.,* 56, 253, 1991.

37. **Sundaram, S.G., Goldstein, P.J., Manimekalai, S., and Wenk, R.E.,** α-Fetoprotein and screening markers of congenital disease, *Clin. Lab. Med.,* 12, 481, 1992.

38. **Greenberg, F., Faucett, A., Rose, E., Bancalari, L., Kardon, N.B., Mizejewski, G., Haddow, J.E., and Alpert, E.,** Congenital deficiency of α-fetoprotein, *Am. J. Obstet. Gynecol.,* 167, 509, 1992.

39. **Hanson, L.A., Adlerberth, I., Carlsson, B., Zaman, S., Hahn-Zoric, M., and Jalil, F.,** Antibody-mediated immunity in the neonate, *Padiatr. Padol.,* 25, 371, 1990.

40. **Goldman, A.S., Goldblum, R.M., and Hanson, L.A.,** Anti-inflammatory systems in human milk, *Adv. Exp. Med. Biol.,* 262, 69, 1990.

41. **Avanzini, M.A., Plebani, A., Monafo, V., Pasinetti, G., Teani, M., Colombo, A., Mellander, L., Carlsson, B., Hanson, L.A., and Ugazio, A.G.,** A comparison of secretory antibodies in breast-fed and formula-fed infants over the first six months of life, *Acta Paediatr.,* 81, 296, 1992.

42. **Gleicher, N. and el-Roeiy, A.,** The reproductive autoimmune failure syndrome, *Am. J. Obstet. Gynecol.,* 159, 223, 1988.

43. **Tung, K.S. and Lu, C.Y.,** Immunologic basis of reproductive failure, *Monogr. Pathol.,* 33, 308, 1991.

44. **Purvis, K. and Christiansen, E.,** Male infertility: current concepts, *Ann. Med.,* 24, 259, 1992.

45. **Harris, E.N.,** Maternal autoantibodies and pregnancy — I: the antiphospholipid antibody syndrome, *Baillieres Clin. Rheumatol.,* 4, 53, 1990.

46. **Moncharmont, P., Juron-Dupraz, F., Doillon, M., Vignal, M., and Debeaux, P.,** A case of hemolytic disease of the newborn infant due to anti-K (Cellano), *Acta Haematol.,* 85, 45, 1991.

47. **Steyn, D.W., Pattinson, R.C., and Odendaal, H.J.,** Amniocentesis — still important in the management of severe rhesus incompatibility, *S. Afr. Med. J.,* 82, 321, 1992.

48. **Wan, M.R.,** Serum ABO immune antibodies in 1944 pregnant women, *Chung-Hua Fu Chan K'o Tsa Chih Chin. J. Obstet. Gynecol.,* 26, 12, 1991 (in Chinese).

49. **Rex-Kiss, B.,** Relationship between blood groups and sex ratio of the newborn, *Acta Biol. Hung.,* 42, 357, 1991.

50. **Trowsdale, J. and Campbell, R.D.,** Complexity in the major histocompatibility complex, *Eur. J. Immunogenet.,* 19, 45, 1992.

51. **Srivastava, R., Ram, B.P., and Tyle, P.,** Immunogenetics of the major histocompatibility complex: an introduction, in *Immunogenetics of the Major Histocompatibility Complex,* Srivastava, R., Ram, B.P., and Tyle, P., Eds., VCH Publishers, New York, 1991, 1.

52. **Krzanowski, J.J.,** Human major histocompatibility complex. Genes and diseases, *J. Fl. Med. Assoc.,* 79, 97, 1992.

53. **Campbell, R.D.,** The molecular genetics of components of the complement system, *Baillieres Clin. Rheumatol.,* 2, 547, 1988.

54. **Simpson, E.,** Minor histocompatibility antigens, *Immunol. Lett.,* 29, 9, 1991.

55. **Bikoff, E.K., Jaffe, L., Ribaudo, R.K., Otten, G.R., Germain, R.N., and Robertson, E.J.,** MHC class I surface expression in embryo-derived cell lines inducible with peptide or interferon, *Nature (London),* 354, 235, 1991.

56. **Verrell, P.A. and McCabe, N.R.,** Major histocompatibility antigens and spontaneous abortion: an evolutionary perspective, *Med. Hypotheses,* 32, 235, 1990.

57. **Redman, C.W.G.,** Immunological aspects of eclampsia and pre-eclampsia, in *Immunological Aspects of Reproduction and Fertility Control,* Hearn, J.P., Ed., MTP Press, Lancaster, 1980, 83.

58. **Redman, C.W.,** Immunological aspects of pre-eclampsia, *Baillieres Clin. Obstet. Gynaecol.,* 6, 601, 1992.

59. **Christopherson, W.A., Kanbour, A., and Szulman, A.E.,** Choriocarcinoma in a term placenta with maternal metastases, *Gynecol. Oncol.,* 46, 239, 1992.

60. **Langman, J.,** *Medical Embryology. Human Development — Normal and Abnormal,* 3rd ed., Williams & Wilkins, Baltimore, 1975.

10 Contraception and Assisted Conception

CHAPTER CONTENTS

I.   INTRODUCTION

Any means to reduce the conception rate of fertile couples is considered contraception. Since the urge to copulate is an integral part of sexual behavior to achieve conception, behavioral contraceptive methods are modalities to hinder reproduction by cognitive power in normal individuals. Periodic abstinence from sex is an example of a uniquely human behavioral rhythm opposite to the natural ovulatory cycle. In seasonal breeders, in contrast, gonadal regression occurs during the quiescent period of their reproductive cycles with conspicuous hormonal changes. As continuous breeders, humans can regulate population growth only by creating reliable methods of fertility control.

Based on a recent report by the World Health Organization (WHO), an article on sex, contraception, abortion, and sexually transmitted diseases appeared on the front page of the *San Francisco Chronicle*.[1] This issue is a public concern. According to the number of live births around the world, there are 910,000 conceptions daily. If a 1:100 fecundity ratio is adopted, sexual intercourse occurs approximately 100 million times per day worldwide. Although this rate includes sexual acts protected by contraceptive methods, about half the conceptions were unplanned.

According to WHO, about 70% of the sexual acts in developed countries such as the U.S. are protected. In the Third World countries, there was an increase from 31 to 381 million people using birth control methods within the past three decades. With the availability of effective contraceptive methods, the fertility rate of women in developed countries dropped from 6.1 to 3.9 children per mother. With some exceptions in developed countries, the most popular contraceptive method is female sterilization (26%), followed by male sterilization (19%), and then oral contraceptives (15%). In Japan, over 70% of the people prefer using condoms.

Abortion is also one form of birth control. Annually, there are 36 to 53 million abortions worldwide. Only 40% of the total number of abortions occur in the 25 countries where abortion laws are most permissive. In about 25% of the total population living in countries where abortion is prohibited, the estimated number of illegal abortions is around 15 to 22 million. About 500 women die of failed abortions per day; most of these operations are performed in illegal settings without proper monitoring.

With methods such as *in vitro* fertilization (IVF) being developed, it is now possible for women to conceive without sexual intercourse. By their own choices, single women can acquire donor sperms and get pregnant by artificial insemination.

For a certain type of infertile couples (e.g., low sperm counts and tubal occlusion), ova from the women can be fertilized *in vitro* and reimplanted before the time of implantation. Alternatively, the preimplantation zygote, even after a long period of storage by freezing, can be transferred to a surrogate mother who can carry the conceptus to term. Evidently, our life span is lengthened because of improved medical care. We need better family planning with more efficient and reliable control of human reproduction. As the primary purpose of medical technology, this clinical practice of fertility control enhances the quality of life for us and for future generations.

II. CONTRACEPTIVE METHODS

One can view the period of reproductive quiescence in seasonal animals as a natural contraceptive effort to ensure labor at an appropriate time. The control is, however, neuroendocrine and endogenous with accompanying physical changes (e.g., gonadal regression). In humans, reproduction is apparently not seasonal at a physiological level; there is no conclusive evidence showing physiological or biochemical changes at different times of the year (see Chapter 11). Without a natural mechanism such as in seasonal animals, humans have to find their own ways to regulate reproduction.

Surprisingly, contraception was made illegal in the U.S. in 1873. In that year, Congress passed the Comstock Law prohibiting the sale of contraceptive devices and the delivery of information on contraception through the mail. In 1966, nearly a century later, this law was completely banned in all states. In some places outside the U.S. such as Ireland, the sale of contraceptives was legalized only recently. The idea that women are entitled to the right of birth control was advocated by Margaret Sanger in the U.S. and Marie Stopes in England. They began their efforts as early as 1915 by helping those women with problematic pregnancies or those whose financial situation did not allow for having more children.

Presently, there are many effective contraceptive methods available, though none are perfect. The concept in some methods is quite analogous to those in ancient times. For example, some believed that sponges placed in the vagina could absorb sperms, while the skin of a halved lemon had been used as a cervical cap to create a barrier for sperms. Many women tried to wash their vaginas after sexual intercourse (douche) or even thought they could prevent conception by jumping up and down. Some men thought that holding their breath during ejaculation might be contraceptive. Penile withdrawal before ejaculation *(coitus interruptus)* and abstinence from sex were the two most popular methods and are still being used today.

There are four basic types of contraceptive methods: behavioral, hormonal, surgical, and the use of devices. Table 10.1 is a brief comparison of different contraceptive methods. The most popular method for temporary contraception is oral contraceptives. Over 60 million women worldwide are users; 38 million of them are in developing countries.[2]

TABLE 10.1.
Failure and Mortality Rates of Various Birth Control Methods

Contraceptive method	Pregnancies/100 women/year (%)	Mortality rate (deaths/10^5 women/year)
None	90	8.3 (birth related)
Rhythm method	10–30	2 (birth related)
Withdrawal method	>16	
Hormonal contraceptives		<1
Oral	1–8	(5.2 for smokers)
Injectables	<1	
Barrier method		1.2 (birth related)
Diaphragm/cap	4–25	
Condom	14–16	
Spermicides alone	26	
Intrauterine devices (IUD)	1–5	1.2
RU486 (with prostaglandin analogs)	1–5	<1
Surgical sterilization or abortion	<1	Dependent on surgical complications

Note: Data from Carr, B.R. and Griffin, J.E., *William's Textbook of Endocrinology,* 7th ed., Wilson, J.E. and Foster, D.W., Eds., W.B. Saunders, Philadelphia, 1985, and Fathalla, M.F., Rosenfield, A., and Indriso, C., Eds., *The F.I.G.O. Manual of Human Reproduction,* Parthenon Publishing Group, Park Ridge, NJ, 1990.

A. BEHAVIORAL CONTRACEPTION

1. Abstinence

Although this contraceptive method is 100% effective, there is a high failure rate because it depends entirely on mutual consent or rejection by one partner. Since the consent to engage in an intimate contact is normally interpreted as an expression of love and affection, the lack of mutual understanding may create psychological tension between partners.

Since pregnancy is almost impossible without penile intromission, sexual intercourse is the only form of act not permitted in this contraceptive method. All other kinds of sexual activities such as kissing and petting need not be prohibited. The problem is that these other activities often lead to one's inability to refrain from penile intromission.

2. Rhythm Method

This is different from the endogenous reproductive cycle. It usually depends on deliberate behavioral synchronization with the menstrual cycle that is monitored by vaginal mucus and basal body temperature. The method is very unreliable and prone to human error. It has been estimated that at least four unexpected pregnancies may result, even when this method is used correctly, throughout one's lifetime. Unexpected pregnancies have been suggested to have a higher chance of congenital abnormalities because the zygotes are usually from aged oocytes.

This method also suffers from the same drawbacks of abstinence from sex. The partners have to exercise periodic abstinence from sex. Mutual consent plays an important role, and the success depends on individual personality. Some couples who are rigid in their lifestyle and prefer scheduled activities may find this method appropriate. Planning sexual activities ahead of time may sometimes be part of the fun. On the other hand, couples who like sexual spontaneity may find the practice aggravating. Anyhow, the reliability is not high.

Figure 10.1 shows a chart of body temperature change during the menstrual cycle. Some women can time ovulation accurately by detecting the midcycle rise in temperature and by examining vaginal mucus. As plasma estrogen concentration increases, cervical secretions become more abundant and clear before ovulation. After ovulation, the progesterone level increases, leading to changes in the cervical mucus. The secretion becomes thick and viscous. Experienced women can usually detect the change in a normal cycle. The failure rate varies greatly from 10 to 30%. The reliability may be enhanced if this method is used concurrently with other methods.

3.   Coitus Interruptus

This is commonly called the withdrawal method. This method is highly unreliable with 16% failure rate per trial. The major problem is that some sperms may be present in the fluid before ejaculation, and partial ejaculation may also occur unconsciously.

B.   HORMONAL CONTRACEPTION

These methods are mostly based on the understanding of the ovarian cycle. Maintaining the level of sex steroids at a constant but low level can inhibit ovulation. Alternatively, there are drugs available for inhibiting implantation and even inducing abortion. In comparison to surgical sterilization, hormonal contraception is safer. Although there are side effects, there is no risk of surgical complications.

1.   Oral Contraceptives

This is the most common method with a failure rate of less than 2%. The failure rate includes human errors such as missing pills. Side effects include obesity and skin changes (e.g., acne). Since not all women are suitable (about 50% may have observable reaction), this is on prescription in the U.S. The data on its connection with cervical and breast cancer are inconsistent, except in women who smoke or are over 35. It may be correlated with a higher incidence of cardiovascular diseases. The overall risk, however, is less than pregnancy or car accidents.

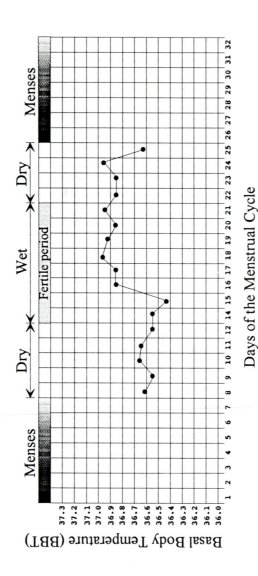

FIGURE 10.1. Changes in basal body temperature during menstrual cycle.

2.   Injectable or Implants

Long-acting injectable hormonal contraceptives were first available in the 1960s. The obvious advantages of using injectables are that they are very effective, are independent of coitus, and have a low frequency of administration. Currently, it is estimated that several million women are using these types of methods worldwide. The contraceptives include depo-medroxyprogesterone acetate (DMPA), norethindrone enanthate (NET-EN), and other progestin-only injectables. Very often, it requires only once-a-month injection, but frequent routine medical checkups are recommended.[3] The major disadvantage of the progestin-only contraceptive is menstrual disruption, which leads to unpredicted bleeding, spotting, and headaches.

For long-term protection against pregnancy, a subdermal implant containing the contraceptive can be used instead of an injection. The first implant system developed was Norplant,[4] a set of six rubber or silastic capsules filled with levonorgestrel and implanted under the skin in the inside part of the upper arm. It is normally effective for 5 years without replacement. The implant releases sufficient levels of medication to protect against pregnancy. The average failure rate is 0.05% per year, compared to a failure rate of 0.2 to 0.5% when standard oral contraceptives are taken. Again, the common side effect of the implant method is menstrual disruption.

The primary mechanism of action in Norplant is suppression of ovulation. No change in carbohydrate metabolism, blood coagulation, or liver function has been reported. Lipid levels have decreased 5 to 15%. After removal of Norplant, fertility returns rapidly, and there have been no adverse effects on infants. A recent clinical study has provided further evidence showing that Norplant does not depend on the termination of early pregnancy.[4] In the same study, hCG production was not detected in all Norplant users.

Norplant is currently approved in 12 countries including the U.S.; clinical trials are being conducted in 37 countries. In addition to this system, permanent or biodegradable subdermal implants, injections, intrauterine and intracervical devices, and vaginal rings are all employed as delivery systems for contraceptive progestins.[5]

C.   BARRIER METHODS

The basic concept of these methods is to create a barrier between sperms and eggs so that the chance of fertilization is reduced. It has only moderate reliability. Failure correlates mostly with accidental loss of the barrier, misuse, or damaged devices. The use of these devices in combination with spermicide improves the reliability.

1.   Vaginal Diaphragm

It is a hollow hemispheric device with a circular coil spring (round or flat) in the outer rim (see Figure 10.2). The diaphragm is inserted into the vagina and placed in front of the cervix. The interior end of the diaphragm is situated at the

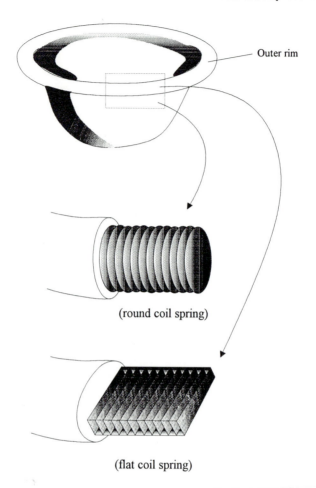

Outer rim

(round coil spring)

(flat coil spring)

FIGURE 10.2.   Vaginal diaphragm.

posterior vaginal fornix, while its outer end is just behind the symphysis pubis. Common diaphragms are usually 65 to 80 mm in diameter. If a diaphragm is properly inserted, it should cover the cervix and most of the anterior vaginal wall. The failure rate varies from 4 to 25%.

2.   Cervical Cap

As its name implies, it is a cap for the cervix (see Figure 10.3). Its size varies from 22 to 31 mm in diameter, and a specific one is required after measuring the diameter of the cervix by physicians. If the size is suitable, it should create a partial vacuum when the cervix is capped properly. In comparison to the diaphragm, it is more effective, but difficult to install and remove. Again, it must be carefully checked as to whether it is secure or not and is best used with spermicidal jelly or cream. In addition, it is recommended that it not be left in the vagina for more than 3 days, otherwise there may be unpleasant odor or even bacterial infection.

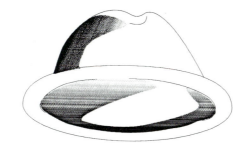

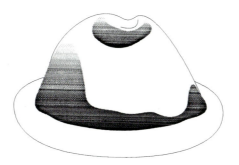

FIGURE 10.3. Cervical cap.

3. Condom

The use of condoms with spermicides may fail to protect against pregnancy at a rate of 14 to 16%. Without spermicides, the failure rate can be up to 26%.[6] Recently, the use of condoms has been advocated for protecting against the HIV infection, though there is no conclusive evidence showing its effectiveness for this purpose. Nevertheless, if everyone is using condoms, as suggested by Gordon,[7] it may contribute to the effort to control the AIDS epidemic.

D. INTRAUTERINE DEVICES (IUDs)

These kinds of devices had been used for centuries, but they became widely accepted and popular only by the early 1960s. The mechanism of action is not well understood. There are two major types of IUDs: medicated and nonmedicated. The most popular nonmedicated IUD is the Lippes loop, which is inexpensive and easy to install (see Figure 10.4). For medicated types of IUDs, copper or hormonal contraceptives are incorporated.

The antifertility effect of the IUD itself may depend on uterine changes leading to impaired sperm and ovum transport as well as the actual fertilization process itself. It may also interfere with the implantation process. Possible biochemical and histological changes in the endometrium may be induced by the IUD. On the

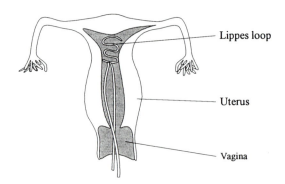

Lippes loop

Uterus

Vagina

FIGURE 10.4. Intrauterine device.

other hand, some believe that these changes are not minor factors only. Sponta-neous expulsion of the device is the major cause of failure. There are cases in which pregnancy occurs even with the IUD in place. The overall failure rate is 1 to 5%.

Copper has been incorporated in some IUDs such as Copper T, Copper 7, and the later TCu-200. They are made of polyethylene T wound with a pure copper wire. Copper is toxic to mouse preembryos *in vitro*, even in the form of a wire.[8] Therefore, the incorporation of copper to an IUD is thought to enhance its contraceptive effect.

Although some clinicians may claim that IUDs are perfectly safe and reliable, it has a correlation with the incidence of pelvic inflammatory disease (PID) in the U.S. (about 2%). Most women in China are using IUDs, but the incidence of PID is low. Another possible complication is uterine perforation, but the number of reported cases is small.

An interesting recent report on ectopic pregnancy in users of copper IUDs has shown that users of progestin-only IUDs had a markedly higher rate of ectopic pregnancy (17.1%) than users of copper IUDs (3.9%). The estimated rate of ectopic pregnancy for users of IUDs having 200 mm^2 of copper was 40% that of noncontraceptive users in the U.S. from 1970 to 1978. For users of devices with more than 350 mm^2 of copper, ectopic pregnancy rates were only 10% those of the noncontraceptive users. Most IUDs protect against ectopic pregnancy, except those with high concentrations of progestin incorporated.[9] It should be noted that the comparison of ectopic pregnancy rates between IUD users and nonusers may not be fair because the total number of pregnancies per year is much reduced in IUD users.

E.   SURGICAL CONTRACEPTION

1.   Tubal Occlusion

Surgically, the oviduct can be occluded in many ways. There are different techniques with different names: Madlener, Uchida, Pomeroy, Irving, and fimbriectomy (removal of the oviducal funnel). The main purpose is to block the passage of sperms or ova. There are also other ways to block the oviduct such as electrocoagulation, thermocoagulation, mechanical devices (e.g., rings and clips), and chemicals (e.g., sclerosing agents, tissue adhesives). All these require surgical procedures to expose the oviduct.

In the Madlener technique, the oviduct is looped and crushed with a crushing clamp. The loop is cut in the case of Pomeroy, and the cut ends are tied by nonabsorbable suture. In the Uchida procedure, the oviduct is cut without making a loop, and the two ends are tied individually. In the more complicated technique of Irving, the distal side of the cut oviduct is tied and secured to the uterine wall. This method may reduce the chance of reanastomosis.

2. Vasectomy

This is a simple 15-min surgical procedure that can be performed under local anesthesia without hospitalization. The purpose is to interrupt the continuity of the vas deferens by removing a short segment of the duct. The vas deferens can easily be felt on each lateral side of the scrotum above the testicle. Bilateral incisions are usually made, and the duct on each side can be picked up by a small clamp (see Figure 10.5).

To ensure discontinuity of the duct, a segment is removed and the cut ends are tied or electrocoagulated. Reanastomosis does occur, but it is less than 1%. Failure may also be due to semen accumulation at the proximal side of the cut point, resulting in rupture and release of sperms. Granuloma is formed at the cut end, and a canal can be created through this structure. Another possibility is the residual sperms left in the distal side of the vas deferens during the first week after the operation can be ejaculated during intercourse. Therefore, the patient is recommended to use another contraceptive method just after the operation.

Complications after vasectomy are rare and usually related to poor surgical techniques or inadequate sterile conditions. Excluding these possibilities, about 1% of the vasectomized men develop antispermic antibodies. So far, vasectomy is considered to have no major effects on the physical or mental health of men.[10] This procedure is routinely performed, mainly in the doctor's office, for over 1000 patients a day worldwide.[11]

Although vasectomy is considered an irreversible sterilization, it is possible to perform an anastomosis procedure. In about 50% of the cases, the fertility can often be restored. Recently, requests for vasectomy reversals are increasing in numbers.[12] Alternatively, this complicated reversal procedure can be avoided if semen samples are frozen and stored prior to the vasectomy.

3. Hysterectomy and Castration

Surgical removal of the uterus is the second most commonly performed major operation (next to cesarean section) in the U.S. The number is up to 650,000 times annually,[13] including therapeutic hysterectomy required for removing neoplasms. For example, total abdominal hysterectomy and bilateral salpingo-oophorectomy

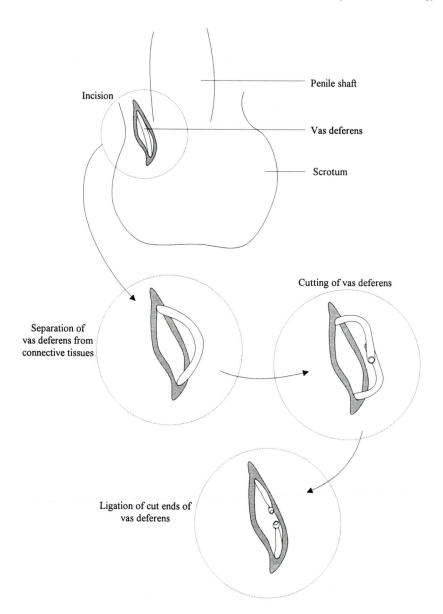

FIGURE 10.5. Vasectomy.

(removal of ovaries) are performed for those with ovarian neoplasms.[14] In a recent Italian article,[15] the trauma linked to hysterosalpingo-oophorectomy was suggested to induce sexuality changes such as a decrease in satisfaction, coital frequency, and desire.

F.   FUTURE METHODS

1.   Melatonin Progestins

The influence of melatonin/progestin combinations on the pituitary-ovarian axis and ovulation has recently been studied in 32 women. In most cases, melatonin combined with norethisterone (NET) suppresses the pituitary-ovarian axis. During the study, LH, FSH, estradiol, and progesterone blood levels were determined at regular intervals. After a 4-month period, daily administration of 300 mg melatonin for 30 days caused significantly decreased mean LH levels. LH and E_2 inhibition reached significant levels in the fourth medication month. Also, treatments of 75 mg melatonin combined with 0.3 mg NET caused a significant decrease in LH, E_2, and P4 levels in the first and fourth medication months. This indicates that melatonin-NET combinations can be an effective oral contraceptive.[16]

2.   Male Hormonal Contraceptives

During the last two decades, possible methods for male fertility control based on hormonal control related to sperm maturation and transport have been studied.[17] The use of condoms has a high failure rate, while vasectomy lacks reversibility despite its high reliability. Hormonal contraceptives for the male may provide all these. There are several approaches currently being tested. First, there is selective inhibition of FSH by antibodies or inhibin. Second, the pituitary-gonadal axis can be inhibited by steroids such as testosterone, progestin-testosterone combinations, and LHRH analogs with and without testosterone substitution. Third, spermatogenesis can be selectively inhibited by a phenolic compound called gossypol extracted from the cotton plant *(Gossypium barbadense)*.

Gossypol possibly reduces sperm motility by inhibiting the Ca^{2+}-ATPase pump on the plasma membrane as shown in studies on human ejaculated spermatozoal plasma membrane vesicles.[18] This potential male contraceptive also inhibits glucose uptake by promoting lipid peroxidation, which subsequently leads to membrane damage.[19] The inhibitory action of gossypol on sperm motility can be observed when the semen is incubated with the drug for more than 15 min. Since no inhibitory effect could be found immediately after mixing with the sperms, it is not suitable for use as a vaginal spermicide.[20]

The antifertility action of gossypol depends on its effect on spermatogenesis, possibly through its inhibition on mitochondrial activity.[21] Although gossypol is a promising oral contraceptive with a high efficacy to inhibit spermatogenesis, it has two adverse side effects: occasional symptomatic hypokalemia and 10% irreversibility of aspermia.[22] In addition, a recent study on rats has demonstrated a dose-response suppression of motivation or interest in seeking and maintaining contact with a receptive female.[23]

3.   GnRH Analogs

With the advances in understanding the mechanism of actions of GnRH in recent years, more than 2000 analogs, agonists, and antagonists have been synthesized. The GnRH gene is located on the short arm of chromosome 8. GnRH requires calcium and its two intracellular receptors, calmodulin and protein kinase C, to produce its physiological effects. Pulsatile GnRH exposure induces an up-regulation of the receptors for LH and FSH, but continuous GnRH or GnRH agonist administration induces a receptor loss and a pituitary desensitization. Although the mechanism of desensitization is unclear, this process is very useful for contraceptive purposes and can be used to induce a reversible medical castration. The agonist causes an initial rise in gonadotrophins and gonadal steroid secretion, but not the bioactive FSH. In contrast, the antagonist competes with GnRH for its receptors, suppressing LH and FSH secretion.[24]

4.   Anti-Zona Pellucida Antibodies

The zona pellucida contains tissue-specific antigens that are conservative among many species, including fish. Polyclonal antibodies against some of these antigens inhibit sperm attachment and cross-react with the zona pellucida of mouse and fish. These antigens are possibly part of the ZP3 fraction in which sperm receptors are found. Although immunization against zona antigens is a promising contraceptive method in humans, such vaccination might require unacceptable adjuvants or large amounts of antigen.[25] Since the ovary contains a large number of oocytes, the antibodies will have a tremendous direct effect on it. In addition, pregnancy could still occur in cases of naturally occurring anti-zona pellucida autoantibodies in humans. This raises the question of effectiveness of this potential contraceptive method.

Nevertheless, the conservative nature of these antigens among vertebrates allows the immunizing use of the zona pellucida from lower vertebrates for raising antibodies against human zona pellucida. If this modality is successful, contraception for about 5 years is available after several immunizing injections. This is a better alternative to subcutaneous implantation of steroids, if the undesirable side effects are well understood.

III.   ABORTION OR CONTRAGESTATION

Since gestation begins immediately after fertilization, any methods interfering with postfertilization events are contragestational or abortive. The method can act on the process of implantation, preimplantation, and/or postimplantation development to terminate the pregnancy. Most abortive methods available today work with a lower risk when done before fetal growth during the first trimester. Surgical abortion is the most traditional method to terminate pregnancy up to 3 months, though the mortality rate is high as compared to medical abortion. New drugs inducing miscarriage up to 7 to 8 weeks are being tested with mild side effects. An IUD can actually be classified in this category because it also interferes with implantation.

A.   MORNING-AFTER PILL

This method is a postcoital oral administration of high-dose ethinylestradiol. Since the steroid is administered after fertilization, the contraception depends on intercepting implantation. A recent electron microscopy report has shown some ultrastructural changes in epithelial cells of the secretory human endometrium.[26] The nucleolar channel system, typically present in the epithelial cell nucleus during the secretory phase of the human endometrium, disappears completely in treated volunteers. Prominent glycogen deposits have been found at the basal membrane and in the apex of the cell. With morphological changes observed by light microscopy, these deposits contribute to the induced failure of implantation.

The morning-after pill may also include those postcoital drugs interfering with implantation or inducing abortion, such as prostaglandins or Mifepristone (RU486) which will be discussed in Sections III.C and III.D. In view of the danger of surgical abortion, chemical abortion becomes a better choice.[27] It should be clarified that RU486 is a synthetic steroid competing with progesterone, whereas the nonmedical term "morning-after pill" usually refers to the oral intake of a double dose of a combined oral contraceptive pill containing 50 µg ethinylestradiol and 0.5 mg norgestrel 72 h after unprotected sexual intercourse.[28] The side effects associated with such an acute dose of oral contraceptives include nausea, vomiting, breast tenderness, and menorrhagia. This method is commonly recommended for rape victims. Unlike RU486, this method is ineffective once the zygote is implanted.

B.   DILATATION AND EVACUATION (D&E)

This is a truly surgical method involving dilatation of the cervix and physical extraction of the fetus. The procedure of surgical evacuation requires special skills that are not always available to all practitioners. The potential danger of this method is uncontrolled bleeding. An estimated 500 women die of abortions (including illegal operations) daily worldwide. In view of the high rates of maternal mortality and morbidity, D&E must be performed skillfully in well-equipped clinics.

C.   INTRAUTERINE ADMINISTRATION OF DRUGS TO INDUCE ABORTION

In recent years, several methods with safer and more effective options are available clinically. Intra-amniotic instillation of hypertonic solutions, particularly saline or urea, proved in many instances to be a good method for pregnancies beyond 15 weeks of gestation. Due to a long latency period after instillation, these agents are often supplemented with an intravenous oxytocin infusion. Extraovular hypertonic saline or ethacridine (Rivanol) have their advocates, particularly in the grey zone of pregnancy ranging from 13 to 15 weeks. In the last two decades, intrauterine prostaglandins were added to the methods in current use. Extra-amniotic prostaglandins (E_2, $F_{2\alpha}$, or 15-methyl $F_{2\alpha}$) were originally given in

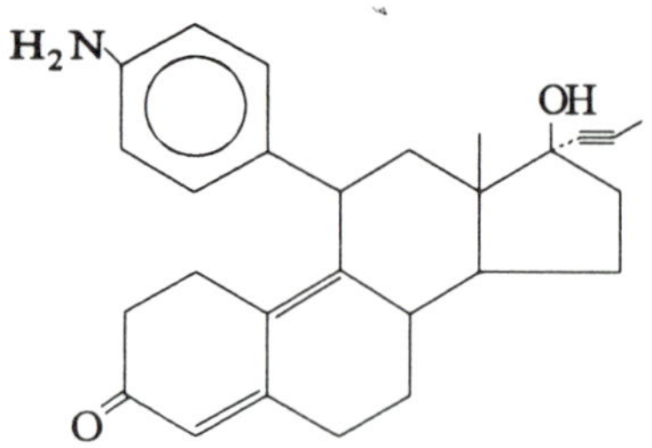

Mifepristone (RU486)

FIGURE 10.6.   Chemical structure of mifepristone (RU486), a progesterone antagonist.

repeated doses or as a continuous local drip, but later a single instillation was used, usually mixing the drug with a viscous solution or gel. Intra-amniotic prostaglandins, in much higher doses, particularly the 15-methyl analog, proved highly effective and relatively safe, especially when combined with laminaria tent insertion in the cervix.[29] In a recent study on the acceptability of the medical and surgical procedures for inducing abortion in Swedish patients, there is a high degree of acceptability for the prostaglandin treatment.[30]

D.   MIFEPRISTONE (RU486)

RU486, a synthetic derivative of norethisterone with an α-side chain and an 11β-ring substitution, is a progesterone antagonist which acts competitively with progesterone at the level of progesterone and glucocorticoid receptors (see Figure 10.6 for chemical structure). It is primarily used as a postcoital contraceptive to terminate pregnancy up to 7 weeks of amenorrhea.[31] The first successful clinical use was in 1982 at University Hospital of Geneva, Switzerland.[32] It is now being used in Europe as an effective alternative to surgical abortion[33] with much less maternal mortality. In addition, it has also been used in trials of menstrual regulation, abortion and induction of labor, during treatment of breast or ovarian cancer, and some forms of hypertension and meningioma.[33]

Progesterone forms a progesterone-receptor (PR) complex by removing a 90-kDa heat shock protein (hsp90) that caps the DNA-binding domain of the receptor. This PR complex binds to a specific DNA region called the "hormone regulatory element" and activates gene expression. RU486 binds to the receptor with a higher affinity and stabilizes its structure.[34] The RU486-receptor complex does not bind DNA and prevents progesterone from binding with the receptor to exert its biological effect. Increasing progesterone concentration can reverse the antagonist effect of RU486.[31]

Since RU486 binds to serum albumin, it has a half-life of about 24 h after oral administration. It also has weak progesterone agonist actions. It induces menstruation by acting directly on the endometrium and modulates LH and FSH secretion by antagonizing the feedback actions of progesterone.[34] The local mechanism of RU486 on the endometrium may involve enhanced synthesis of

$PGF_{2\alpha}$ and PGE_2, and it also increases the sensitivity of the myometrium to prostaglandins.[35,36] Therefore, when RU486 is used in combination with prostaglandin analogs, gemeprost or sulprostone, the success of terminating an early pregnancy is 95 to 99%.[31]

Although RU486 is mainly used as a postcoital contraceptive, it has potential value in other medical treatment. Besides its possible beneficial effect of reducing breast or ovarian cancer, it is a safe method to treat ectopic pregnancy. With all the clinical trials and actual uses, further improvement of RU486 will provide a safe alternative to surgical abortion or a hormonal contraceptive that needs to be taken once a month.[31] At present, the best available method is the combination of an antiprogesterone (RU486) and a low dose of prostaglandin, either in an injection (sulprostone) or in a vaginal pessary (gemeprost). With further improvement of the treatment schedules, these types of medical abortions will be the future safe methods of choice.[37] This method is especially important for rape victims who may react to morning-after pills or are late in reporting the incident.

IV. ASSISTED CONCEPTION

Infertility is considered a form of disease requiring medical attention. Recent advancement in the techniques of aided conception has made the cure of some forms of infertility possible. In the U.S., the number of visits to infertility clinics increased from 600,000 in 1968 to 2 million annually in the 1980s. The estimated annual cost spent on medical care related to infertility is over $1 billion. Infertility can be caused by the male or female. Causes of male infertility can be oligospermia (low sperm counts) and defective sperms, while causes of female infertility can be irregular menstrual cycle and oviduct occlusion. There are various methods available to overcome these reproductive deficiencies.

A. HORMONAL CONTROL OF THE REPRODUCTIVE CYCLE

1. Regulated Cycle

Amenorrhea is the most common type of female infertility. It is a condition involving menstrual acyclicity and anovulation. Hyperprolactinemia is a frequent cause of anovulatory sterility, although spontaneous pregnancy may occur occasionally. Dopaminergic treatment is highly effective for the treatment of both idiopathic and tumoral hyperprolactinaemia.[38] Bromocriptine, a dopamine agonist, is being used to restore ovulation in over 90% of the cases. This drug is normally used for treating hyperprolactinemia caused by suppressed release of dopamine from hypothalamic dopaminergic neurons. According to most reports, both spontaneous and drug-induced pregnancies are not associated with any increase in abortion, twins, or malformations.

Clomiphene citrate is an orally active nonsteroidal agent commonly used to induce ovulation in patients with normal endogenous levels of estrogens. It does not stimulate ovulation directly, but it causes an increase in peripheral serum FSH and LH as in a normal menstrual cycle. It is effective in patients with less than four to five cycles per year. The initial dose is one tablet of 50 mg daily for 5 days. If ovulation occurs, the dose is maintained until pregnancy. Otherwise, the dose is increased in small increments up to 250 mg daily. Over 50% of the appropriate patients respond to this ovulation induction.

If clomiphene treatment fails to induce ovulation within six ovulatory cycles, therapy using menotropins and pulsatile GnRH should be considered for women with hypogonadotrophic anovulation. Very often, pretreatment with GnRH analogs may reduce premature luteinization and result in higher pregnancy rates.[39]

2.   Superovulation

Patients undergoing human menopausal gonadotrophin (hMG) superovulation have been found to have a 54.5% multiple pregnancy rate after intrauterine artificial insemination.[40] This indicates that, as in mice, multiple oocytes are ovulated when induced by hormonal stimulation in humans. In addition, a higher norepinephrine (NE) content in the follicular fluid of these superovulated patients is found.[41] This has been suggested to be related to the ovulatory mechanism, postovulatory tubal motility, and progesterone secretion.

Superovulation is routinely used in experimental reproductive biology. The major advantages are the more accurate timing of ovulation and the increased number of oocytes ovulated. If an 8- to 12-week-old mouse is injected intraperitoneally with 5 I.U. pregnant mare serum gonadotrophin (PMSG) on day 1 followed by 5 I.U. hCG on day 3 (about 46 to 48 h), the expected ovulation time is day 4 (see Figure 10.7). If the number of ovulated eggs is too high, a high percentage of them with a lower quality can be found. There are conflicting reports showing the presence and absence of abnormalities in superovulated oocytes.

Mice used in embryo culture studies are commonly superovulated to maximize the yield of preimplantation zygotes; normally over 20 two- to four-cell zygotes can be obtained per mouse. Those zygotes that can successfully form blastocysts may be transferred to the uterus of pseudopregnant mice. If the embryo transfer procedure is performed correctly, over 50% of them develop to full term with a delay of about 24 h in the developmental schedule (see Figure 10.7). Alternatively, the blastocysts can be maintained *in vitro* beyond the attachment stage to assess their developmental potentials. In humans, clomiphene citrate is used instead of PMSG. In some patients who are mildly superovulated, the surviving newborns of multiple pregnancies are apparently normal. Therefore, the dosage calculation is important for an individual patient to avoid superovulation.

B.   ARTIFICIAL INSEMINATION FROM DONOR (AID)

For male infertility caused by defective sperms, AID is the only alternative. This procedure is also known as therapeutic donor insemination (TDI). Very often, the male has a low sperm count in his semen and IVF may be an alternative (discussed in Section IV.C). Therefore, it is important to perform semen analysis at least twice, about 2 months apart, before diagnosis. The normal range of sperm

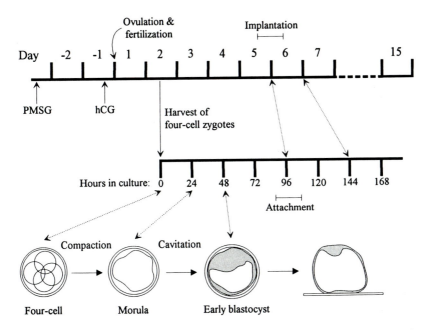

FIGURE 10.7. Superovulation and collection of preimplantation zygotes for embryo culture in mice. Note the differences between the *in vivo* and *in vitro* developmental schedules.

counts varies from 10^6 to 6×10^6 sperms per milliliter, and 2×10^6 is usually taken as the lower limit.[42] The following is a list of normal values for an ejaculate taken after 2 to 5 days of abstinence from sexual activity.

1. Volume: 2 to 6 ml
2. Viscosity: liquefaction within 60 min
3. Count: $\geq 2 \times 10^6$ sperms per milliliter
4. Motility: $\geq 50\%$ motile within 2 h after ejaculation
5. Morphology: $\geq 60\%$ normal

The fertilizing ability of the sperm can also be evaluated by the Hamster Test or the Sperm Penetration Assay (SPA).[43] The usefulness of the test is limited because of the variability among laboratories. In principle, it is a test of the ability of the sperm to penetrate a zona-free hamster oocyte. A correlation between infertility and low SPA scores can be found. However, cases of spontaneous pregnancies for men with their sperms showing no penetration and of sperms with high SPA scores showing low fertilization rates in IVF have been reported. Recent studies have demonstrated that sperm motility and morphology are better predictors correlative with the success rate, while SPA has no predictive value.[44,45]

When the sperms are abnormal with all tests failed, sperms from donors have to be used. There are guidelines for screening donors and their semen analysis. According to the American Fertility Society, all frozen semen samples should be quarantined for 180 days and the donor tested for diseases including HIV before the samples are released. The personal and family history of the donor are also important. For example, being a relative may pose future emotional problems.

Insemination can be performed intrauterinely or intracervically, though the results are not statistically different.[46] If cervical mucus is not sufficient at ovulation time, intrauterine AID may be a better choice. Normally, the success rate is about 10 to 20% per cycle or 85% within 6 months. If pregnancy does not occur after this time, other tests for possible female infertility have to be considered, such as hormonally stimulated ovulation. With close monitoring of hormone and ultrasound parameters following ovarian stimulation by clomiphene citrate and hMG, there is a higher success rate of AID.

There are other new or variant methods of AID such as intraperitoneal insemination[47] and the Fallopian tube sperm perfusion (FSP).[48] FSP is a method combining ovarian stimulation, ovulation induction, and intrauterine insemination with a 4-ml volume of sperm suspension.

C.   *In Vitro* Fertilization (IVF) and Embryo Transfer (ET)

Robert G. Edwards spent more than 20 years studying oocyte maturation and developing the IVF techniques before the birth of the first "test-tube baby" Louise Brown on July 25, 1978.[49] Her birth proved the successful combination of IVF and ET based on laparoscopy developed by his long-term collaborating clinician Patrick C. Steptoe. The mother had a history of infertility for 9 years with tubal occlusions and unsuccessful salpingostomies. Laparotomy was performed prior to the IVF procedure to remove the distorted tubal remnants. The abnormal ovarian adhesions were excised to position the ovaries for oocyte recovery. Laparoscopic recovery of oocytes was performed on November 10, 1977, followed by IVF and embryo culture. The fertilized egg was allowed to develop into an eight-cell morula and transferred to the uterus on the second day. The IVF-ET procedure is now a routine method for treating infertility worldwide. In the U.S., the overall live delivery rates in 1990 were 14% for IVF (based on 16,405 retrievals), 22% for gamete intrafallopian transfer (GIFT; based on 3750 retrievals), and 16% for zygote intrafallopian transfer and related practices (based on 1370 retrievals). The delivery rates for frozen ET cycles and IVF with donor egg cycles were 9 and 22%, respectively.[50]

To enhance the success rate of IVF, the fertilizing capacity of the husband's sperms must be evaluated properly. The tests used in AID are useful for this purpose. Recently, cryopreserved aged human oocytes have been used as in the Hamster Test.[51] In this study, oocytes arising from assisted conception cycles and showing no signs of fertilization 48 h postinsemination were used and frozen by a slow method using propanediol as the cryoprotectant with a survival rate of 60%. After removing the zona pellucida enzymatically with pronase, these oocytes were inseminated with spermatozoa from a fertile donor or from men previously exhibiting fertilization failure in an IVF treatment cycle. The rate of pronuclear formation in the patient group was significantly lower than in the donor group (45 vs. 89%, respectively; $p < 0.02$).

Induced ovulation or superovulation is normally performed to have a more accurate time for oocyte retrieval. GnRH analogs prevent premature luteinization in hMG-induced IVF and GIFT cycles, resulting in lower cancellation rates and improved oocyte quality.[39] In addition, the method for ovulation detection is also important and is now routinely done by ultrasound. Recently, a new biochemical method of testing urinary glycosaminoglycans (GAG) has been proposed to be an accurate method.[52] Interestingly, urinary GAG content showed a characteristic pattern of fluctuations during normal and hormonally induced cycles. There is a distinct peak at ovulation (106.7 ± 46.2 µg/ml urine). All types of GAGs except heparin have been detected with chondroitin sulfate C as the major component at ovulation. In hormonally induced menstrual cycles, a noticeable increase in GAG concentration (70%) was observed.

D. GAMETE INTRAFALLOPIAN TRANSFER (GIFT)

There are some cases of male infertility such as azoospermia or severe oligoaestenospermia with an indication for using donor semen. The female partner must first be investigated with no major cause found to account for the couple's infertility. Then, using the basic clomiphene citrate and hMG protocol, it is possible to achieve a pregnancy rate of 56% per GIFT cycle.[53] If these attempts are unsuccessful, the couples are offered GIFT. In comparison to conventional infertility treatment in 174 couples with different causes of infertility except tubal factors,[54] it was concluded that GIFT is more cost effective than conventional infertility treatment in patients with endometriosis and anovulation. In patients with idiopathic infertility, immunologic infertility, a cervical mucus factor, and multifactorial infertility, induction of ovulation followed by intrauterine artificial insemination or normal intercourse proved to be more cost effective. However, the results in another prospective study to compare the outcomes of GIFT and IVF-ET suggest that GIFT did not have significant advantage over IVF-ET for the treatment of nontubal infertility.[55]

V. ETHICS AND IMPACT OF FERTILITY CONTROL

Most young couples use contraceptives only to control the timing of conception without an intention to prevent pregnancy permanently. The idea is analogous to natural mechanisms of gonadal regression or delayed implantation in seasonal breeders responding to unfavorable conditions. The advent of reliable methods for reversible fertility control has made this idea feasible in humans. Steroidal contraception is an effective way to induce anovulation reversibly, while embryo cryopreservation allows one to control the timing of implantation.

As an animal species, humans have the fundamental right to perpetuate. All animal species must slaughter plants and/or other animals for food. One species may even alter the population growth of another to enhance its chance of survival. Without exception, the human species must also kill for food and destroy habitats of other species for shelter. We may also regulate the population growth of other species in ways beneficial to human existence and the welfare of the ecosystem.

Undoubtedly, we have successfully developed the necessary tools to achieve these purposes. Many methods of contraception and assisted conception have been applied to pets, wild animals, insects, and plants. This powerful capability has a strong impact on the ecosystem. The outcome can be destructive or constructive, depending on our insights and decisions. It is imperative to establish laws and ethical standards to govern these practices based on a thorough understanding of reproductive biology and ecology.

Intraspecific slaughtering is a common strategy in many species to control population growth. These "natural" methods of population control are considered unethical by most people. Although the human species has somewhat evolved to avoid this method, homicides and wars are still common. The only method available is to control the birth rate; the ethical issue is at what level.

Contraceptive and contragestative methods can be classified according to four different levels at which the birth rate is regulated (see Figure 10.8). The lowest level is gamete maturation (Level I). The most common type of control is to prevent ovulation. The ovary can be surgically removed by salpingo-oophorectomy for sterilization. Oral contraceptives are reversible alternatives by inhibiting ovulation. Equivalent methods in the male include orchectomy, vasectomy, and the use of male contraceptives to inhibit spermatogenesis.

Many methods operate at Level II. For example, the rhythm and withdrawal methods reduce the chance of fertilization by controlling sexual behavior. Vaginal douching and barrier methods serve a similar purpose using physical methods. Spermicides are used to reduce the number of viable sperms after ejaculation and thus lower the chance of fertilization. Fertility control at Level III inhibits preimplantation development and/or reduces the chance of implantation. IUDs containing copper are detrimental to preimplantation zygotes and inhibitory to their implantation. Both morning-after pills and RU486 prevent the preimplantation zygote from implanting. Surgical and chemical abortions work after implantation to inhibit early postimplantation development and organogenesis (Level IV). The risk to the mother is increased if the abortion is performed beyond the eighth week of pregnancy.

The ethical decision depends on how one defines the beginning of a human individual. It is almost universal that citizenship is not given to a fetus, even hours before birth. Legally, only a newborn has the right to be a person whose activities are still subject to parental discretion. Ignoring this legal definition, one may consider a fertilized oocyte or a normal fetus with a recognizable human face as an individual. If a fetus without unique human features is classified as a person with the right to decide, Level IV methods are unacceptable. Level III methods would be unethical only if preimplantation zygotes are considered human individuals. Using Levels I and II methods would be an act of slaughtering for those who view unfertilized oocytes or sperms as human individuals. Furthermore, if altering the chance of procreation is unlawful, no contraceptive method should be used.

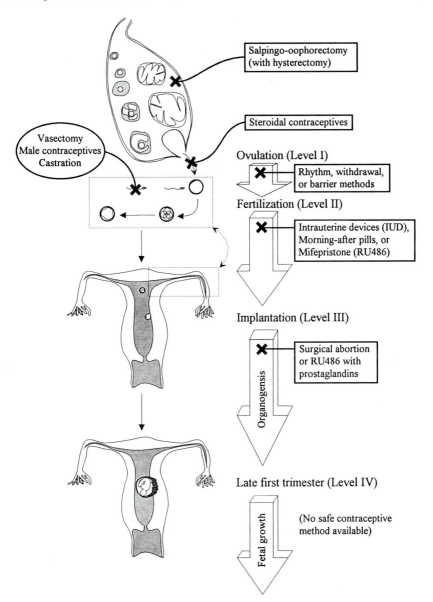

FIGURE 10.8. An overview of contraceptive methods operating at four different levels of the reproductive process.

REFERENCES

1. **Chronicle Wire Services,** The world has sex 100 million times daily, *San Francisco Chronicle,* June 25, 1992, A1.
2. **WHO Scientific Group on Oral Contraceptives and Neoplasia,** Oral contraceptives and neoplasia: report of a WHO scientific group, World Health Organization, Geneva, 1992.
3. **Bardin, C.W.,** Long-acting steroidal contraception: an update, *Int. J. Fertil.,* 34(Suppl.), 88, 1989.
4. **Segal, S.J., Alvarez-Sanchez, F., Brache, V., Faundes, A., Vilja, P., and Tuohimaa, P.,** Norplant implants: the mechanism of contraceptive action, *Fertil. Steril.,* 56, 273, 1991.
5. **Darney, P.D.,** Subdermal progestin implant contraception, *Cur. Opinion Obstet. Gynecol.,* 3, 470, 1991.
6. **Jones, E.F. and Forrest, J.D.,** Contraceptive failure in the United States: revised estimates from the 1982 National Survey of Family Growth, *Fam. Plan. Perspect.,* 21, 103, 1989.
7. **Gordon, R.,** A critical review of the physics and statistics of condoms and their role in individual versus societal survival of the AIDS epidemic, *J. Sex Marital Ther.,* 15, 5, 1989.
8. **Brinster, R.L. and Cross, P.C.,** Effect of copper on the preimplantation mouse embryo, *Nature (London),* 238, 398, 1973.
9. **Sivin, I.,** Dose- and age-dependent ectopic pregnancy risks with intrauterine contraception, *Obstet. Gynecol.,* 78, 291, 1991.
10. **Thonneau, P. and D'Isle, B.,** Does vasectomy have long-term effects on somatic and psychological health status?, *Int. J. Androl.,* 13, 419, 1990.
11. **Rajfer, J. and Bennett, C.J.,** Vasectomy, *Urol. Clin. North Am.,* 15, 631, 1988.
12. **Marmar, J.L.,** The status of vasectomy reversals, *Int. J. Fertil.,* 36, 352, 1991.
13. **Miyazawa, K.,** Technique for total abdominal hysterectomy: historical and clinical perspective, *Obstet. Gynecol. Surv.,* 47, 433, 1992.
14. **Jones, D.R., Vasilakis, A., Pillai, L., and Timberlake, G.A.,** Giant, benign, mucinous cystadenoma of the ovary: case study and literature review, *Am. Surg.,* 58, 400, 1992.
15. **Giannone, R., Bernorio, R., Poli, M., Panizzardi, G., and Piacezzi, C.,** Changes in sexual behavior of women receiving substitution therapy after surgical menopause and women in physiological menopause, *Minerva Ginecol.,* 44, 165, 1992.
16. **Voordouw, B.C., Euser, R., Verdonk, R.E., Alberda, B.T., de Jong, F.H., Drogendijk, A.C., Fauser, B.C., and Cohen, M.,** Melatonin and melatonin-progestin combinations alter pituitary-ovarian function in women and can inhibit ovulation, *J. Clin. Endocrinol. Metab.,* 74, 108, 1992.
17. **Frick, J. and Aulitzky, W.,** Male contraception, *Hum. Reprod.,* 3, 147, 1988.
18. **Kanwar, U., Batla, A., Sanyal, S., Minocha, R., Majumdar, S., and Ranga, A.,** Gossypol inhibition of Ca^{2+} uptake and Ca^{2+}-ATPase in human ejaculated spermatozoal plasma membrane vesicles, *Contraception,* 39, 431, 1989.
19. **Kanwar, U., Kaur, R., Chadha, S., and Sanyal, S.,** Gossypol-induced inhibition of glucose uptake in human ejaculated spermatozoa may be mediated by lipid peroxidation, *Contraception,* 42, 573, 1990.
20. **Hong, C.Y., Huang, J.J., and Wu, P.,** The inhibitory effect of gossypol on human sperm motility: relationship with time, temperature and concentration, *Hum. Toxicol.,* 8, 49, 1989.
21. **Kramer, R.Y., Garner, D.L., Ericsson, S.A., Wesen, D.A., Downing, T.W., and Redelman, D.,** The effect of cottonseed components on testicular development in pubescent rams, *Vet. Hum. Toxicol.,* 33, 11, 1991.
22. **Woolley, R.J.,** Contraception — a look forward, Part II: Mifepristone and gossypol, *J. Am. Board Fam. Practice,* 4, 103, 1991.
23. **Taylor, G.T., Griffin, M.G., and Bardgett, M.,** Search for a male contraceptive: the effect of gossypol on sexual motivation and epididymal sperm, *J. Medico,* 22, 29, 1991.
24. **Schaison, G.,** GnRH and its analogs — structure, mechanism of action and therapeutic applications, *J. Steroid Biochem.,* 33, 795, 1989.

25. **Caudle, M.R. and Shivers, C.A.,** Current status of anti-zona pellucida antibodies, *Am. J. Reprod. Immunol.,* 21, 57, 1989.
26. **van Santen, M.R., Haspels, A.A., Heijnen, H.F., and Rademakers, L.H.,** Interfering with implantation by postcoital estrogen administration. II. Endometrium epithelial cell ultrastructure, *Contraception,* 38, 711, 1988.
27. **Soller, P.C.,** Third World birth control — is it abortion? Drug combination gains support as alternative to surgical abortion, *Med. Law,* 10, 241, 1991.
28. **Henzl, M.R.,** Contraceptive hormones and their clinical use, in *Reproductive Endocrinology: Physiology, Pathophysiology and Clinical Management,* 3rd ed., Yen, S.S.C. and Jaffe, R.B., Eds., W.B. Saunders, Philadelphia, 1991, 807.
29. **Toppozada, M. and Ismail, A.A.,** Intrauterine administration of drugs for termination of pregnancy in the second trimester, *Baillieres Clin. Obstet. Gynaecol.,* 4, 327, 1990.
30. **Rosen, A.S.,** Acceptability of abortion methods, *Baillieres Clin. Obstet. Gynaecol.,* 4, 375, 1990.
31. **Avrech, O.M., Bukovsky, I., Golan, A., Caspi, E., and Weinraub, Z.,** Mifepristone (RU486) alone or in combination with a prostaglandin analogue for termination of early pregnancy: a review, *Fertil. Steril.,* 56, 385, 1991.
32. **Herrmann, W., Wyss, R., Riondel, A., Philibert, D., Teutsch, G., Sak, G.E., and Baulieu, E.E.,** Effect d'un steroid antiprogesterone chez la femme, interruption du cycle menstruel et de la prosesse au debut, *C.R. Acad. Sci. Paris,* 294, 933, 1982.
33. **Healy, D.L.,** Progesterone receptor antagonists and prostaglandins in human fertility regulation: a clinical review, *Reprod. Fertil. Dev.,* 2, 477, 1990.
34. **Baulieu, E.E.,** RU486 (an anti-steroid hormone) receptor structure and heat shock protein mol. wt 90,000 (hsp 90), *Hum. Reprod.,* 3, 541, 1988.
35. **Hamm, J.T. and Allegra, J.C.,** New hormonal approaches to the treatment of breast cancer, *Crit. Rev. Oncol. Hematol.,* 11, 29, 1991.
36. **Bygdeman, M., Gemzell, K., Gottlieb, C., and Swahn, M.L.,** Uterine contractility and interaction between prostaglandins and antiprogestins: clinical implications, *Annu. N.Y. Acad. Sci.,* 626, 561, 1991.
37. **Kovacs, L.,** Future direction of abortion technology, *Baillieres Clin. Obstet. Gynaecol.,* 4, 407, 1990.
38. **Crosignani, P.G. and Ferrari, C.,** Dopaminergic treatments for hyperprolactinaemia, *Baillieres Clin. Obstet. Gynaecol.,* 4, 441, 1990.
39. **Blacker, C.M.,** Ovulation stimulation and induction, *Endocrinol. Metabol. Clin. North Am.,* 21, 57, 1992.
40. **Hurst, B.S., Tjaden, B.L., Kimball, A., Schlaff, W.D., Damewood, M.D., and Rock, J.A.,** Superovulation with or without intrauterine insemination for the treatment of infertility, *J. Reprod. Med.,* 37, 237, 1992.
41. **Bodis, J., Bognar, Z., Hartmann, G., Torok, A., and Csaba, I.F.,** Measurement of noradrenaline, dopamine and serotonin contents in follicular fluid of human graafian follicles after superovulation treatment, *Gynecol. Obstet. Invest.,* 33, 165, 1992.
42. **Glass, R.H.,** Infertility, in *Reproductive Endocrinology: Physiology, Pathophysiology and Clinical Management,* 3rd ed., Yen, S.S.C. and Jaffe, R.B., Eds., W.B. Saunders, Philadelphia, 1991, 689.
43. **Rogers, B.J.,** The sperm penetration assay: its usefulness reevaluated, *Fertil. Steril.,* 41, 5, 1984.
44. **Marshburn, P.B., McIntire, D., Carr, B.R., and Byrd, W.,** Spermatozoal characteristics from fresh and frozen donor semen and their correlation with fertility outcome after intrauterine insemination, *Fertil. Steril.,* 58, 179, 1992.
45. **Claassens, O.E., Menkveld, R., Franken, D.R., Pretorius, E., Swart, Y., Lombard, C.J., and Kruger, T.F.,** The Acridine Orange test: determining the relationship between sperm morphology and fertilization *in vitro, Hum. Reprod.,* 7, 242, 1992.
46. **Johnson, L., Hemmings, R., and Tulandi, T.,** Comparison of intrauterine insemination, intracervical insemination, and timed intercourse in women treated with human menopausal gonadotrophin, *Int. J. Fertil.,* 37, 218, 1992.

47. **Karlstrom, P.O., Bakos, O., Bergh, T., and Lundkvist, O.,** Hormone and ultrasound parameters in ovarian stimulation cycles for direct intraperitoneal insemination, *Hum. Reprod.*, 7, 813, 1992.

48. **Kahn, J.A., von During, V., Sunde, A., and Molne, K.,** Fallopian tube sperm perfusion used in a donor insemination programme, *Hum. Reprod.*, 7, 806, 1992.

49. **Steptoe, P.C. and Edwards, R.G.,** Birth after the reimplantation of a human embryo, *Lancet*, 2, 366, 1978.

50. **SART,** *In vitro* fertilization-embryo transfer (IVF-ET) in the United States: 1990 results from The IVF-ET Registry, Medical Research International. Society for Assisted Reproductive Technology (SART), The American Fertility Society, *Fertil. Steril.*, 57, 15, 1992.

51. **Morroll, D.R., Critchlow, J.D., Matson, P.L., and Lieberman, B.A.,** The use of cryopreserved aged human oocytes in a test of the fertilizing capacity of human spermatozoa, *Hum. Reprod.*, 7, 671, 1992.

52. **Carranco, A., Reyes, R., Huacuja, L., Guzman, A., and Delgado, N.M.,** Human urinary glycosaminoglycans as accurate method for ovulation detection, *Int. J. Fertil.*, 37, 209, 1992.

53. **Macfoy, D., Hewitt, J., Barker, E., and Francis, W.A.,** Successful treatment of failed AID cases by use of gamete intra-fallopian transfer using donor semen (GIFT/D), *Eur. J. Obstet. Gynecol. Reprod. Biol.*, 43, 35, 1992.

54. **Wessels, P.H., Cronje, H.S., Oosthuizen, A.P., Trumpelmann, M.D., Grobler, S., and Hamlett, D.K.,** Cost-effectiveness of gamete intrafallopian transfer in comparison with induction of ovulation with gonadotrophins in the treatment of female infertility: a clinical trial, *Fertil. Steril.*, 57, 163, 1992.

55. **Toth, T.L., Oehninger, S., Toner, J.P., Brzyski, R.G., Acosta, A.A., and Muasher, S.J.,** Embryo transfer to the uterus or the fallopian tube after *in vitro* fertilization yields similar results, *Fertil. Steril.*, 57, 1110, 1992.

56. **Carr, B.R. and Griffin, J.E.,** Fertility control and its complications, in *William's Textbook of Endocrinology*, 7th ed., Wilson, J.E. and Foster, D.W., Eds., W.B. Saunders, Philadelphia, 1985, 452.

57. **Fathalla, M.F., Rosenfield, A., and Indriso, C., Eds.,** Reproductive health, global issues, in *The F.I.G.O. Manual of Human Reproduction*, Parthenon Publishing Group, Park Ridge, NJ, 1990.

11 The Environment and Reproduction

CHAPTER CONTENTS

I. INTRODUCTION

Environmental factors are classified into two types: abiotic and biotic. Temperature, humidity, atmospheric pressure, and electromagnetic waves including ultraviolet and visible lights are abiotic factors. The characteristics of these factors depend on the earth's physical attributes such as air and soil composition, its distance from the sun, and its speed of axial rotation. The reproductive process of all living species must have evolved to interact with these abiotic factors and reproduce successfully.

Biotic factors are attributed to the activities of living organisms. The characteristics of these factors depend on the interactions among individuals of the same or other species. For example, pheromones may alter sexual behavior to enhance sexual union (see Chapter 7), while animal excretions may enrich the soil and enhance plant growth. Genital infections in humans drastically alter the reproductive process (see Chapter 12). Living organisms may also change the characteristics of abiotic factors. Pollution is an example of the impact of human activities on abiotic factors.

The reproductive success of a species depends on how it can cope with both abiotic and biotic factors specific to the habitat. Despite the periodic changes in these factors, the species must be able to determine the optimal time of reproduction. The characteristics of some abiotic factors may fluctuate and become unfavorable to the species. Phototoxicity, for instance, refers to the harmful effect of light. Exposure to strong sunlight is extremely hazardous, and yet seasonal breeders evolved to adopt it as a regulatory factor for biorhythms.

An interactive mechanism between the reproductive process of a species and the environment is the key to its evolutionary success. This regulatory system is driven by the balance between optimal and hostile environmental conditions encountered by the species. While the environment plays a regulatory role in biorhythms, it can also disrupt reproductive physiology. These two contradictory roles of the environment are studied in two separate disciplines: chronobiology and reproductive toxicology.

II. LIGHT-DARK CYCLE AND BIORHYTHM

The light-dark cycle is a periodic fluctuation of light intensity because of the earth's axial rotation. There is a continually changing duration of exposure to

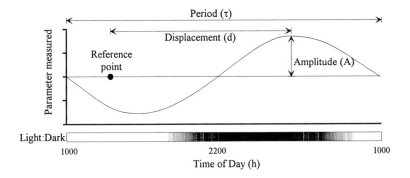

FIGURE 11.1. A hypothetical diurnal rhythm represented as a chronogram.

sunlight throughout the year. Accompanying this change, temperature also fluctuates generally with a higher temperature when the day length is longer. These changes pose a difficult problem for living organisms to cope with, especially for their reproductive activities.

A.   BIORHYTHMS

Biorhythms (or biological rhythms) are endogenous to living organisms; they evolved to cope with the varying length of the light-dark cycle each year. These endogenous biorhythms are synchronized and closely associated with the light-dark cycle or temperature fluctuations.

1.   What Is a Rhythm?

A rhythm is a regular recurrence of a characteristic that can be measured in a system. When the change in the expression of the characteristic is measured as a response variable against time, the regularity can be defined mathematically by three basic parameters: amplitude, period, and displacement. The amplitude is the height of the peak response, while the period is the interval between two adjacent peaks. Displacement is the interval between a reference timepoint and the first peak that follows (see Figure 11.1).

2.   Definitions of Biorhythms

Circadian rhythm is a free-running, endogenous rhythm, which persists in constant darkness with a period slightly longer than 24 h. Daily rhythm is a biorhythm with a period of exactly 24 h after synchronization with the light-dark cycle environment of 24-h periodicity.

Diurnal rhythm is a biorhythm of biological activity with observable differences during the day between sunrise and sunset or during the illuminated portion of an artificial light-dark cycle. Nocturnal rhythm is a biorhythm of biological activity with observable differences during the night between sunset and sunrise or during the dark portion of an artificial light-dark cycle.

3.   Time-Series Analysis of a Biorhythm

The period governs the frequency of the rhythm; shorter periods are found in rhythms of higher frequencies and vice versa. The displacement is the position of the peak relative to a reference timepoint. The hypothetical rhythm shown in Figure 11.1 is a chronogram showing the diurnal rhythm of a parameter measured and can be represented by the following equation.

$$Y(t) = \beta_0 + \beta_1 t + \beta_2 \cos\left(\frac{2\pi t}{\tau}\right) + \beta_3 \sin\left(\frac{2\pi t}{\tau}\right)$$

The first two terms are components of the long-term trend, which is the axis of the rhythm, and is often called the secular trend line. The third and fourth terms are components contributing to the cyclic effect varying according to the time (t) and period (τ). The amplitude (A) and displacement (d) are determined by the coefficients (β_0, β_1, β_2, and β_3). These are only basic terms for this simple mathematical model. Additional terms can be added to the equation to model an actual biorhythm that deviates from this basic pattern. These terms can also be combined to simplify the equation. If we take $\omega = 2\pi/\tau$ as the angular frequency, we have $Y(t) = M + A\cos(\omega t + \phi)$, where M is the rhythm-adjusted mean called mesor ϕ and is the acrophase. With this equation, a chronogram can be transformed into another rhythmic representation called cosinor if the time of day on the X axis is converted to degrees (see Figure 11.2).

Cosinor representation is very useful for comparing peaks of different rhythms. In Figure 11.2, peaks P_1 and P_2 with amplitudes A_1 and A_2 occur at different timepoints. If midnight is 0° at the origin of the chronogram, the positions of the peaks can be defined as ϕ_1 and ϕ_2 in the unit of degrees. The entire 24-h period is 360°. These parameters are conveniently shown in a cosinor diagram. Besides, the 95% confidence intervals of A and ϕ are transformed into an ellipse for each peak. The sizes and positions of the ellipses can easily be compared. Although the cosinor method is a very useful tool for quantifying these parameters, there are cases where the representation is inadequate. Information is lost during transformation from a chronogram to cosinor, such as the asymmetry of the peak or plateau.

Time-series analysis is a general statistical procedure to model the changes in a response variable with time.[1] Although the technique is widely used in seasonal trends in econometrics and physical sciences, it is seldom applied to annual rhythms. A recent paper by Boklage et al. studied the annual and subannual rhythms in human conception rates by time-series analyses. They demonstrated statistically significant annual and weekday but not monthly rhythms in human conception rates.[2] This statistical procedure is an appropriate test for data taken at multiple timepoints.

In the analysis of daily rhythms, time-series analysis may not be adequate if the experimental design is only limited to four sampling timepoints within one 24-h cycle. For example, in studying the daily rhythm of hormonal concentrations such as melatonin,[3] a minimum number of timepoints with small sample sizes are necessary to reduce the number of animals used. The animals at each timepoint

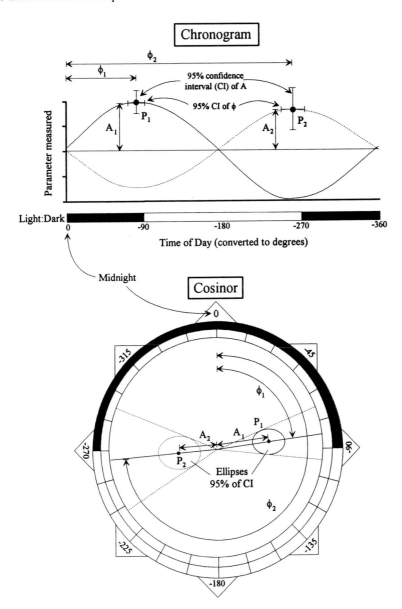

FIGURE 11.2. Transformation of a chronogram into cosinor.

are considered as a treatment group exposed to a unique time of day. Analysis of variance (ANOVA) is applied to test whether there is a difference among groups at different timepoints. The peak is then located by pairwise comparisons. Since the timepoints are selected by the experimenter before the experiment, the amplitude and displacement may vary from one report to another if the data are analyzed by ANOVA.

The ANOVA method does have its drawbacks. For example, the treatment groups at different timepoints are essentially separate experiments performed within 24 h. In contrast to time-series analysis, ANOVA provides no analysis on the trend from one timepoint to another with the assumption that the variances are homogeneous across different groups. Therefore, prior to ANOVA, it is recommended to run Bartlett's tests for homogeneity of variances.

In a recent report, a computer program called COSIFIT has been written in BASIC for biorhythm analysis.[4] It is an interactive nonlinear least-squares analysis for simultaneous multioscillator cosinor analysis of time-series data. The program computes optimal frequency, mesor, amplitude, and phase with standard errors of measurement and both parametric and nonparametric estimates of goodness-of-fit. In addition, ANOVA was also employed to show statistical differences between the parameter values of selected curves.

4. Types of Biorhythms

The period of biorhythms varies greatly from several seconds to many years. For example, in the smooth muscle of the digestive tract in human and other mammals, there are rhythms in mechanical and electrical activity with periods ranging from 2 s to 2.5 h.[5] Based on period length, there are four common classes of reproductive rhythms: annual, daily, infradian, and ultradian.

The infradian and ultradian rhythms are those with periods longer or shorter than 24 h, respectively. When the period length is much more than 24 h but less than 1 year, the rhythms are called subannual. There are weekly and monthly rhythms found in human activities. As discussed in Chapter 4, there are ultimate and proximate causes, but both are external. Some rhythms are apparently driven by external causes, while others may have endogenous cyclicity. The menstrual cycle is an excellent example of an endogenous monthly cycle altered by extrinsic factors.

If the period length is about 1 year, it is known as circannual rhythm. Although the circannual rhythm is endogenous and persists in a constant environment, it needs to be synchronized, in the real world, with the annual cycle in seasonal animals. Seasonality in humans is controversial. Details will be discussed in Section II.B.

It should be noted that there are true periodic and pseudoperiodic biorhythms. Periodic biorhythms are rhythms with regular cycles such as estrous cycles and many hormonal rhythms. They are said to be generated by "accurate pacemakers." Some biorhythms such as serum LH are not well defined in their periodicity and are called pseudoperiodic biorhythms. The irregular patterns may be produced by "sloppy pacemakers."[6] Although time-series analysis has been used to describe these biorhythms as random fluctuations with a mean frequency, a well-defined mathematical model is necessary to accomplish more reliable analyses.

B. CIRCADIAN RHYTHMS

As defined rigorously earlier, a circadian rhythm is an endogenous rhythm that persists in constant darkness. If it is synchronized with the light-dark cycle, it

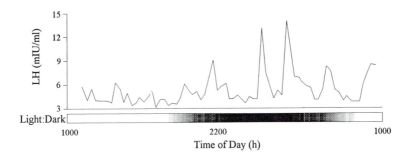

FIGURE 11.3. A diurnal rhythm of luteinizing hormone (LH). (Modified from Kapen, S., et al., *J. Clin. Endocrinol. Metab.*, 39, 293, 1974.)

becomes indistinguishable from a diurnal rhythm. If a diurnal rhythm does not persist in constant darkness, it is not circadian. Since most well-defined diurnal rhythms are normally circadian, the term circadian is often used, though less accurately, to describe diurnal rhythms observed under natural or artificial light-dark cycles.

Circadian rhythms can be demonstrated in most biochemical, physiological, and behavioral processes related to reproduction. The ultimate purpose of these rhythms is to provide a time-sensitive regulatory mechanism for temporal organization of reproductive events. It is a clock mechanism interacting with the light-dark cycle that provides cues or *Zeitgeber* (time sense) for resetting the clock. Such a mechanism is probably a prerequisite for all plants and animals, including humans, to survive on earth.[6]

The circadian system consists of multiple oscillators operating at different levels and frequencies. They are coupled with each other in response to the ambient light-dark cycle and other physical factors such as temperature. As discussed in Chapter 3, the universal pacemaker SCN located in the hypothalamus orchestrates the rhythmicity of the neuroendocrine system. In humans, hormonal biorhythms may play crucial roles in reproductive functions, despite the lack of a true physiological seasonality. Some features of the human circadian system may be clinically significant.[7] For example, the responsiveness to drug treatment fluctuates with the light-dark cycle. Also, the characteristics of physiological events and hormonal biorhythms have diagnostic values. A healthy person usually has a high degree of temporal sequence.

1. Gonadotrophins

LH and FSH are pseudoperiodic with no clear-cut diurnal property, though rhythms of serum gonadotrophin levels have been reported in some mammalian species. In humans, there is no marked diurnal fluctuation of LH and FSH in men, and the plasma LH rhythm is modulated by the menstrual cycle in women (see Figure 11.3). Diurnal changes in gonadotrophin release have weak rhythmicity, and the nocturnal rise may be sleep related.

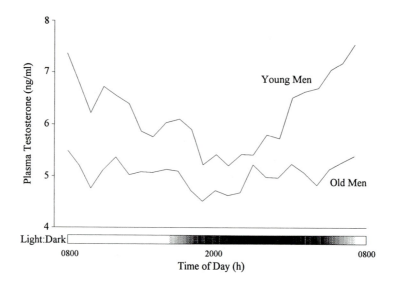

FIGURE 11.4.   Diurnal rhythms of plasma testosterone in young and old men. (Modified from Bremner, W.J., Vitiello, M.V., and Prinz, P.N., *J. Clin. Endocrinol. Metab.*, 56, 1278, 1983.)

2.   Prolactin

The serum prolactin level exhibits a distinct diurnal rhythm in many species including humans. The diurnal rhythm in humans is bimodal. A trough occurs at noon and an increased secretion in the afternoon. A major peak appears at the onset of sleep. Since it is difficult to conduct experiments in humans to determine whether the rhythm is truly circadian or not, it is possible that the prolactin rhythm is driven by the sleep-wake cycle. Studies on "jet-lag" subjects have shown that in a delayed sleep-wake cycle, sleep onset did not induce a sustained elevation of prolactin level. This still does not prove that the rhythm persists in constant darkness.

3.   Steroids

Diurnal rhythms of testosterone in young men and of estrogen and progesterone in young women have been observed. The testosterone rhythm in old men is lower than that in young men (see Figure 11.4). Aging probably induces a loss of diurnal rhythmicity. These rhythms become less conspicuous in aged individuals. In women, the diurnal fluctuations of estrogen and progesterone are more pronounced around the time of ovulation. There are reports showing variable fluctuations during other phases of the menstrual cycle. In addition, it has been suggested that the steroid rhythms may be associated with the cortisol rhythm which exhibits a well-defined diurnal rhythm.[5]

4.   Melatonin

The most well-defined circadian rhythmicity is the melatonin rhythm. Melatonin is a neural hormone secreted by the pineal gland into the general blood circulation. It is also synthesized in extrapineal tissues such as the retina.[3] Figure

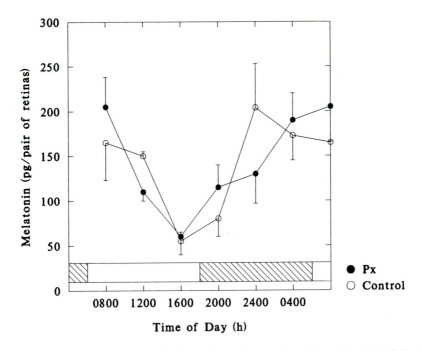

FIGURE 11.5. Diurnal rhythms of retinal melatonin in normal and pinealectomized (Px) rats. (From Yu, H.S., *Melatonin: Biosynthesis, Physiological Effects, and Clinical Applications,* Yu, H.S. and Reiter, R.J., Eds., CRC Press, Boca Raton, FL, 1993, 365. With permission.)

11.5 shows a well-defined diurnal rhythm of retinal melatonin which is endogenous to the eye. Although melatonin function is still uncertain in humans, its role in the reproductive physiology of seasonal breeders is well documented. The melatonin rhythm plays an important role in the time-keeping mechanism for the hypothalamo-hypophyseal-gonadal axis. This rhythm is a major component for internal signaling of photoperiodic changes, leading to the expression of the seasonality of the physiological state.[8]

III. ANNUAL CYCLE AND SEASONALITY

In contrast to circadian rhythm, circannual rhythm depends very much on external factors, though the oscillator is known to be endogenous. Two possible origins of this circannual oscillator in mammals have become apparent. First, it was established in response to the annual cycle during mammalian evolution. Second, it had to be present before the emergence of mammals. Since nonmammalian animals also possess the circannual oscillator, the second possibility is favored. On the other hand, the first possibility is also reasonable since the circannual rhythm is very sensitive to proximate and ultimate factors. Perhaps, both are possible. Early mammals 65 million years ago might have the inherited primitive circannual oscillator from their nonmammalian ancestor. In response to environmental changes, this primitive system might have evolved into a wide range of circannual rhythms in today's mammals.

There are now over 4000 mammalian species. They occupy different niches in different habitats with unique sets of proximate and ultimate factors. Seasonal fluctuations of these factors vary from one niche to another. The reproductive process must be finely tuned in harmony with the microenvironment. With an appropriate neuroendocrine pathway, they evolved to adapt these factors with unique patterns of seasonal reproductive physiology. The ultimate control is located in the brain (see Chapter 3). The circannual oscillator is an extremely complex system involving the pineal gland, SCN, and GnRH pulse generator.[9] These enable detection of changes in food availability, ambient temperature, photoperiod, pheromonal cues, nonspecific aversive emotional stimuli, etc.

A.   CIRCANNUAL AND SEASONAL RHYTHMS

Circannual rhythms are endogenous biorhythms with a period of about 1 year. Like circadian rhythms, circannual rhythms will be free running without environmental cues. The annual cycle of varying environmental cues on earth because of its orbiting around the sun provides a resetting mechanism for circannual rhythms. In mammals, there are different environmental cues used as signals for seasonal changes. The major ones are the changing light-dark cycle, temperature, and food availability. When a circannual rhythm is synchronized with the annual cycle, the reproduction of the animal is seasonal. This feature is known as seasonality.

Like the difference between the definitions of "diurnal" and "circadian," "seasonal" is not equivalent to "circannual." Seasonality refers to the seasonal responses of animals to the annual cycle. In most seasonal mammalian species, their annual reproductive cycles are truly driven by the endogenous circannual rhythm synchronized with the annual cycle. Natural selection favors such a synchrony because it provides a mechanism to time an appropriate set of environmental conditions for reproduction. It has been suggested that all different forms of mammalian seasonality were evolved from a single ancestral mechanism for annual time keeping.[10] Since it is mostly regulated by a photoperiodic mechanism, this annual time-keeping mechanism is linked with the circadian oscillator.

B.   THE INTEGRATIVE MODEL OF SEASONALITY

For seasonality in mammals, Bronson[9] has proposed an integrative model in which most environmental factors are considered. The interaction among the factors produces the resultant effect. The GnRH pulse generator, which regulates the secretion of LH and FSH, is the central core of the mechanism. Photoperiod, temperature, food availability, social primers, and nonspecific emotional stimuli are the major external factors affecting the pulse generator directly or indirectly via negative-feedback sensitivity. Social primers are those associated with pheromones and are stress related to the social status found in rodents and primates. Nonspecific emotional stimuli refer to those factors evoking physiological responses which alter the hormonal secretion.

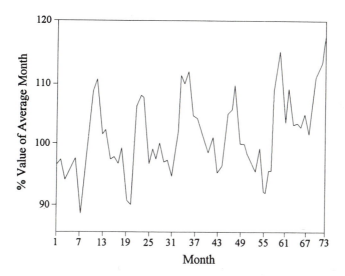

FIGURE 11.6.　Seasonality of birth in humans. (Modified from Boklage, C.E., Zincone, L.H., and Kirby, C.F., Jr., *Hum. Reprod.*, 7, 899, 1992.)

C.　SEASONALITY IN HUMAN REPRODUCTION

Based on epidemiological studies in several geographical areas, seasonality exists in human natural conception and birth rates. It is well documented that the rate of natural conception in women varies annually with a peak during winter in warm areas worldwide.[11] In the U.S., two significant decreases in births occur in early spring and early autumn (see Figure 11.6). The bimodal trend has been explained by the changes in sperm quality, ovulation, and conception rates throughout the year. During a hot summer, the sperm quality is poor, resulting in low conception rates. Therefore, the birth rate is low in spring and this is especially pronounced in southern areas such as San Antonio, TX.[12] On the other hand, if the temperature is too low during the winter, the ovulation and conception rate may be reduced.[13] Therefore, the birth rate is low in autumn, about 10 months after the month with low-temperature records.

In Third World countries where food availability varies seasonally, seasonality in natural conception is probably associated with food supply, seasonal employment, sociocultural factors, and health conditions. It may not be similar to the circannual rhythm of seasonal breeders where the highest birth rate occurs at the time of high food availability. The factors involved are less complicated than in developed countries. The practice of contraception, variable lifestyles, modern diets, stress-induced physiological changes, etc. are additional factors. The following is a list of major factors suggested, though there are others that may exist.

1.　Light-Dark Cycle

The ovulation rate is enhanced by a longer period of light exposure in animals and humans. It is well known in the poultry industry that extra light exposure at night during winter enhances egg production in hens.[14] In humans, stimulatory and inhibitory responses induced by light and dark periods, respectively, are observed. During the winter season, there is a higher incidence of anovulation, leading to endometrial hyperplasia. This is thought to be caused by exposure to short light periods.

In correlation with its effect on the ovulation rate, the light-dark cycle also influences the menstrual cycle. Continuous nocturnal light has been shown to reduce the cycle length in women having irregular menstrual cycles. Seasonality of the human menstrual cycle exists with longer cycle periods in winter,[15] while seasonality in endometrial receptivity may be associated with endogenous rhythms of steroids.

2. Temperature

The most pronounced effect of temperature is on semen quality. It seems to occur in many mammalian species including humans.[11] Sperm production may be reduced in areas with higher temperature and relative humidity. It is well known that spermatogenesis is inhibited when scrotal temperature is raised to body temperature.

Figure 11.7 shows an interesting correlation between temperature and sexual violence in two selected locations in Georgia and Illinois. Four types of violent crimes were investigated: assaults, rapes, robberies, and murders. The crime rate was expressed as the mean number of occurrences per month. In both locations, increased crime rates were mostly associated with higher temperatures during summer. Temperature alone may not have a direct effect on human aggressiveness. It is also difficult to correlate with reproductive activity, but behavioral seasonality does exist in humans.

3. Behavior

Behavior is an important factor in humans. For example, a lower frequency of sexual intercourse would seem likely to reduce the conception rate during summer. Yet this is not so because seasonality is also observed in the conception rate following artificial insemination (AID). The seasonal cycle of conception rate in AID patients is not altered by the number of donors or inseminations. This provides good evidence against the factor of frequency of sexual intercourse.

4. Endogenous Rhythms

The menstrual cycle is certainly an endogenous rhythm. Oocyte maturation, ovulation rate, and endometrial receptivity are part of the menstrual cycle. The survival of preimplantation zygotes is also affected by changes in maternal physiology related to the menstrual cycle. In humans, there is no evidence showing seasonality in oocyte maturation *in vivo* or *in vitro* and in early embryonic loss.

D. EVOLUTION OF SEASONALITY

To study the possible seasonality in human reproduction, we must understand the mechanisms involved in seasonal breeders in clear annual rhythmicity. Seasonality is closely linked to photoperiodism with a strong genetic basis. There

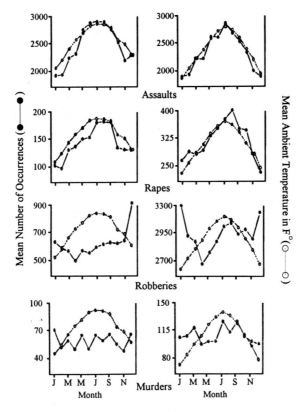

FIGURE 11.7.   Seasonality of sex and violence in humans. (Modified from Michael, R.P. and Zumpe, D., *Am. J. Psychiatry,* 140, 883, 1983.)

are significant species differences in photoperiodic responsiveness with a varying degree of seasonality. Exposure to different environmental conditions is the main driving factor for the evolution of seasonality. Domestication, for example, is known to reduce seasonality.

In humans, the seasonality is probably diminished by domestication. In developed countries, food supply and environmental conditions can almost be controlled with high constancy. Seasonal reproduction in such an environment becomes less important, and humans are apparently sexually active throughout the year. The seasonality observed is likely to be residual responses to environmental factors associated with some endogenous behavioral rhythms. It is unlikely that seasonality in human reproduction can be eliminated since we are still responsive to the light-dark cycle.

IV.   REPRODUCTIVE TOXICOLOGY

As part of the interaction between the reproductive process and the environment, some factors evoke toxic responses from the organism under specific conditions. If the toxic response is expressed as reproductive failure or even permanent sterility, the interaction is not only detrimental to the individuals, but also to the whole population. Apart from natural toxic factors such as radiation and toxins produced by other organisms, a major concern is the reproductive hazard of industrial chemicals. The effects are widespread, and very often the reproductive processes of both humans and animals are affected.

There are different levels at which toxic substances can act. For example, sexual behavior may be changed because of brain intoxication. The substances' toxicity on the neuroendocrine systems can alter the physiology. Toxic substances may directly damage the gonad, rendering the individual infertile. Oocytes and sperms can be exposed and mutations may occur. The fetus may be affected, leading to birth defects. Suppressed postnatal development may reduce also the reproductive capacity of the adult. Studies on lead toxicity were one of the early examples of reproductive toxicology in the late 19th century. It was found that women working in industries where lead was involved had a much higher rate of infertility, spontaneous abortions, neonatal deaths, and malformations. Despite these early reports on lead toxicity on workers, actions were not taken to protect workers at that time. Since then, reproductive toxicology has become a unique discipline bridging reproductive biology and toxicology with social and economic importance.

In recent years, there have been more concerns about fertile or pregnant women in an environment associated with high reproductive and teratogenic risks. According to recent studies, there are many risk factors such as solvents, different types of pollution, anesthetic agents, and even video display terminals.[16] With an increasing use of drugs, a better and stringent screening process is required. Toxicological testings with higher sensitivities are necessary.[17]

A. HISTORY

Congenital anomalies in infants have been known for a long time; the Babylonians, as early as 2000 B.C., recorded 62 human malformations. Hippocrates (ca. 400 B.C.), the father of medicine, showed knowledge of hydrocephalus, while Aristotle (340 B.C.) described in detail congenital malformations with many of his speculations that had dominated for more than 2000 years.

During the 17th century, malformed children were treated as monsters acted upon by supernatural powers. In 1651, Harvey published his important work on the concept of developmental arrest as a cause of malformation and the significance of experimental influences upon prenatal development. Some of his hypotheses are still essentially valid today.[18] In 1768, Haller attempted to describe more accurately the malformations and to challenge many previous erroneous interpretations.

In 1822, Geoffroy Saint-Hilaire published *Philosophie Anatomique* and coined the word "teratology," which is defined as the study of birth defects. He proposed the theory of "amniotic adhesions" as the cause of malformations. He could experimentally produce anencephaly and spina bifida in chick embryos. Ten years later, his son published the *Traite de Teratologie* and advanced the theory further. This publication contains many descriptions of congenital abnormalities with systematics and interpretations that are still being cited today.[18]

The first experimental approach to elucidate developmental mechanisms was adopted in Roux's experiment on the frog embryo in 1888. In his experiment, malformations were induced in the frog zygote after manipulation because he did not remove the damaged blastomeres. Shortly before his report, Dareste already had introduced methods for experimental teratology. He could induce malformations in the chick embryo by varying the incubation conditions of the eggs, and he had accurately classified and described his experimental results.

More than half a century later, the rubella virus is the first environmental factor recognized to be a cause of human malformation.[19] In the last 30 years, toxicological and teratological studies have become increasingly important, especially after the incidence of an astonishing tragedy brought about by thalidomide.[20] Although this over-the-counter sedative had been shown to be harmless to many animal species, it specifically causes congenital malformations in humans. The incident has also implied the differential responses of different species to a teratogen and has drawn the attention of physicians to the potential hazards of drugs and environmental factors to pregnant women.[18]

Since birth defects are obvious signs of toxicity, early studies on reproductive toxicity are teratological. There is so much information available in teratology that several books are necessary to give a complete account of the discipline. In the discussion of reproductive toxicity, teratology is only a component. There are many other points of the reproductive process which can be affected by toxic substances. A toxic substance may not cause birth defects if it is embryotoxic or causes infertility. Without gross abnormalities, early studies failed to uncover these substances.

The most famous example is diethylstilbestrol (DES), which has deleterious effects on both male and female fetuses, causing reproductive dysfunction in these individuals.[21] From late 1940s to 1970s, there were almost three million women taking DES for reducing the likelihood of spontaneous abortions. Later, this therapeutic effect of DES was found to be unreproducible. Most of the women exposed to DES *in utero* developed clear cell adenocarcinoma in the cervicovaginal area. They experienced higher frequencies of spontaneous abortions, ectopic pregnancies, and premature labor, though these individuals were perfectly normal morphologically and anatomically. This incidence raises a question on the long-term risk of exposure to a possible reproductive toxin.

B.   WHAT IS A REPRODUCTIVE TOXIN?

Despite the simplicity of this question, it is extremely difficult to give a confident answer. A toxin is a substance interfering with the normal physiology of a cell, tissue, organ, or entire organism. Reproductive toxins are limited to those directly or indirectly affecting the reproductive process. Without specifying necessary conditions such as concentration and treatment duration, almost anything can be a reproductive toxin. For example, pure distilled water is obviously toxic

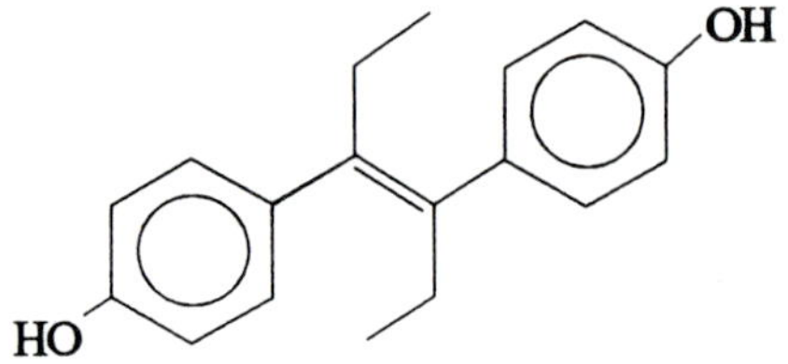

FIGURE 11.8.   Chemical structure of diethylstilbestrol (DES).

to sperms and embryos. Therefore, the expression of toxicity depends on the conditions and testing methodology.

Since the establishment of the causal link between thalidomide and limb abnormalities,[20] there is an extensive search for systemic methods for screening new compounds, and rules were implemented for drugs and other chemicals in many countries. According to the U.S. Food and Drug Administration (FDA) Guidelines,[22] there are three basic types of investigations: general reproductive studies, teratological studies, and perinatal/postnatal studies. These guidelines are still widely accepted.[18]

Perhaps, it was due to the impact of the thalidomide incident that the FDA became extremely cautious in drug approval. It may take several years to pass evaluation. The recent issue of RU486 not being approved by the FDA is possibly caused by, in addition to the political issue, the fear of an incidence similar to the thalidomide disaster. Since RU486 combined with prostaglandins acts by interfering with postimplantation development, its possible teratogenic effects on fetuses which fail to be aborted must be thoroughly studied.

For a new chemical without previous teratological evaluation, there are variations between countries in their guidelines, such as the number of treatment groups, sample number per treatment, duration of treatment, selection of doses, and the number of different species used.

C.   MECHANISMS OF REPRODUCTIVE TOXICITY

There is no general mechanism of toxicity; a toxin may act at a single site or multiple sites. There are only two types of actions: direct and indirect. A toxin with direct effects may have a chemical structure similar to an endogenous compound specifically involved in a process. These toxins are commonly agonists or antagonists of hormones such as DES, a nonsteroidal estrogen (Figure 11.8). In other words, these toxins interact with receptors directly responsible for the process being affected. Direct actions may also include other levels such as levels of gene expression and protein synthesis. These compounds may be simple molecules (e.g., cadmium) or complex proteins (e.g., mitomycin C). They can be mutagenic, carcinogenic, or chemically reactive.

Reproductive toxins with indirect effects may require metabolic activation after entering the organism or may alter physiological control governing some steps in the reproductive process. There are different types of indirect actions. The toxin may be metabolized into a compound with direct toxic effects. Cyclophosphamide (Cytoxan), a therapeutic agent for kidney diseases, is metabolized by microsomal monoxygengases into active toxic metabolites. The toxin may alter synthesis, secretion, or degradation of steroids. Pesticides such as DDT are good examples of this type of indirect toxins.

D. TOXICITY ON GONADS AND GAMETES

Ovary and testis are vulnerable to many reproductive toxins, direct or indirect. Direct toxins alter the process of gametogenesis, while indirect toxins induce changes in the endocrine functions of gonads. In both cases, if gametogenesis is altered, the reproductive potential of the individual is affected.

1. Ovarian Toxicity

The ovary is central to the control of the female reproductive cycle. The normal running of the ovarian cycle is essential for a timely supply of Graafian follicles for ovulation. Reproductive toxins may act on different locations of the ovary at different times. The indirect toxicity may be through actions on blood supply, affecting the follicular development. For direct effects on follicles, there is a differential follicle complex toxicity.[23]

Different toxins may act on follicles of different stages. If a toxin destroys matured follicles specifically, fertility is reduced immediately until the removal of the toxin. If a toxin kills primary and secondary follicles specifically, reduced fertility will not be observed immediately. After the removal of the toxin, it will take a much longer time to restore fertility. Obviously, if primary follicles are affected, there will be an increased rate of atresia. Since there is a fixed number of follicles after birth, the loss of primary follicles will lead to premature ovarian failure or early menopause. This results in a reduction of the female reproductive lifespan.

2. Testicular Toxicity

In contrast to oogenesis, the entire process of spermatogenesis occurs in the adult testis. Spermatogonia lying along the basement membrane of the seminiferous tubule mitose maintain the stem cell population. While type A spermatogonia continue to divide mitotically, type B spermatogonia derived from some of their daughter cells, intermediate spermatogonia, further divide into primary spermatocytes. Each primary spermatocyte undergoes meiosis and differentiates into a sperm. Since it takes about 64 days for a spermatogonium to form a matured sperm, spermatogenesis can easily be disrupted at any point by toxins.

If the toxin does not wipe out all spermatogonia and the exposure time is short, the damage is often reversible. There is only a temporary loss of fertility if the remaining spermatogonia can resume normal mitosis. Ionizing radiation and alkylating agents (e.g., cyclophosphamide and nitrogen mustards) are toxic to dividing spermatogonia but nontoxic to resting spermatogonia, resulting in transient infertility. The male reproductive lifespan is seldom affected if the resting spermatogonia are not permanently damaged.

It should be noted that the time required for spermatogenesis is apparently a constant.[24] Almost all toxic agents tested failed to alter the rate of differentiation of individual spermatogonia. The toxic response of each spermatogonium is all or none; it may continue to differentiate on schedule or degenerate. With millions of differentiating sperms having a varying degree of toxic response to the same treatment, the overall toxic response is a decreased rate of sperm production.

Although spermatogenesis is a process more sensitive to reproductive toxic agents, matured sperms before and after ejaculation are also vulnerable to environmental insults. As an explanation for the seasonality of human reproduction discussed earlier (see section III.C.2) sperms have lower fertilizing capability during the hot summer. A hostile environment in the vagina or uterus can create a barrier for sperms to achieve fertilization. Spermicidal contraceptives are good examples.

There are many chemicals known to induce testicular toxicity either directly or indirectly. They include analgesics such as indomethacin and morphine; androgens and their antagonists; antibiotics such as amphotericin B; insecticides such as DDT and parathion; some food additives such as cyclamates, metanil yellow, and caffeine; heavy metals such as cadmium and mercury.

3.   Effects of Toxicants on Fertilization

Fertilization is another stringent screening checkpoint along the reproductive process. In contrast to external fertilization in lower vertebrates, internal fertilization in mammalian reproduction is already a better guarantee of success. If the gametes are healthy and the microenvironment in the female reproductive tract is normal, the chance of successful fertilization is high. With the medical technology achieved today, the rate of fertilization *in vitro* is always over 50% under conditions found optimal in the laboratory.

Even if gametes are normal, there are crucial factors required for the process of fertilization to be performed successfully. Before the actual union of male and female nuclei, there is a series of necessary events: sperm transport in the female reproductive tract, sperm capacitation and the maintenance of sperm motility, penetration of the cumulus oophorus, acrosome reaction, sperm binding and fusion with vitellus, and the cortical reaction in the oocyte. Different compounds have been found to act on these steps specifically, while some affect all of them nonspecifically.[25] In any case, fertilization can be inhibited or the fertilized oocyte can fail to develop further.

E.   EMBRYOTOXICITY AND TERATOGENICITY

Once the oocyte is successfully fertilized, it enters the stage of preimplantation development, leading to another stringent screening checkpoint, implantation. It has been estimated that only about 40% of preimplantation zygotes can implant successfully under normal conditions.[26] Implantation is a crucial step to eliminate possible abnormal zygotes to avoid babies with birth defects later.

There are numerous chemicals interfering with implantation.[27] After fertilization, the zygote needs to be properly transported to the uterus by the oviduct while it continues to cleave. In addition to the oviduct-driven egg transport, the intraoviducal environment must be maintained optimally for preimplantation development. A reproductive toxin upsetting this maternal environment inhibits implantation. On the other hand, if the toxicant is embryotoxic, the abnormal development of preimplantation zygotes also leads to implantation failure.

The process of implantation requires proper interactions between progesterone and estrogen. Analogs of LHRH and steroids or other compounds interfering with progesterone or estrogen are found to affect implantation. For example, DDT analogs and polychlorinated biphenyl compounds are insecticides with estrogenic properties. In mice, they have been shown to prolong pregnancy or reduce the number of implantation sites. Ions of heavy or transition metals such as cadmium, copper, and zinc inhibit the binding of estrogen, leading to implantation failure.

If the toxicant does not lead to implantation failure, there are three possibilities for the fate of the implanted zygote. First, in spite of the damage, the embryo continues to develop and restore the damaged parts of the zygote. If the toxicant is removed or not toxic to postimplantation zygotes, the embryo may succeed in developing into a normal fetus. Second, the toxicant may not be toxic to postimplantation zygotes. The damage to the zygote before or during implantation was too extensive so that the subsequent embryonic development is abnormal. A malformed fetus may be formed and later resorbed or become a newborn with congenital abnormalities.

For the third possibility, the toxicant may also be toxic to the postimplantation zygote. Depending on the specificity of its toxic action, malformation or abortion may occur at any point during postimplantation development. If the toxicant leads to newborns with birth defects, it is teratogenic. If it kills the embryo eventually, it is embryotoxic. The developmental system fails to eliminate malformed embryos exposed to teratogenic toxicants. Most malformed newborns die shortly after birth, while others may survive but be burdened with congenital anomalies.

F. TOXICITY ON OTHER STRUCTURES RELATED TO REPRODUCTION

Although some toxicants directly or indirectly toxic to the gonad are reproductive toxins, other toxicants benign to the gonad may also be reproductive toxins if they are toxic to structures associated with the reproductive process. Alternatively, they may be toxic to both the gonad and related structures. For example, there are a number of xenobiotic chemicals found in the human seminal plasma such as pesticides, heavy metals, antibiotics, and alcohol. This indicates that accessory genital glands are also susceptible to environmental insults. Even if the gametes produced are normal, the presence of toxicants in the seminal plasma imposes risks on the reproductive process.

It should be mentioned that prostate cancer is the second leading cause of cancer mortality in men.[28] About 10% of American men will develop prostate cancer with an annual incidence of 20,000 prostate cancer cases in men under the age of 65. In addition to possible predisposed genetic factors for prostate cancer, environmental factors are suspected to play a role. Early diagnosis is imperative when the disease is still pathologically organ-confined so that treatment is possible.[29] The prostate function is at least partially lost. This may become a factor leading to sexual dysfunction.

Since sexual behavior plays a crucial role in mating, some drugs affecting the brain are known to induce reproductive failure. For example, drugs inhibitory to steroid biosynthesis such as alcohol and narcotics or those blocking steroid receptors such as cyproterone acetate and spironolactone are found to lower libido and sexual performance.[30] Drugs including alcohol have detrimental effects both prenatally and postnatally.[31] Besides morphological anomalies, damages to the CNS not discernible immediately during sexual differentiation and development may occur. If the damages are irreversible, the affected individual may suffer from abnormal permanent sexual behavior that may jeopardize reproductive capability. Drugs may also induce a transient change in sexual behavior. Although the change is transient, the change in sexuality does affect the reproductive outcome. For example, the effects of alcohol on human sexuality have been demonstrated in psychological studies.[32]

G. Species and Gender Differences in Toxic Responses

Species differences in toxic responses pose complex problems in reproductive toxicology, especially in the area of toxicity assessment. Depending on specific mechanisms, a reproductive toxin may be extremely safe in one species, but a powerful toxicant in another. Thalidomide is an excellent example. Since differences between rats and mice or even among different strains of mice can be observed, toxicological testings using animal models do not provide a reliable extrapolation to humans. So multiple toxicological testings across different species including nonhuman primates and *in vitro* testings using human cell lines are necessary prior to clinical trials.

Another concern is the gender difference in toxic responses. In humans, differences in immune responses between men and women have been established. Although it is still uncertain whether there is a gender difference in toxic responses, it is always beneficial to take the sex of the subject into consideration during studies. In addition, there are other important variables such as developmental stages or age. For some toxicants, their actions may be more effective at a certain time of the reproductive process. For example, galactose or azathioprine are toxic to the developing ovary before birth. In contrast, they are nontoxic to postnatal ovaries.[33]

H. Reproductive Toxicity of Selected Compounds

1. Steroids and Related Compounds

Hormonal contraceptives are steroid analogs that alter gonadotrophin release. The risk of voluntarily taking oral contraceptives has been discussed in Chapter 10. The dosage used for contraception is maintained at a low daily level (e.g., 50 μg).

However, occupational exposure to these preparations for female workers is hazardous to their reproductive health. Impaired ovarian function is often observed in women exposed to dust containing mestranol or ethinylestradiol, leading to reduced fertility.[34] Occupational exposure to androgens is also a concern to women. The exposed individuals may have an enlarged clitoris, increased hair growth, and masculinization.

Obviously, steroids and their analogs also have pronounced effects on men. In the sporting world, the use of anabolic-androgenic steroids has become an epidemic,[35] though their use is prohibited by the International Olympic Committee. Since their uses are more popular even among recreational and adolescent athletes, the problem is now a public health issue. If the use of steroids is supervised correctly with supplements at optimal dosages under supervision, the treatment may improve muscular performance. Since steroids are easily available even through mail, the control of abused uses is difficult; very often, commercial advertisements are misleading.[36] Some health risks associated with overdosage may be irreversible and life threatening, especially when they are used in combination with other drugs.

2. Heavy Metals

Lead, mercury, and cadmium are common heavy metals known to impair the reproductive process. Both prenatal and postnatal exposure to these heavy metals are detrimental. They can be presented in various forms such as chloride, sulfates, or organic complexes. The toxicity of the metal depends on its form. For example, chlorides vary greatly in aqueous solubility; lead chloride is sparingly soluble, while cadmium chloride is highly soluble in aqueous solutions. Lead is more toxic in the form of acetate or organic complexes such as tetramethyl or tetraethyl lead because these forms are highly lipid soluble. Cadmium chloride, on the other hand, is highly toxic in aqueous solution, but the inorganic cadmium ion is difficult to cross the cell membrane.

Figure 11.9 shows the *in vitro* toxic effects of 5 µg/ml cadmium chloride on mouse preimplantation zygotes 24 h after treatment. Vacuolation in the cytoplasm of the blastomeres could be observed in the cadmium-treated morulae. If a day-8 pregnant mouse is treated with 0.1 mg cadmium chloride in 0.9% saline intraperitoneally, some of the fetuses on day 15 become exencephalic (see Figure 11.10). This malformation is caused by a cadmium-induced delay in the development of the brain and skull. In humans, a similar ancephalic malformation also occurs in 0.1% of newborns for some unknown reasons.

The source of these heavy metals is usually industrial.[37] For example, organic lead is a component of antiknock mix, while inorganic mercury is used in barometers and other electrical machinery. Cadmium is found in batteries, electroplating, and as amalgam in dentistry. A recent study on workers exposed to cadmium in smelters or to lead in a battery factory in Belgian has shown that the fertility of these workers was reduced.[38] In another study on women in areas with high lead and cadmium content in soil, there were fewer women with three or more pregnancies, and the number of preterm deliveries was higher.[39]

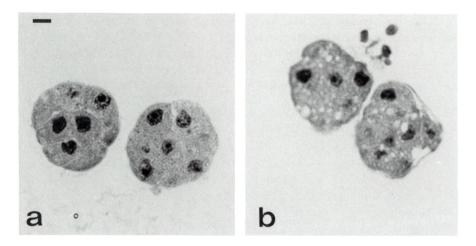

FIGURE 11.9.   Cadmium toxicity on mouse preimplantation zygotes. A four-cell zygote was cultured for 24 h in (a) the control medium and (b) a medium containing 5 μg/ml cadmium chloride. Note the vacuolated cytoplasm of blastomeres in the cadmium-treated zygotes.

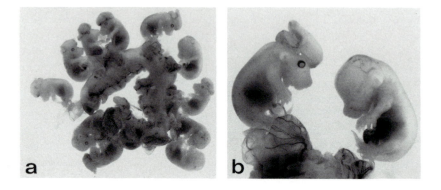

FIGURE 11.10.   Cadmium teratogenicity on mouse fetuses. A day-8 pregnant mouse (F1 hybrid of C57 and A_2G) was treated intraperitoneally with 0.1 mg cadmium chloride in 0.9% saline. On day 15, a litter of 11 fetuses with 4 normal and 7 exencephalic fetuses was found (see a). Note the absence of the skull and a malformed brain in the ancephalic fetus (see b).

Both prenatal and postnatal exposure to these heavy metals are detrimental as shown in studies on rodents. Prenatal exposure often results in birth defects such as ancephaly, and in mild situations, as with cadmium, gonadal formation is impaired. During the postnatal development establishment of the hypothalamic-hypophyseal-ovarian-uterine axis, treatment of these heavy metals results in ovarian atrophy, decreased fertility, and altered cycles.

3.   **Pesticides**

Common pesticides used are dibromochloropropane (DBCP), DDT, and, the previously popular one, chlordecone (kepone). There are many different pesticides and herbicides used in agriculture. They are mostly organic compounds. DBCP was the first pesticide reported in 1977 to have reproductive toxicity.[40] It was associated with occupational exposure in workers of a manufacturing company. Male workers reported impotence or decreased libido with elevated FSH levels. There was a loss of germ cells, leading to azoospermia or oligospermia and eventually to reduced fertility.

In laboratory animals, DBCP has also been shown to induce severe testicular degeneration in males and irregular estrous cycles in females. DDT also causes a marked reduction in fertility in mice with its possible estrogenic actions. However, in contrast to DBCP, the reproductive toxicity of DDT on humans has not been clearly demonstrated. Chlordecone (Kepone) is also associated with reduced sperm count and motility and with an increased number of abnormal sperms in humans. Workers exposed to high levels of this pesticide have symptoms such as nervousness, tremor, and visual problems.[37] Interestingly, this pesticide can also be found in breast milk, indicating that it may also affect the infant.

4.   **Organic Solvents**

In contrast to pesticides, organic solvents are simpler molecules. Examples are ethylene glycol, toluene, benzene, hexane, etc. Almost all organic solvents studied have reproductive toxicity; they either reduce gonadal function or interfere with the embryonic development. Since organic molecules are lipophilic, they can pass through the cell membrane easily. They diffuse readily through the uterine wall, placenta, or the blood-gonadal barrier. In highly industrialized countries, there are numerous types of organic solvents used. It becomes a health concern not only for workers involved in the industrial process but also for the public.

Ethylene glycol ethers are commonly used as antifreeze in automobile coolant. They have been shown to induce testicular degeneration in rats, though there has been no documented reproductive toxicity in humans. Toluene is a common solvent in paints. Some women exposed to toluene occupationally suffer from menstrual disorders. In pregnant women, there is a decrease in fetal growth and newborn weight among those exposed to toluene, which is embryotoxic rather than teratogenic.

5.   **Alcohol and Nicotine**

In a recent study on prepubertal female rats, alcohol induces an increase in the hypothalamic content of GHRH and LHRH with a concomitant decrease in serum GH and LH.[41] These results support earlier studies showing that alcohol causes a delayed onset of puberty in female rats.[42] The alcohol-treated rats have a delay in vaginal opening and decreased uterine weight and ovarian functions. A clinical study on pregnant women who drink twice a week or more shows that about 50% of cases of spontaneous abortions may be attributed to alcohol consumption.[43] The mean alcohol intake per drink was 0.72 to 2.50 oz in absolute amount, but a chronic consumption of 6 oz per day is agreed to constitute a high risk.[44] Also, spontaneous abortion is a natural screening mechanism to eliminate malformed fetuses.

Some fetuses may not be aborted in pregnant women who start to drink late in their pregnancies. A few may develop to apparently normal babies, while others may develop fetal alcohol syndrome (FAS). At least several hundred children are born each year with FAS and thousands more with some alcohol-induced defects.[44] The syndrome includes microcephaly, mental retardation, cardiac abnormalities, and other neural defects. Alcohol possibly induces fetal growth retardation and neural tube defects.

Despite the possible effects of alcohol on the reproductive system, psychological studies in humans have shown that alcohol alters sexual behavior.[32] Alcohol at low doses disinhibits psychological sexual arousal and at higher doses suppresses physiological responses to sexual stimulation. Perhaps, alcohol indirectly affects sexual behavior through altering the cognitive function transiently.

Alcoholic mothers very often smoke or even take illegal drugs. The teratogenic effects are compounded. Infants of smoking mothers have a lower mean birth weight. Nicotine is the main causative agent. As a potent vasoconstrictor, it reduces uteroplacental blood flow and causes fetal growth retardation.[45] Through nicotinic receptors, nicotine stimulates uterotubal motility. Nicotine also increases norepinephrine release and oxytocin secretion from the pituitary.[33] Nicotine may also suppress fetal tissue growth directly.[45] Smoking alone has been proven to increase the chance of spontaneous abortion, but no conclusive evidence is available to show its teratogenic effects.

V. REPRODUCTIVE TOXICITY OF THE ENVIRONMENT

To reproduce successfully, an organism must determine the optimal time, duration, and location to initiate the reproductive process. If environmental conditions are predictable, the organism can use these daily or annual changes in physical factors as cues to regulate its reproductive physiology. Circadian systems and seasonal cycles are evolved in those species that can adapt to this rhythmic fluctuation and reproduce. When they become acclimated to these conditions, unpredictable changes in the environment may disrupt the normal regulatory mechanism of reproduction. In other words, the factors in this new environment are "toxic" to their reproductive process. Some may develop toxic responses to cope with these hostile conditions, while others fail to survive. The reproductive toxicity of an agent, either chemical or physical, depends on the magnitude of its deviation from the optimum. A drastic change elicits vigorous toxic responses from organisms not used to the environmental change.

Our ancestors experienced many unpredictable changes during evolution. Since the human species survived, it is not surprising to find that humans have basic mammalian time-keeping mechanisms. Human behavior is still very much circadian and seasonal. We have learned to improve our quality of life by domestication. Technology is being developed to predict or even control the climate, to treat toxic wastes, and to restore environmental conditions suitable for life. This capability of controlling environmental changes is the key to human survival and is beneficial to all the life on earth. Unfortunately, some of these technologies have led to pollution problems, creating hostile environmental conditions. It is imperative to understand reproductive toxicology while developing new technology. Substances nontoxic to somatic cells may be reproductive toxins. Some agents benign to most species may be highly teratogenic to humans.

As discussed in previous chapters, the reproductive process consists of major components including the differentiation of proper sexual behavior, normal gametogenesis, successful fertilization, and implantation, as well as punctual embryonic and neonatal development. Many timepoints along this developmental continuum are sensitive to hostile environmental factors. Disruption at any one of them jeopardizes the reproductive success. Our medical technology allows us to remove these hostile environmental factors or to restore damages caused by toxicants. New procedures enhance the survival of premature babies and malformed newborns.

Nevertheless, the sensitivity of the reproductive process to environmental stress serves as a stringent screening mechanism to select the best newborn. With improved medical technology, delivery can occur during the seventh month of gestation. Infertile couples can now pass their genes to the next generation through artificial insemination or *in vitro* fertilization. We can now overcome barriers imposed by the stringent screening mechanism of the reproductive process. Our children may become more dependent on an artificial environment and medical assistance. It could be catastrophic if, one day, we cannot tolerate unpredictable environmental changes without the necessary technology that may become unavailable.

REFERENCES

1. **Wei, W.W.S.,** *Time Series Analysis: Univariate and Multivariate Methods,* Addison-Wesley, Reading, MA, 1990.
2. **Boklage, C.E., Zincone, L.H., and Kirby, C.F., Jr.,** Annual and sub-annual rhythms in human conception rates: time-series analyses show annual and weekday but no monthly rhythms in daily counts for last normal menses, *Hum. Reprod.,* 7, 899, 1992.
3. **Yu, H.S.,** Melatonin in the eye: functional implications, in *Melatonin: Biosynthesis, Physiological Effects, and Clinical Applications,* Yu, H.S. and Reiter, R.J., Eds., CRC Press, Boca Raton, FL, 1993, 365.
4. **Teicher, M.H. and Barber, N.I.,** COSIFIT: an interactive program for simultaneous multioscillator cosinor analysis of time-series data, *Comput. Biomed. Res.,* 23, 283, 1990.
5. **Edmunds, L.N., Jr.,** *Cellular and Molecular Bases of Biological Clocks: Models and Mechanisms for Circadian Timekeeping,* Springer-Verlag, New York, 1988.
6. **Turek, F.W. and van Cauter, E.,** Rhythms in reproduction, in *The Physiology of Reproduction,* Knobil, E. and Neill, J., Eds., Raven Press, New York, 1988, 1789.

7. **Aschoff, J.,** Circadian rhythms in man, in *Biological Timekeeping,* Brady, J., Ed., Cambridge University Press, Cambridge, 1984, 143.

8. **Goldman, B.D. and Nelson, R.J.,** Melatonin and seasonality in mammals, in *Melatonin: Biosynthesis, Physiological Effects, and Clinical Applications,* Yu, H.S. and Reiter, R.J., Eds., CRC Press, Boca Raton, FL, 1993, 225.

9. **Bronson, F.H.,** Seasonal regulation of regulation in mammals, in *The Physiology of Reproduction,* Knobil, E. and Neill, J., Eds., Raven Press, New York, 1988, 1831.

10. **Goldman, B.D. and Nelson, R.J.,** Melatonin and seasonality in mammals, in *Melatonin: Biosynthesis, Physiological Effects, and Clinical Applications,* Yu, H.S. and Reiter, R.J., Eds., CRC Press, Boca Raton, FL, 1993.

11. **Rojansky, N., Brzezinski, A., and Schenker, J.G.,** Seasonality in human reproduction: an update, *Hum. Reprod.,* 7, 735, 1992.

12. **Levine, J.R., Matthew, R.W., Chenault, B.C., Brown, M.H., Hurtt, M.E., and Bently, K.S.,** Differences in the quality of semen in outdoor workers during summer and winter, *N. Engl. J. Med.,* 323, 12, 1990.

13. **Kauppila, A., Kivela, A., Pakarinen, A., and Vakkuri, O.,** Inverse seasonal relationship between melatonin and ovarian activity in humans in a region with a strong seasonal contrast in luminosity, *J. Clin. Endocrinol. Metab.,* 65, 823, 1987.

14. **Warren, D.C. and Scott, H.M.,** Influence of light on ovulation in the fowl, *J. Exp. Zool.,* 74, 137, 1936.

15. **Sundararaj, N., Chern, M., Gatewood, L., Hichman, L., and McHugh, R.,** Seasonal behavior of human menstrual cycles: a biometric investigation, *Hum. Biol.,* 50, 15, 1978.

16. **Persaud, T.V.,** The pregnant woman in the work place: potential embryopathic risks, *Anat. Anz.,* 170, 295, 1990.

17. **Sullivan, F.M.,** Reproductive toxicity tests: retrospect and prospect, *Hum. Toxicol.,* 7, 423, 1988.

18. **Persaud, T.V.N.,** Brief history of teratology, in *Basic Concepts in Teratology,* Persaud, T.V.N., Chudley, A.E., and Skalko, R.G., Eds., Alan R. Liss, New York, 1985, 1.

19. **Gregg, N.M.,** Congenital cataract following German measles in the mother, *Trans. Ophthalmol. Soc. Aust.,* 3, 35, 1941.

20. **McBride, W.G.,** Thalidomide and congenital abnormalities, *Lancet,* 2, 1358, 1961.

21. **Stillman, R.J.,** In utero exposure to diethylstilbestrol: adverse effects on the reproductive tract and reproductive performance in male and female offspring, *Am. J. Obstet. Gynecol.,* 142, 905, 1982.

22. **U.S. Food and Drug Administration (FDA),** Guidelines for reproduction studies for safety evaluation of drugs for human use, FDA, Washington, D.C., 1966.

23. **Mattison, D.R.,** Clinical manifestations of ovarian toxicity, in *Reproductive Toxicology,* Dixon, R.L., Ed., Raven Press, New York, 1985, 109.

24. **Desjardins, C.,** Morphological, physiological, and biochemical aspects of male reproduction, in *Reproductive Toxicology,* Dixon, R.L., Ed., Raven Press, New York, 1985, 131.

25. **Gwatkin, R.B.L.,** Effects of chemicals on fertilization, in *Reproductive Toxicology,* Dixon, R.L., Ed., Raven Press, New York, 1985, 209.

26. **Kline, J. and Stein, Z.,** Very early pregnancy, in *Reproductive Toxicology,* Dixon, R.L., Ed., Raven Press, New York, 1985, 251.

27. **Wu, J.T.,** Chemicals affecting implantation, in *Reproductive Toxicology,* Dixon, R.L., Ed., Raven Press, New York, 1985, 239.

28. **Carter, B.S., Carter, H.B., and Isaacs, J.T.,** Epidemiologic evidence regarding predisposing factors to prostate cancer, *Prostate,* 16, 187, 1990.

29. **Scardino, P.T., Weaver, R., and Hudson, M.A.,** Early detection of prostate cancer, *Hum. Pathol.,* 23, 211, 1992.

30. **Eliasson, R.,** Clinical effects of chemicals on male reproduction, in *Reproductive Toxicology,* Dixon, R.L., Ed., Raven Press, New York, 1985, 161.

31. **Hoegerman, G., Wilson, C.A., Thurmond, E., and Schnoll, S.H.,** Drug-exposed neonates, *West. J. Med.,* 152, 559, 1990.

32. **Crowe, L.C. and George, W.H.,** Alcohol and human sexuality: review and integration, *Psychol. Bull.,* 105, 374, 1989.

33. **Mattison, D.R. and Thomford, P.J.,** Mechanisms of action of reproductive toxicants, in *Toxicology of the Male and Female Reproductive Systems,* Working, P.K., Ed., Hemisphere Publishing Corp., New York, 1989, 101.

34. **DeMorales, A.V., Rivera, R.O., Harrington, J.M., and Stein, G.F.,** The occupational hazards of formulating oral contraceptives: a survey of plant employees, *Arch. Environ. Health,* 33, 12, 1978.

35. **Kleiner, S.M.,** Performance-enhancing aids in sport: health consequences and nutritional alternatives, *J. Am. Coll. Nutrit.,* 10, 163, 1991.

36. **DiPasquale, M.G.,** Beyond anabolic steroids, in *Drugs in Sports Series,* M.G.D. Press, Warkworth, 1990.

37. **Barlow, S.M. and Sullivan, F.M.,** *Reproductive Hazards of Industrial Chemicals,* Academic Press, London, 1982.

38. **Gennart, J.P., Buchet, J.P., Roels, H., Ghyselen, P., Ceulemans, E., and Lauwerys, R.,** Fertility of male workers exposed to cadmium, lead, or manganese, *Am. J. Epidemiol.,* 135, 1208, 1992.

39. **Laudanski, T., Sipowicz, M., Modzelewski, P., Bolinski, J., Szamatowicz, J., Razniewska, G., and Akerlund, M.,** Influence of high lead and cadmium soil content on human reproductive outcome, *Int. J. Gynaecol. Obstet.,* 36, 309, 1991.

40. **Whorton, D., Krauss, R.M., Marshall, S., and Milby, T.H.,** Infertility in male pesticide workers, *Lancet,* 2, 1259, 1977.

41. **Les Dees, W., Skelley, C.W., Hiney, J.K., and Johnston, C.A.,** Actions of ethanol on hypothalamic and pituitary hormones in prepubertal female rats, *Alcohol,* 7, 21, 1990.

42. **Bo, W.J., Krueger, W.A., Rudeen, P.K., and Symmes, S.K.,** Ethanol-induced alterations in the morphology and function of the rat ovary, *Anat. Rec.,* 202, 255, 1982.

43. **Kline, J., Shrout, P., Stein, Z., Susser, M., and Warbuton, D.,** Drinking during pregnancy and spontaneous abortion, *Lancet,* 2, 176, 1980.

44. **Brent, R.L. and Beckman, D.A.,** Principles of teratology, in *Reproductive Risks and Prenatal Diagnosis,* Appleton and Lange, Norwalk, 1992, 43, chap. 3.

45. **Werler, M.M., Pober, B.R., and Holmes, L.B.,** Smoking and pregnancy, *Teratology,* 32, 473, 1985.

46. **Kapen, S., Boyar, R.M., Finkelstein, J.W., Hellman, L., and Weitzman, E.D.,** Effect of sleep-wake cycle reversal on luteinizing hormone secretory pattern in puberty, *J. Clin. Endocrinol. Metab.,* 39, 293, 1974.

47. **Bremner, W.J., Vitiello, M.V., and Prinz, P.N.,** Loss of circadian rhythmicity in blood testosterone levels with aging in normal men, *J. Clin. Endocrinol. Metab.,* 56, 1278, 1983.

48. **Michael, R.P. and Zumpe, D.,** Sexual violence in the United States and the role of season, *Am. J. Psychiatry,* 140, 883, 1983.

12 Human Reproduction and Sexuality

CHAPTER CONTENTS

I. INTRODUCTION

Most mammals are seasonal breeders, with a few exceptions such as some domesticated animals (e.g., guinea pigs, pigs, and laboratory rats and mice) and primates (e.g., apes, colob and macaque monkeys, baboons, and humans). In humans, seasonality in natural conception and birth rates has been observed (see also Chapter 11). Possible causal factors include the deterioration in sperm quality during the hot summer months and the seasonality of the ovulation rate.[1] Without consistent neuroendocrine data, any seasonal reproductive patterns found in humans are believed to be behavioral. Food availability and shelter are still significant factors affecting the reproductive process in humans, especially in developing countries.

Humans are always sexually active, and the control of sexual behavior relies on cognitive functions (see also Chapter 7). With effective contraceptive methods, human sexual behavior becomes less associated with the reproductive process. Most sexual activities are nonreproductive. The decision process to interact sexually does not necessarily involve the intention to reproduce. The terms "sexual values," "sexual morality," and "family values" have been created to describe different reference points in the decision process. These reference points are constraints established based on the sociocultural norm of a community. It is a dynamic control mechanism of behavior in social groups which governs human sexuality and eventually our reproductive pattern. The institution of marriage is clearly, at least in part, a mechanism to regulate human sexual activities.

The purpose of marriage, at least for some couples, is to create lifelong relationships during which the heterosexual couples can reproduce. Despite this original intent, about 50% of marriages are not lifelong, and these couples often remarry with others. Metaphorically, a series of marriages in humans resembles a period of several years in seasonal breeders with annual reproductive cycles. The period of each "marital cycle" varies greatly from one couple to another. In the U.S., more marriages break up within the first 3 years and around the 7th and 20th years. This pattern cannot be explained in terms of neuroendocrine physiology. An understanding of marriage is necessary in the discussion of human reproduction and sexuality.

II. MARRIAGE

Although the concept of marriage is unique to humans, we can find similar phenomena in other social animals. Two major features of a human marriage, pair bonding and parental care, are observed in the mating style of some birds and nonhuman mammals. In humans, these two features are extremely important for the uniquely long duration of postnatal dependence.

To avoid confusion, the term "marriage" will not be used to describe pair bonding in nonhuman species. Also, human marriage is rigorously defined in legal terms. Sexual partners without marriage recognition (e.g., certificate or ceremony) legalized by the community at the place of residence are not considered married; they are classified as cohabitors. This definition is necessary for a clear distinction of premarital, marital, and extramarital activities.

A. MONOGAMY AND POLYGAMY

The definitions of monogamy and polygamy are only related to the union of female and male gametes. Sexual activities without reproduction are not considered. In a monogamous species, one female mates with a male to produce offspring during her lifetime and vice versa. Interestingly, the two sexes in these species are commonly similar in body shape and size. The lack of sexual dimorphism is probably caused by the balanced pressure between inter- and intrasexual selection for mating. Well-known examples of monogamous primates are the marmoset and gibbon. Without examining their external genitalia, one finds it difficult to identify males from females.

In a polygamous species, one female mates with many males and vice versa. As in monogamy, inter- and intrasexual selection pressures for mating are balanced, resulting in a lack of sexual dimorphism. The chimpanzee is a rare example among primates to be truly polygamous. Both females and males can mate freely with one another without intense competition. Very often, they are described as promiscuous. It should be clarified that promiscuity is the behavior and polygamy refers to the reproductive result. Polygamous species are promiscuous, but promiscuity can be found in a monogamous species if the sexual interaction outside the monogamous pair is nonreproductive.

There are two variant forms of polygamy: polygyny and polyandry. In a polygynous species, only one male can mate with several females. This inequality leads to an obvious sexual dimorphism caused by aggressive competition among males. This is a typical mating system in primates such as gorillas, orangutans, macaques, and baboons. The male is sometimes twice the size of a female. This dominating male must be able to defend his territory and his females against rival males. Polyandry is the opposite, with a female having several males. Although it is rare, this mating system exists even in some human societies. The behavior is still promiscuous in both polygynous and polyandrous species, at least in one sex. Figure 12.1 summarizes the effect of sexual selection in different mating systems.

With a high incidence of divorce and remarriage, many have multiple reproductive partners throughout their lifetimes, though one can have only one legal spouse at a time. These statistics are based on legal marriages only. Reproductive partners in unrecorded marriages, cohabitation, and extramarital relationships are excluded. If polygamy is the behavior of having multiple reproductive partners in one's lifetime, then almost 50% of Americans are polygamous. True monogamy should be limited to those, as all monogamous animals, who reproduce with only one partner.

Astonishingly, "legal" polygamy predominates in different human societies as reviewed by van den Berghe (1979).[2] In a study of 800 human societies by Murdock in 1967, 83% were polygynous, 16% were monogamous, and 0.5% were polyandrous. In another study of 93 societies by Whyte in 1980, 61% were polygamous. There are many other examples that can be found in different cultural communities. In Pahari, northern India, wives are expensive, so brothers share one first and buy another later when they can afford her. In Tibet, brothers can take a common wife. Polyandrous marriages are also found in other tribes where the number of males is less.

In the early 19th century, plural marriage was allowed among members of the Mormon Church in the U.S. Each man may have had four wives (polygyny).

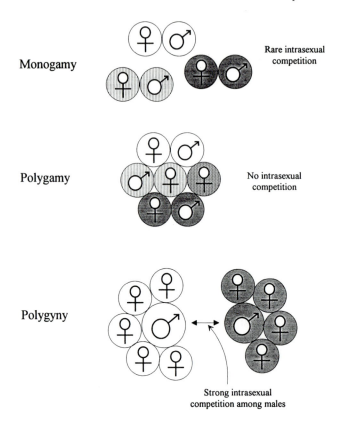

FIGURE 12.1. Effects of sexual selection in different mating systems.

However, on September 24, 1890, Wilford Woodruff, the president of the Mormon Church, issued the Manifesto to disapprove plural marriages officially.[3] Monogamy was strongly enforced in the U.S. over a century ago. Interestingly, it is more important to forbid polygamy than, say, to infringe the right of the people to keep and bear firearms. Should marital arrangement be regarded as highly private and personal choices among consenting adults?

Other famous examples of polygamy are the experiments of group marriage in the U.S. with unsuccessful outcomes. An earlier experiment is the Oneida community created by John Humphrey Noyes in the 1880s as a religious communist ideal.[2] They were fundamentalistic Christians who settled in Oneida, NY from 1847 until 1881 with a peak of 500 community members. With the ideal of economic communism, Noyes' followers were willing to share almost anything from clothing and toys to land and business. Although there was no economic class, the male-dominated society was hierarchical with Noyes as the ruler who imposed laws and ethical standards. Monogamy was prohibited with no family structure. Children were raised communally with designated fathers. Although polygamy was advocated, the system was polygynous in practice. The contraceptive method was *coitus reservatus*, sexual intercourse without ejaculation. Men were allowed to ejaculate when they wanted to have babies or were having sex with postmenopausal women.[2]

In the 1870s, the Oneida community began to disintegrate as the children became matured. Noyes forbade them to identify with their biological parents. He even became obsessed with being the first husband of pubescent girls in the community. With increasing opposition, Noyes escaped in 1879 to avoid rape charges. In 1881, the community became an incorporated company called Oneida Ltd., which is still a large stainless steel manufacturer in the U.S. In recent years, there were other experimental group marriages, which usually lasted for short periods of time. Long-term polygamy is obviously not an appropriate model for human marriage.

Sexual practices in the human species are diversified. Examples of polygyny, polyandry, and true monogamy can be found. Humans are polygamous in nature if the genetic exchange between generations is examined (see Chapter 7, Figure 7.8 and Figure 12.2) A special term "serial monogamy" is created for humans as a compromise between monogamy and polygamy. It is possible that humans are evolving from polygamy to monogamy. Monogamy has an advantage of superior parental care, and the quality of offspring may be enhanced. This is particularly appropriate for the human species with a long gestation period and extended infant dependence.

If the major purpose of monogamy is to provide superior parental care for the offspring, a discordant marriage may not be able to achieve this purpose. On the other hand, this purpose is served when the offspring becomes independent. The pair bonding in both cases may be ended. With our long lifespan, the purpose of having lifelong monogamy is therefore beyond providing parental care. It is the philosophy of marriage to create a family structure with genetically confined individuals in the first progeny, and these individuals are bonded by love. Perhaps, this is the family value of a lifelong monogamous and formal pair bonding between one male and one female with several children. Unfortunately, this type of family is not the majority in the human society.

The genetics of the offspring in a serially monogamous relationship is dramatically different. Figure 12.2 is a comparative account of the mating trees in lifelong and serial monogamy. A binuclear family is created when, say, only the father has one previous marriage with children, while the ex-wife of this man has also remarried with new children. The genetic variability of this man's children is the same as that of a polygynous male, while the ex-wife is essentially polyandrous.

With the advent of efficient contraceptive methods, reproduction in serially monogamous or polygamous relationships can be controlled effectively. If the offspring produced under this type of reproductive pattern are as competitive as those from lifelong monogamous parents, this mating system persists.

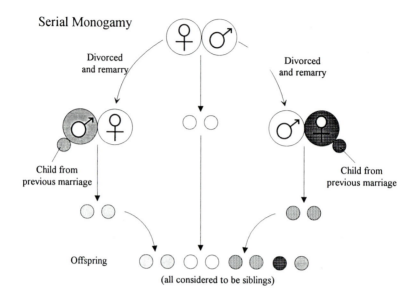

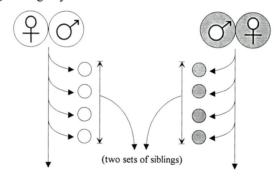

FIGURE 12.2.   Comparison of serial and lifelong monogamy.

B.   PREMARITAL RELATIONSHIP

Figure 12.3 shows the trend of the average age of marriage from 1890 to 1990 reported by the U.S. Bureau of the Census.[4] The recent figure of about 25 is similar to that of a century ago. There was a dip to about age 20 in the 1950s after World War II. Baby boomers were born during this period. The mean age of marriage did not change drastically, mostly in the early twenties. The time from late puberty to marriage is the premarital period, during which mating selection occurs. According to a report by Greeley,[5] about 50% of men and women from age 18 to 24 have premarital sex. This figure includes those who have sexual intercourse with someone other than their prospective spouses.

Some premarital sexual partners have a stronger commitment. They view the premarital relationship as a prelude to marriage. This type of premarital sexual

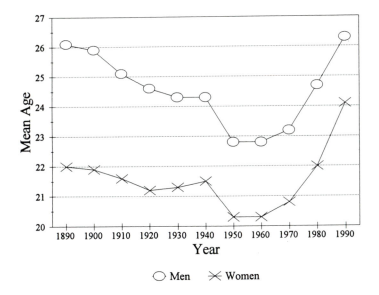

FIGURE 12.3. Mean age of first marriage in the U.S. (Data from U.S. Bureau of the Census, Current Population Reports, Series P-20, No. 461, U.S. Government Printing Office, Washington, D.C., 1992.)

bonding is a significant type of relationship called cohabitation. It is essentially similar to marital agreement, and the characteristics of the relationship are comparable to a formal marriage. It is an alternative to marriage without all traditional social burdens of a formal marriage, though some have created some types of ceremonies (e.g., move-in parties). Today, this lifestyle has been shown to increase from 10% of older couples over age 65 to 40% of younger couples from age 18 to 24. However, cohabitation does not reduce the divorce rate in the subsequent marriage.[5] It can be considered part of the marriage.

Since cohabitation is usually nonreproductive, it cannot be characterized as a monogamous or polygamous relationship. It can be described as promiscuous or nonpromiscuous. There are couples who like lifelong nonpromiscuous cohabitation or treat cohabitation as a prelude to marriage. These couples may eventually be lifelong monogamous. Some may view cohabitation as a selection process for a stable mating partner. If the intention to find a stable mate is genuine but the relationship fails later, the serial cohabitation resembles serially monogamous relationships. If the cohabitation is brief and unintentional, the relationship is causal and the individuals are promiscuous.

Although we should not ignore some long-term relationship starting from teenage romance, teenage sexuality is usually considered as causal. Another important aspect is also the age and financial independence. In Sweden, despite the high incidence of sexual intercourse in this age group, the teenage pregnancy rate is low. The phenomenon is reversed in the U.S.; the incidence of teenage pregnancy is high despite the lower incidence of sexual intercourse among teenagers. Good education about sex and contraception is crucial. American teenagers may be exposed to contradictory messages about sex from the media including news, movies, music, stories, talks, etc. On one hand, sex is romance, love, commitment, affection, enjoyment, and proof of adulthood. The worst message is that having sexual experience is an evidence of attractiveness. On the other hand, adults are visibly casual about sex. Many parents are divorced or separated but still involved in sexual relationships. One piece of information is missing. How can they prevent pregnancy? Wearing a condom before sex is rarely a part of a romantic scene, except in comedies.

Another message is "Good girls should say no," but it usually happens to say "Oh! No! I did it...that's bad." On the other hand, they experience a strong peer pressure to engage in sex as evidence of attractiveness and adulthood. If this is the pattern of teenager sexuality, it is illogical to ask them to change their behavior to solve the pregnancy problem. It may be an easy task for adults to say no or yes. During puberty, it may be a very biological need and curiosity about sex. Their developing cognitive power to control may fail, leading to an occasional inability to say "no" with a real "no" in action. After puberty, most would learn to exercise their cognitive power, but only to find out that they misbehaved while young. Unfortunately, they have already created the teenage pregnancy problem. Therefore, the pregnancy problem must be solved first before teaching them how to develop the cognitive control of their sexual behavior.

C. MODELS OF MARRIAGE

In 1963, Cuber and Harroff suggested five distinct types of relationships in over 400 Americans studied.[6] They are total, vital, conflict habituated, passive congenial, and devitalized. Since these classifications were based on successful marriages at the time of the study, the marital style might not correlate with their stability. Because of the differences in personalities, the couple had to adapt to each other to create a successful marriage. The concept of these marital models, with some modifications, is still widely accepted by contemporary experts in the field.[7]

The ultimate biological purpose of marriage is to achieve sexual reproduction and raise offspring. According to the traditional concept, marriage is also a heterosexual relationship. At present, marriage refers to a legalized relationship between a man and a woman. A homosexual relationship is considered as an alternative lifestyle since the sexual interaction is homogametic. Homogametic sexual interaction in humans is nonreproductive. Figure 12.4 is an overview of all the different lifestyles in humans, including homosexual and polygamous relationships. Heterosexual marriage is the major reproductive force, including serially monogamous individuals. Polygamous, mostly polygynous, individuals in developing countries also contribute significantly to population growth. According to the U.S. Bureau of the Census,[4] about 10% of the population age 18 or less was born to parents who never married.

The five marital models can be extended to characterize cohabiting couples or other types of sexual relationships. With recent data, all marriages fall into three categories (see Figure 12.4): intrinsic, utilitarian, and open.[7]

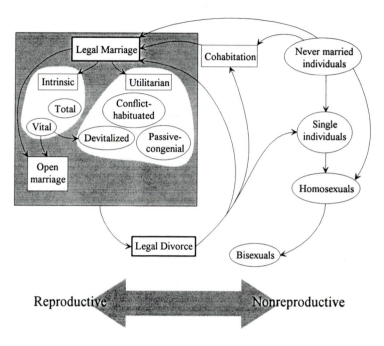

FIGURE 12.4. An overview of human reproduction and sexual lifestyles.

1. Intrinsic — The involvement between the two partners is intrinsic. Their primary concern in life is each other with deep feelings. Sexual activity is important in these couples.

   - Total — "Total" refers to the mutual and voluntary requirement of constant togetherness. Since the couples share almost all activities, their personal growth is locked.
   - Vital — They are highly involved with each other but not restrictive. Unlike the total relationship, they also enjoy individual growth. They share and communicate with each other on the basis of interests.

   According to marital therapists, couples of the intrinsic type are rare among their patients. Perhaps these couples are less problematic or they do not seek therapy. However, no formal study on the stability of intrinsic marriages has been reported.

2. Utilitarian — This is also a successful type, but couples prefer to be not so involved with each other. They spend more time for themselves individually to achieve their important goals such as establishing careers and raising children. The style is more traditional with defined sex roles. They want their responsibilities to be socially good husbands and wives instead of intense involvement.

- Conflict habituated — The couples communicate through fighting, argument, and disagreement. They can tolerate this way of communication because the conflicts are eventually resolved. Although this is a successful type of marital style, it is the type where couples require frequent visits to therapists.
- Passive congenial — The couples have well-defined roles with the traditional responsibilities of a husband and wife. Although they know they have to love each other, they are never intensely involved and never have conflicts.
- Devitalized — It is a marital style that changes from the vital type in early marriage to the passive congenial. If both have agreed to the change, the transition will not disrupt the marriage.

Utilitarian marriage is the norm for Americans. The intense involvement in intrinsic marriages is time-demanding for those who are busy with careers, social events, and raising families. More Americans prefer a less involved but functional and comfortable relationship.

3. Open Marriage — This has evolved from vital marriages in which the couple has intense involvement with each other. They allow individuality to such an extent that extramarital sex is permissible. Fidelity for them is an unconditional commitment to each other without sexual exclusiveness. Mutual respect for the spouse's judgment and behavior is the key to this type of marriage. They do not place restrictions on each other's activities and discuss matters openly, including any extramarital affairs.

All these types of marriages are also applicable to cohabiting individuals. The success and happiness of the marriage do not depend on what model it is. There is also no guarantee of success if one belongs to a certain type, and it may not be possible for one to choose a model for practice. It is suggested that a mixed type may be more unstable, e.g., a traditional husband and an open wife, or that a change of type at a certain time may lead to marital discord.

D. SEXUAL ACTIVITY OF MARRIED INDIVIDUALS

Generally, the frequency of sexual activity decreases with the duration of the marriage. A marked decrease occurs after the first 2 years. As traditionally claimed, recent studies have shown that men predominantly initiate sexual activities (51% of the husbands studied and 12% of wives initiated). Couples having an equal incidence of sex initiation and refusal claimed to have a happier marriage. The frequency of sexual intercourse is also affected by a change in the mode of life, for example, the birth or death of a child. It is often associated with emotional changes such as loss of a job or occurrence of extramarital affairs. Although sexual activity plays an important role in marital happiness, the character of the partners and their compatibility are significant factors too (see Figure 12.5).

Data on the incidence of extramarital sex are variable, and the figures are usually underestimated. Generally, 40 to 50% husbands and 25 to 35% of wives admitted having at least one episode of extramarital intercourse. When sexual

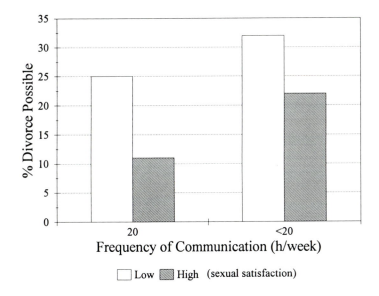

FIGURE 12.5. The role of verbal communication and sexual satisfaction in marital stability. (Data from Greeley, A.M., *Faithful Attraction,* Tom Doherty Associates, New York, 1991.)

intercourse occurs outside the marriage, the individual is considered to have committed adultery. Previously, adultery had been classified as a crime in the law of many cultures. Despite the incompatibility of the polygamous nature of humans, prohibiting adultery is the best guarantee for genetic purity of the offspring in a monogamous marriage.

The second reason is the stability of the pair bonding. Occurrences of adultery are often associated with marital discords. The cause and effect are difficult to separate. If adultery is the cause of instability, the major issue is the infidelity that causes marital problems instead of the sexual act itself. In one study, 50% of the husbands studied admitted extramarital sex; 20% of them told their wives after the incidence and 8% of them actually told their wives before the incidence.

If infidelity is the issue, marital stability may also be affected even if the extramarital affair occurs without sexual intercourse. The statistics are usually based on the occurrence of the sex act. Any degree of intimacy between the spouse and the extramarital partner can pose a problem when they fail to communicate openly before or shortly after the incidence. A happy marriage with open communication is resistant to problems caused by extramarital affairs that, perhaps, may never have a chance to occur.

III. DIVORCE

Divorce is a formal procedure to end a legal marriage. It does change the legal status of an individual who is then classified as "divorced" instead of "single." Previously, proof of adultery was often necessary for the court to grant a divorce.

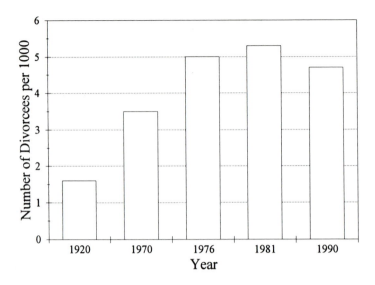

FIGURE 12.6. Divorce rates from 1920 to 1990 in the U.S. (Data from Lasswell, M. and Lasswell, T., *Marriage and the Family,* 3rd ed., Wadsworth Publishing Co., Belmont, CA, 1991 and Current Population Reports, Series P-20, No. 461, U.S. Government Printing Office, Washington, D.C., 1992.)

With more permissive divorce laws, divorce has become a popular solution to unresolvable marital problems. Thus, the incidence of divorce has increased in the past three decades.

A. INCIDENCE

In the U.S., the divorce rate is around 5.0 to 5.5 per 1000, with a steady increase from 1920 to 1981 (see Figure 12.6). After 1982, there was a decrease in the number of divorces because of an increase in cohabiting couples. These data are misleading for two major reasons. First, individuals at all ages are included. An increase in the number of children under 15 will lower the divorce rate. Second, there is no account of the number of marriages for an individual; the probability of having a divorce is different in subsequent marriages of an individual. For example, the divorce rate may be higher in second or subsequent marriages in comparison to the first.

Therefore, the divorce ratio is created by the U.S. Bureau of the Census. It is defined as the number of currently divorced persons per 1000 currently married persons living together. The courts in the U.S. dissolve over 3000 marriages daily. Nearly half the marriages today will end in divorce. This is expected to be a plateau, and the rate may fluctuate or even decline if more couples prefer cohabitation and late marriages.

B. FACTORS AFFECTING THE DIVORCE RATE

There is no single cause of divorce, and there are specific reasons in different cases. Studies in this area are often based on random samples taken at some selected locations during a certain period. Several important factors have to be considered: randomness, sample size, and systematic biasedness in responses to the survey questionnaire. In contrast to journalism, the aim of research studies is to make generalizations based on the norm. An interesting story of a special case presented on television may almost be impossible to occur, though it may provide a role model for an immature audience to follow. Similar nonrandomness can sometimes be found in survey reports.

Even for research studies with proper statistical analyses, sampling errors and response biasedness are inevitable. Therefore, a comparative account of different studies is crucial. The following is a list of conclusions from different studies.

1. Age — Teenage couples have twice the probability of being divorced.
2. Education — College-educated couples have lower divorce rates, but they usually marry late. Amazingly, women with 17 or more years of education (i.e., graduate students) have a slightly higher divorce rate than those who have only 4 years of college.
3. Religion — Exogamous Catholics have a higher divorce rate (24.3%) than endogamous Catholics (6.1%). Similar findings have been reported in other religious groups.
4. Population — In the U.S., there is a variation of divorce rates among different regions and states. The divorce rate is generally higher in urban than rural areas. In descending order, the divorce rate decreases from western, south, north central, and northeast states. There is a multitude of factors involved. The role of geographical factors such as weather is highly speculative. It may be related more to education, religion, and tradition. Couples frequently relocating and those in a rapidly developing environment have more labile marriages.
5. Intergenerational influence — In one study, the chance of couples divorcing is correlated with whether their parents are divorced or not. If neither parents are divorced, the divorce rate is 15%. If either set of parents is divorced, the divorce rate is increased to 24%. If both sets of parents are divorced, the divorce rate is as high as 38%.[7]

C. CAUSES OF MARITAL PROBLEMS

As mentioned in the preceding section, the reasons for divorce are specific. Generalizations are made based on the norm. No two marital pairs are exactly alike, and some couples can never learn to become the norm. Since specific causes have to be identified in different cases, professional help is often recommended.

1. Compatibility — This is related more to the personality that contributes to which type of marriage style. Usually, mixed marriage models are problematic. A marriage with marked differences in philosophies about important aspects (e.g., sexuality, child education, religion) has consistently less satisfaction and marital happiness. Even though personality compatibility is important, sexual satisfaction is also a crucial factor. Sexual problems are often linked to daily conflicts as an expression of disagreement.

2. Extramarital affairs — This is a cause and effect problem. A serious extramarital affair often emerges when the marriage becomes problematic. The extramarital partner acts as an outlet for one of them and as a signal of the problem. A healthy, happy couple is usually not vulnerable to extramarital affairs. When it is the cause of marital problems, the reason is not the affair itself, but it is the infidelity and betrayal.

3. Domestic violence — This is a serious problem. According to statistics in 1977, about 6 million women are victims of domestic abuse annually. In studies on couples living together, 3.5 million wives and 0.28 million husbands experience severe beatings by their spouse. The figures are expected to increase.

   Child abuse is serious, too. There are almost 2 million reported cases each year; 8% were kicked, bitten, or punched, while 3% were threatened with a gun or knife! It is well established that children from these problematic families will usually become involved in unhappy marriages of a similar kind. Couples are encouraged to seek professional help when repetitive domestic violence occurs. Although this is one of the factors leading to divorce, it is suspected that many of these problematic marriages are continuing.

IV. ALTERNATIVE SEXUALITY

Although most American couples are heterosexual and about 50% can maintain true lifelong monogamous relationships, there is a significant number of individuals who have other sexual preferences. In contrast to views several decades ago, some sexual relationships previously prohibited are now considered part of human sexuality. If the sexual conduct does not interfere with others, sexual preferences other than heterosexual monogamy are classified as alternative sexuality. It should be noted that sexual activities other than heterosexual interactions are nonreproductive (see Figure 12.4).

A.   SINGLE LIFESTYLE

According to the U.S. Bureau of the Census,[4] the number of never-married adults age 18 or above rose from 21 million (16.2%) in 1970 to 41 million (22.6%) in 1991. The number of currently divorced persons tripled from 4.3 million (3.2%) in 1970 to 15.8 million (8.6%) in 1991. Considering the increase in the total adult population from 133 to 184 million during these two decades, there is a noticeable increase in the number of people who voluntarily prefer to be single. Widowed persons represent a consistent 7 to 9% of the total adult population. Therefore, about 30% are currently unmarried (see Figure 12.7).

Another interesting comparison is the men and women age 20 to 24. In 1991, the percentage of never-married men (80%) was higher than women (64%), and the total percentage rose during the past two decades (55 and 36% in 1970, respectively; see Figure 12.8). This indicates that men prefer to marry later, and more individuals of both sexes prefer late marriage nowadays. The obvious reason is the career requiring a longer education time in a complex and advanced society.

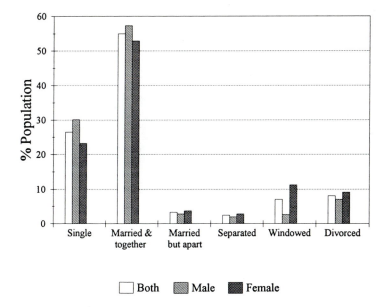

FIGURE 12.7. Marital status of Americans age 18 or above. Note that most married couples are living together; less than 5% of them are apart (e.g., for job-related reasons). (Data from U.S. Bureau of the Census, Current Population Reports, Series P-20, No. 461, U.S. Government Printing Office, Washington, D.C., 1992.)

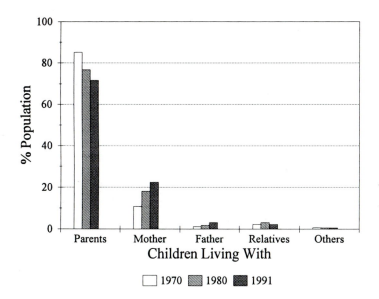

FIGURE 12.8. Percentage of never-married young Americans in two age groups. (Data from U.S. Bureau of the Census, Current Population Reports, Series P-20, No. 461, U.S. Government Printing Office, Washington, D.C., 1992.)

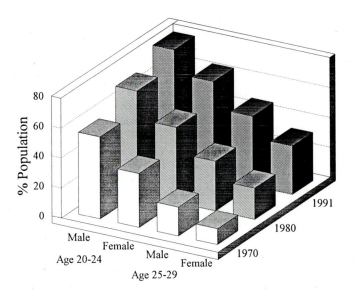

FIGURE 12.9. Living arrangement of American children under age 18. (Data from U.S. Bureau of the Census, Current Population Reports, Series P-20, No. 461, U.S. Government Printing Office, Washington, D.C., 1992.)

Intuitively, the burden of a family reduces the freedom of choice in a career. The preference of cohabitation instead of marriage should also be considered a major contribution to the increase in the number of never-married individuals.

Sexual activities in single individuals are presumably nonreproductive. Interestingly, data suggests an increasing trend of single parenthood (see Figure 12.9). Among children age 18 or less, the percentage of those living with one parent increased from 12% in 1970 to 26% in 1991. Out of the 26%, only 3.1% of the children stayed with the father only. Most children lived with their mothers. This trend is natural because the mother is the one giving birth to the child and having the necessary maternal behavior.

Among one-parent children, 37% are raised by divorced parents, while 33% are born to a parent who had never married. The later category is the typical case of single unmarried mothers as in the "Murphy Brown" television show. In other words, almost one in ten children age 18 or less in the U.S. are the result of premarital sex with one or both parents preferring to stay single. Women are the majority in this category. It may be difficult for a never-married man to have a child with a woman and raise the child alone.

Despite the visible single lifestyle with sexual activities, the attitude toward premarital sex remains nonpermissive. It is much more permissive toward unmarried sex of more matured individuals than teenagers. For divorced individuals at the age of 55 in some studies, most of them are sexually active and may have several partners in a year.[7] In addition, there is a double standard in the permissiveness. Premarital or nonmarital sex is more acceptable for men than for women.

Celibacy is a type of single lifestyle of those who prefer not to have sexual activity with another person. Priests and nuns of certain religions are examples; they take vows not to perform sexual activity with others and even not to masturbate or have sexual fantasies. Despite some successful celibates who really enjoy being asexual, there are others who violate their vows from time to time and engage in heterosexual or homosexual activities.

B. HOMOSEXUALITY AND BISEXUALITY

Individuals with an exclusive preference for the same sex are homosexual. According to Kinsey's reports and other studies,[7a] about 4% of the total population are exclusive homosexuals. About 30% have at least one homosexual experience, which is defined clearly by the evidence of sexual activity with the same sex. This later group is not exclusively homosexual and has varying degrees of heterosexuality. Therefore, there is a continuous spectrum of sexual preference from exclusive homosexuality to exclusive heterosexuality. Those individuals in the transition zone are bisexual. It should be noted that in a recent survey,[7b] only 1% of men admitted that they were gay. This shows the variable results in different studies, possibly caused by sampling population variance. Although exclusive heterosexuality is obviously not the majority, bisexuality is a significant part of human sexuality. Thus, homosexuality was deleted in the list of psychological disorders by the American Psychiatric Association in 1973.

There are some homosexual or bisexual individuals who prefer to seek psychiatric treatment. Using therapeutic methods such as psychoanalysis and aversion therapy, their sexual preference can be changed to heterosexual. Recent treatment methods are actually helping them to adapt to homosexual or bisexual lifestyles instead of altering their sexual orientation. Since sexual values are highly personal, the way to handle one's private sexual behavior is his or her own freedom of choice.

Despite the private nature of sexual preference, homosexuality has become a political issue in recent years. Some people like to classify themselves and others as "straight," "gay," or "lesbian." In contrast to racial classification based on skin color, no physical attribute is available for objective identification of sexual preferences. Besides, sexual preference is dynamic; one can never guarantee to be a lifelong exclusive homosexual or heterosexual. The promise can only be as reliable as the marital commitment to have lifelong monogamy.

If sexual preference is so personal and private, no law should exist to govern one's sexual preference. Everyone should have the freedom of choice to accept or reject another's sexual preference. Perhaps the only law necessary is one that prohibits acts interfering with others' activities directly. For example, an individual having a particular sexual preference should not repeatedly impose another to accept. If heterosexuality, bisexuality, and homosexuality are genetically determined, it would be futile to change each other's sexual orientation.

C. GROUP MARRIAGE AND SWINGING

As discussed earlier about polygamy, the Oneida community is an example of a large-scale group marriage. Smaller group marriages may occur whenever more than two persons are involved in a consensual sexual relationship. In group marriages, the interaction is beyond sexual; children are also involved with a more complicated family structure. It is a truly polygamous, polygynous, or polyandrous relationship.

Except in cases of marital experiments and polygamous cultures, group marriages often evolve from combined relationships of marital and extramarital partners. It may be an alternative to binuclear families after divorce. Initially, one or more extramarital partners may become more emotionally and sexually involved with one or both of the marital partners. If the marriage survives and the sexual interaction becomes consensual, the relationship stabilizes and family restructuring occurs.[8]

Consensual extramarital sex does not necessarily lead to polygamy if no child birth occurs. For bisexual individuals, sexual interactions with the same sex outside of marriage are also extramarital sex. If the incidence of extramarital sex in both sexes is high, these types of consensual extramarital sex are expected to occur in many of them. There is a spectrum of intensity from those occasional extramarital sexual encounters in vital marriages to the more permissive views in open marriages. Extreme cases are found in swinging couples engaging in mate swapping.

D. VARIANT SEXUAL BEHAVIORS

Previously, homosexuality was classified as a type of abnormal sexual behavior. Since a significant proportion of the human population is found homosexual or bisexual, homosexuality is now discussed as a separate topic of alternative sexuality. Therefore, we become more cautious to label a certain type of sexual behavior as "abnormal," and we do not even use the word "deviant." To describe sexual behaviors different from the norm, the word "variant" is used. It indicates that these sexual behaviors occur only in a small percentage of our population. Since bisexuality is currently not the norm, it can still be called a type of variant sexual behavior.

It is possible that humans may evolve into a bisexual species if bisexuality is not a behavior prohibiting sexual reproduction. Based on the principle that sexual activities involving consenting individuals are lawful, bisexuality is not prohibited. Since heterosexual activities occur in bisexuals, they are reproductive and continue to pass their genes to the next generation. Similarly, the variant sexual behaviors described in Sections IV.D.1 to IV.D.5 may be considered lawful if the activities do not interfere with reluctant individuals. If the action is unlawful, we may call it "abnormal." With the varying permissiveness of the legal system in different societies, the distinction line between variant and abnormal sexual behaviors is vague.

1. Transsexualism

True transsexuals are individuals who suffer from the feeling that their gender should be opposite to their biological sex. This condition occurs in both men and women, but it is rare. The cause is uncertain. In these individuals, the sexual differentiation of the brain may not correlate with the development of body sex despite the committed genetic sex. It should be mentioned that many transsexuals express their gender confusion since early childhood. The genetic program in these individuals creates a discrepancy between body sex and brain sex (see also Chapter 1).

Sexual preference of transsexuals is different from homosexuals. Although transsexuals and homosexuals are both attracted to the same sex, transsexuals consider the attraction heterosexual. For example, a transsexual man attracted to another man considers himself a woman and has a strong desire to become a woman physically. They even show hostility to homosexuals who are comfortable with their body sex and are not inclined to change their sex surgically.

2. Transvestism

Transvestic individuals prefer to wear clothing of the opposite sex to gain sexual excitement. Transsexuals are sometimes called transvestites because they are fond of cross-dressing. Interestingly, some homosexuals also cross-dress, though the action is not necessarily sexually stimulating and they do not refer to themselves as transvestites. They are merely female impersonators and act as "drag queens" for fun. This also occurs in lesbians, but it is not as common as in gay men.

True transvestites should be distinguished from transsexuals and homosexuals because they are primarily heterosexual in preference. Very often, transvestites gain sexual excitement through cross-dressing or fantasizing cross-dressing during heterosexual encounters. In contrast to transsexuals, they have no desire to have sex-change operations. Apparently, there is a severity continuum of transvestism from homosexuality to transsexualism. Extreme homosexuals are not transvestic at all, while extreme transvestites are transsexuals who want their body sex to be reversed completely.

3. Fetishism

"Fetish" refers to an idol or an object with magical power. Fetishism in sexual behavior is a condition in which an individual is sexually aroused by an object. In rare cases of complete fetishism, such an object can lead to orgasm without additional sexual acts. In most cases, fetishism is partial, and the fetish object only enhances sexual gratification during masturbation or sexual intercourse. Fetishism is generally considered male specific, though it may also occur in women as subtle forms of perversion, which may be unnoticed.[9]

The cause, as in other variant behaviors, is unknown. Psychiatric treatment may help. A recent case report has shown that drug treatment may be effective. For example, buspirone hydrochloride has been reported to be successful in the treatment of a patient with an atypical paraphilia and transvestic fetishism.[10] Another interesting case showing its association with multiple sclerosis and hypersexuality has been reported in a patient with frontal and temporal lesions demonstrated by magnetic resonance imaging (MRI).[11]

4. Sadism and Masochism

Sadism is the experience of sexual pleasure by inflicting pain on others, while masochism is sexual arousal by experiencing pain. Collectively, it is called sadomasochism or algolagnia. In Kinsey's report of 1953 and more recent reports in 1974,[7a] about 3% of females and 10% of males practiced sadomasochism. About 25% of both sexes have some form of mildly violent acts such as biting during sexual foreplay.[8]

Frequently, the male inflicts the pain and the female is the recipient. The usual examples are activities of being tied (bondage) or whipped. Some devices are available in "adult" stores. Since a certain degree of violence is involved in these sexual practices, the legality is sometimes controversial (see also Section V.A).

5. Others

There are other types of variant sexual behaviors classified as harmless if individuals involved consent fully. For example, erotic pleasure can be derived from various sources: klismaphilia (from enemas), coprophilia (from feces), coprophagia (from eating dirty substances), coprolalia (from using filthy language), mysophilia (from nonfecal dirt), and urophilia (from urine). These types of erotic pleasure are relatively rare.[8]

The more common types are sexual analism and urethralism observed in individuals who gain erotic pleasure from stimulating the anus or urethra, respectively. Nymphomania and satyriasis are extreme cases of promiscuity in females and males, respectively.

V. SEX AND CRIME

The attitude toward different kinds of sexual activities changes from time to time. The legality of some controversial sexual activities is being revised frequently. Oral sex between married couples, for instance, had long been classified as illegal. It is interesting to know that there were laws to prohibit private sex acts showing love and affection between husband and wife. Nowadays, in most civilized communities, whether the sex act is legal seems to rely on the consent of individuals involved in the sexual activity. The action can be illegal if one partner is involved without consent, even among married couples. Sometimes, the acts involving consenting individuals are illegal such as incest and sex with children. There are indeed many other controversial acts that may be unethical but not illegal, such as the marriage to a godparent or even an in-law. The law varies from one state to another, and the penalty differs.

A. VIOLENCE

Violence is the major factor in determining the legality of the sexual activities, especially without the consent of the partner. As discussed earlier in sadomasochism, there are sexual activities with a certain degree of violence between two consenting partners. It is extremely difficult to draw a distinct line between legal and illegal sex with violence. In most reported cases, the success of prosecution depends on whether the nonconsent of one partner can be established or not. Even in rape cases, the reasonable doubt in the possible consent of the victim can jeopardize the prosecution. The problem is attributed to the recognition that the act of inflicting pain during consensual sexual activity is legal. Minor injuries in a rape case therefore are not sufficient to establish the case if the victim might have been forced to consent by violence.

Women sexually assaulted by men is the most common sexual violence reported. Reports to the police are possibly underestimated and skewed. According to survey among college female students, over 15% had been sexually assaulted, and 53% of these victims were raped by acquaintances. Less than 1% of these cases among dates were reported to the police.[12] Sexual assaults by strangers are more likely to be reported. Another category is domestic sexual assault; nearly 10% of women had been forced to have sex by their husbands with violence. In many states, these domestic rape victims are not protected by laws even if they do not keep the incidence secret. Surprisingly, the legal definition of sexual assault in many states is still stated as "a sexual intercourse with a woman not his wife." It is an obvious marital exemption. There are also influences by tradition and religion that wives should not refuse their husbands' sexual advances even when the action becomes violent.

Sexual assault also occurs in men by women, men by men in gay communities, and women by women among lesbians.[12] The sexual assault is not necessarily limited to penile-vaginal intercourse, but also oral and anal penetration. The word "assault" should be used in a broader sense than "rape." Sexual assault should also include unsuccessful attempts to penetrate or be penetrated. The assault can be a verbal threat, though it usually refers to violent physical attacks that can be assessed medically. Sexual assaults among lesbians, for example, may involve other parts of the body besides the vulva. These are indistinguishable from domestic violence involving all types of relationships. With this broad definition, victims of sexual assault can be infants, children, and seniors showing medically discernible signs of physical abuses.

In the U.S., there is no unified way to deal with sex crime and domestic violence, especially when freedom of sexual expression is advocated. As it is extremely difficult to determine what acts of sexual violence are legal or not, the mutual consent becomes the major issue. If the law prohibits one to inflict medically discernible physical injuries to another without documented consent, then it becomes the responsibility of the individuals involved to establish a legal consent before the action. Couples fond of sadomasochism may benefit from having a legal contract and routine medical examinations by their physicians who are informed about their sexual practices. In this way, it becomes possible to prosecute all those who willfully inflict physical injuries to anyone during any kind of sexual activities without documented consent if the victim wishes to take legal action.

Mental or verbal assaults associated with sexual activities are nonviolent and may be called sexual coercion. In a study on college students, nearly half the women said that they were forced to have unwanted sex with their partners because of arguments, threats, or powerful verbal abuses, though actual physical violence had not been used. Commonly, verbal assaults may be preludes to physical violence. Victims are encouraged to report these activities to physicians or others as early as possible.

B.   DRUGS AND ALCOHOL

Drug and alcohol abuses are often associated with sexual assaults. Obviously, sexual assaults associated with illegal drugs are clearly prohibited. Sexual assaults associated with alcohol intoxication are not considered a serious crime. If the individuals are intoxicated, the rapists are less responsible, while the victims are held more responsible.[13]

C.   DEVIANT OR UNUSUAL SEXUAL BEHAVIORS

There are other kinds of sexual behaviors that are often prohibited, though the degree of legality varies in different states. Voyeurism (or peeping-Tomism as commonly called) is a condition of a person who has an urge to view others' naked bodies, sex organs, or sex acts for sexual gratification. The person is called a voyeur (or peeping Tom). As a note of interest, the original "peeping Tom" was a Coventry tailor called Tom who was struck blind after peeping at Lady Godiva in a town called Mercia, now part of England. According to the legend occurring in the 11th century, Lady Godiva was trying to protest against her husband's proposed tax raise for his tenants. She got herself naked and rode through the town. Everybody tried not to look at her except Tom.

Peeping can sometimes be classified as a criminal act. Peepers may be sexually aroused because of the forbiddance; they usually have no interest to go where nudity is permitted (e.g., nude beaches).

"Inappropriate" nudity in public, as Lady Godiva did, is illegal in most areas of the U.S. At some public beaches in the U.S., nudity is allowed, though nearby residents may sometimes complain if nudists step beyond the area. Interestingly, some are willing to pay to view nudity, while others complain about seeing nudists. Why do some people like to be nude in public? Why do some people want to prohibit others from being nude in public? As in the legend of Lady Godiva, if you have a problem with nudity, just do not look at the nudist. For very young children, nudity is natural; they have not learned to associate nudity with sex. If almost all people in our society prefer wearing clothes in public, it is appropriate to educate our children that nudity is associated with sex and privacy. Being private may be the source of pleasure when one enjoys nudity and sex with loved ones. If nudity in public is employed as a means to express resentment often political in nature, as Lady Godiva did, then it becomes difficult to judge whether the act can be permitted as a form of expression.

When an individual performs nudity in public without an apparent reason, the act is usually considered socially "inappropriate," and the individual is called an exhibitionist. The definition varies greatly from nudists at nude beaches to pathological exhibitionists. Some may even label Playboy girls as exhibitionists, while others have no problem seeing naked people walking around in parties. It depends on the moral judgment of the observer. A more restricted definition is necessary for law enforcement or clinical management.

Therefore, an exhibitionist is defined as an individual exposing his or her genitalia in public to another person who does not agree with the act. Although about 86% of reported cases are premeditated, there are others instances where the offenders have no control over their acts. So it is vague to classify exhibitionists as pathological or not; the only comment is that they have unusual sexual behavior. Nearly all exhibitionists are males who expose themselves to female strangers. Most of the first offenders are less than 30 years old, and less than one third of them are married. Exhibitionists account for about 35% of all arrests of sex offenders.[8]

Finally, sex in public among consenting individuals is usually forbidden since the audience usually does not give consent to the observation of sexual interaction. This is also very dependent on the preference of the observers. The general rule seems to be that the sexual act should be terminated if there are others complaining about it. Part of the unique human tradition contributing to the joy of intimacy is galvanized, through our own choice, by the privacy of the sex act.

VI. SEXUALLY TRANSMITTED DISEASES

Sexually transmitted diseases (STDs) are mostly transferred from one person to another through body fluid exchange during sexual contact. The spread of STDs is attributed to those having multiple sexual partners or sexually active travelers.[14] STDs include traditional venereal diseases such as gonorrhea, chlamydial urethritis, syphilis, chancroid, and herpes simplex infection, as well as recent ones such as hepatitis B, hepatitis C, and HIV-1. It should be noted that intimate contact is likely to increase the chance of getting infectious diseases that are not classified as STDs.

In the U.S., there are about 12 million STD cases reported annually, including mostly chlamydia (33%) and gonorrhea (12%), human papillomavirus (8%), genital herpes (4%), syphilis (1%), and over 45,000 cases of AIDS.[15] There are many that are difficult to diagnose and asymptomatic. There may be even a greater number of unreported cases.

A. BACTERIA

In a healthy asymptomatic woman, there is a dynamically changing ecosystem of vaginal microflora of anaerobic and aerobic bacteria, mostly lactobacilli that can maintain their dominance through the secretion of metabolites.[16] Such a condition can be destroyed because of contracting infections through sexual contact. Bacterial pathogens account for a significant portion of the current STD epidemic in the U.S. Gonorrhea, syphilis, and chancroid are especially rife in the nation's poverty pockets. Chlamydial infection, the most common bacterial STD, is prevalent at all socioeconomic levels.[17]

In the past decade, there has been a 34% increase in the incidence of syphilis in the U.S. The actual number is about 30,000 new cases per year. At the same time, the incidence of congenital syphilis also increased, resulting in spontaneous abortions, stillbirths, and neonatal morbidity.[18] There is about 1 in every 10,000 pregnancies. In infants with congenital syphilis, the diagnosis is often obscured by the lack of signs of infection.[19] In France, there is also a rise in congenital syphilis, though it is usually more frequent in developing countries. The neonatal death rate is around 10% within 10 days even in cases with treatment of penicillin G at 50,000 U/kg/day.

Syphilis has a number of stages, including a latent one that may be overlooked. Primary syphilis is characterized by the presence of a painless ulcer known as a chancre.[19] Adequate penicillin treatment during the primary stage results in a very high cure rate. Secondary syphilis often shows constitutional symptoms and a maculopapular rash. There is also an asymptomatic latent stage that may last for years, during which time the patient may still give birth to a child with congenital syphilis. Symptomatic neurosyphilis occurs more often in men than women.[20]

Chancroid is a bacterial disease similar to syphilis, but unlike syphilis, the chancre is painful and unresponsive to penicillin treatment. The number of cases has been rising also in recent years.[21] Bacterial vaginosis is another clinical entity involving primarily lactobacilli which change from aerobic to a predominantly anaerobic flora. The patients in over half the cases are asymptomatic but not entirely benign.[22] The predominant organisms in the healthy vagina are replaced by a mixed flora including species like *Prevotella*, *Porphyromonas*, *Mobiluncus*, and *Peptostreptococcus*. These organisms except the *Mobiluncus* species are members of the endogenous vaginal flora.[23]

B.   VIRUSES

Viruses known to be spread by sexual contact in humans include herpes simplex viruses (HSV), human papillomaviruses (HPV), human immunodeficiency virus (HIV), hepatitis B virus, and cytomegalovirus.[24] Although HSV and HPV are considered epidemically serious, HIV is a retrovirus suspected to cause the most devastating STD, AIDS. By 1991, AIDS was a fatal disease ranked just behind accidents, heart disease, and cancer.[25] Over half a million AIDS cases were diagnosed by 1993 in the U.S. alone. By the year 2000, there will be a cumulative total of over 40 million HIV infections in men, women, and children worldwide.[26] Despite a great improvement in the understanding of the HIV virus, there is still no known method to combat it. Currently, medical care is mainly provided to cure opportunistic infections in AIDS as the immune system of the patient deteriorates. Zidovudine (AZT), once demonstrated to be a possible drug to cure AIDS, loses its antiretroviral effect around 12 to 18 months.

Retroviruses are single-stranded RNA viruses with three characteristic nucleotide sequences called *gag*, *pol*, and *env* (see Figure 12.10). After entering host cells, their RNA genome initiates cDNA synthesis catalyzed by reverse transcriptase. This single-stranded cDNA forms another DNA strand complimentary to itself and becomes double-stranded DNA. After integration with the host genome, this DNA is transcribed by the host machinery, and the viral genes are expressed. The first human tumor retrovirus was isolated in 1980 and was called the human T-cell leukemia virus type (HTLV-1). In addition to another type called HTLV-2, two types of HIV retroviruses (HIV-1 and HIV-2) also have been identified. All of them are transmitted sexually, maternal to fetal, or through prolonged exchange of body fluids or blood.[27]

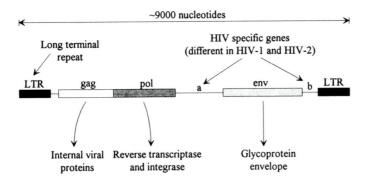

FIGURE 12.10. Genome of HIV viruses.

HTLV-1 is clearly associated with T-cell leukemia/lymphoma among populations in southwest Japan, Taiwan, sub-Saharan Africa, the Caribbean, southern U.S., Central and South America, Australia, Papua New Guinea, Solomon Islands, and western Asia. HTLV-2 is similar with a lower level of endemicity in populations of central Africa and Central and South America. Both are being spread epidemically among intravenous drug users in the U.S. Although HTLV is the cause of many cases of fatal tumor disease in humans, both HTLV-1 and HTLV-2, unlike HIV retroviruses, have no significant effect on the immune system.[27]

There are also two types of human immunodeficiency viruses: HIV-1 and HIV-2 with minor differences in nucleotide sequences (see Figure 12.10). HIV-1 was previously thought to be transmitted mostly through homosexual contact in males. Now heterosexual transmission has become the major mode of transmission worldwide.[28] Spreading among lesbians has also been reported, and there are other nonsexual forms of transmission through contacts with infected blood or even serum products. In comparison to HIV-1, HIV-2 is less infectious and causes less immunosuppression, spreading slowly mostly in west Africa.[27]

In addition to the *gag, pol,* and *env* segments common to all retroviruses as shown in Figure 12.10, the HIV-1 RNA genome specifies at least six additional proteins that regulate the virus life cycle. For example, *tat* and *rev* specify two regulatory proteins essential for replication. These proteins bind to specific sequences of newly synthesized virus RNA and profoundly affect virus protein expression. *Tat* and *rev* are prototypes of novel eukaryotic regulatory proteins. These two genes may play a central role in regulating the rate of virus replication. Three other viral genes, *vif, vpu,* and *vpr,* affect the assembly and replication capacity of newly made virus particles. These genes may play a critical role in the spread of the virus from tissue to tissue and from person to person.[29]

Interestingly, a recent report suggests the presence of nucleotide sequences related to HIV-1 in human, chimpanzee, and rhesus monkey DNAs from normal uninfected individuals.[30] In the same report, methods were presented for the isolation and characterization of two of these endogenous HIV-1-related sequences, EHS-1 and EHS-2, using 5′ and 3′ HIV-1-derived probes. Clone EHS-1 shows sequence similarity with the domain of the envelope cellular protease cleavage site of HIV-1, while EHS-2 is similar to the overlapping reading frame for Rev and gp41. Horwitz et al. suggested that most of the HIV-1-related sequences identified in primate DNA might share a common core of nucleic acid sequence found in both EHS-2 and *rev* and that some of these HIV-1-related sequences have additional larger regions of sequence similarity to HIV-1.[30]

HIV-1 infection is often associated with an increased incidence of Kaposi's sarcoma (KS), and the risk is further enhanced by oral/fecal contact.[31] Originally, KS was a very rare and obscure neoplasm, but now it has become an epidemic in immunosuppressed patients. Clinically, unlike classical KS, lesions are found anywhere on the skin or oral mucosa in AIDS patients with occasional visceral lesions. This special version of KS, however, is rarely the cause of death in AIDS patients and becomes a concurrent disease entity transmitted sexually.[32]

Genital infections by HSV are a common viral STD, which are often a nuisance though not lethal. There are also two types of viruses: HSV-1 and HSV-2. The latter type occurs more frequently as an STD. Unlike retroviruses, the genetic material of HSV is a double-stranded DNA instead of RNA. Characteristic clinical features include prodrome, vesicles, and erosions; oral or intravenous acyclovir has been used as treatment. For mild cases, personal hygiene, use of condoms, and notifying partners are recommended for general management.[33] In pregnant women with primary genital herpes, almost half of their infants become infected. If the mothers are only suffering from recurrences, the chance of perinatal transmission of HSV reduces to 5%.[34]

C.   YEAST AND OTHER GENITAL DISEASES

Vaginitis is a collective term for various common types of vaginal disorders associated with yeast or bacterial infections.[35] A simple evaluation in the doctor's office with a careful microscopic examination of the vaginal secretions for hyphae, budding yeast forms, and clue cells is usually sufficient. In a study on 2153 Malaysian women, common yeast species isolated include *Candida albicans, C. glabrata, C. famata,* and *C. parapsilosis. C. albicans* was isolated from 27% of pregnant women with vaginitis, 14% of pregnant women with no overt vaginitis, 15% of nonpregnant women with vaginitis, and 3% of nonpregnant women with no vaginitis.[36] Among 144 healthy American college students in a study, yeasts were isolated from 42 (29.2%). Only 4 (22%) of 18 women with positive fungal cultures had fungal elements visualized microscopically. Vulvovaginal itching and irritation were reported by 28 (67%) of 42 women whose cultures contained yeast and by 22 (22%) of 102 women whose cultures were not colonized by yeast.[37]

Amazingly, there was a reported case in which the patient acquired a vulvovaginal infection caused by *Saccharomyces cerevisiae*, a yeast used extensively in the baking and brewing industries. Her partner was also infected, and the source of the yeast was suspected to be from bread making. Both patients were cured by oral and topical treatment with nystatin.[38]

STD is the most common risk factor for pelvic inflammatory disease (PID) in which the upper female genital tract is involved. PID can be classified as gonococcal or nongonococcal if it is associated with anaerobic or aerobic organisms, respectively.[39] As discussed in Chapter 10, the use of an IUD is highly correlated with PID. It is possible that the use of foreign devices inside the uterus may increase the chance of transferring sexually acquired or endogenous lower genital tract microorganisms to the upper genital tract. Another concern is postoperative febrile morbidity after caesarean section because of endometritis.[40] The chance is high as a caesarean is often performed in an emergency without skillful assistants. In most cases, aerobic and anaerobic bacteria from the vagina are the causal organisms and antibiotic treatment is the usual therapy.

It appears that the majority of genital infections are described in women. Actually there are related STDs found in men. In addition to the well-known HIV and syphilis, there are some other lesions found in asymptomatic male partners of women with genital condyloma or intraepithelial neoplasia.[41] There are other kinds of bacterial or fungal infections found in the male genital tract. Current treatment protocols allow a rate of 95% cure by easily applicable outpatient treatment modalities even in HPV cases. Although recurrent bacterial and yeast infections are quite a common problem, the most devastating STDs are those associated with HIV. Abstinence from sex without prior medical examination of intended sexual partners should be the safest recommendation to prevent STD spread.

REFERENCES

1. **Rojansky, N., Brzezinski, A., and Schenker, J.G.,** Seasonality in human reproduction: an update, *Hum. Reprod.,* 7(6), 735, 1992.
2. **van den Berghe, P.L.,** *Human Family Systems: An Evolutionary View,* Elsevier/North Holland, New York, 1979.
3. *The Book of Mormon: the Doctrine and Convenants,* Church of Jesus Christ of Latter-Day Saints, Salt Lake City, 1981.
4. **U.S. Bureau of the Census,** Marital status and living arrangements, in Current Population Reports, Series P-20, No. 461, U.S. Government Printing Office, Washington, D.C., 1992.
5. **Greeley, A.M.,** *Faithful Attraction,* Tom Doherty Associates, New York, 1991.
6. **Cuber, J.F. and Harroff, P.,** The more total view: relationships among men and women of the upper middle class, *Marriage Fam. Living,* 25, 140, 1963.
7. **Lasswell, M. and Lasswell, T.,** *Marriage and the Family,* 3rd ed., Wadsworth Publishing Co., Belmont, CA, 1991.
7a. **Reinisch, J.M. and Beasley, R.,** The Kinsey Institute New Report on Sex. What you must know to be sexually literate. St. Martin's Press, New York, 1990.
7b. **Connell, C.,** Only 1% of men say they're gay, study says, *San Francisco Examiner,* April 15, 1993. A1.

8. **DeLora, J.S., Warren, C.A.B., and Ellison, C.R.,** *Understanding Sexual Interaction,* 2nd ed., Houghton Mifflin, Boston, 1981.

9. **Raphling, D.L.,** Fetishism in a woman, *J. Am. Psychoanal. Assoc.,* 37, 465, 1989.

10. **Fedoroff, J.P.,** Buspirone hydrochloride in the treatment of an atypical paraphilia, *Arch. Sex. Behav.,* 21, 401, 1992.

11. **Huws, R., Shubsachs, A.P., and Taylor, P.J.,** Hypersexuality, fetishism and multiple sclerosis, *Br. J. Psychiatry,* 158, 280, 1991.

12. **Muehlenhard, C.L., Goggins, M.F., Jones, J.M., and Satterfield, A.T.,** Sexual violence and coercion in close relationships, in *Sexuality and Close Relationships,* McKinney, K. and Sprecher, S., Eds., Lawrence Erlbaum Associates, Hillsdale, NJ, 1991.

13. **Richardson, D. and Campbell, J.L.,** The effect of alcohol on attribution of blame for rape, *Pers. Soc. Psychol. Bull.,* 8, 468, 1982.

14. **Parenti, D.M.,** Sexually transmitted diseases and travelers, *Med. Clin. North Am.,* 76, 1449, 1992.

15. **Kassler, W.J. and Cates, W., Jr.,** The epidemiology and prevention of sexually transmitted diseases, *Urol. Clin. North Am.,* 19, 1, 1992.

16. **Redondo-Lopez, V., Cook, R.L., and Sobel, J.D.,** Emerging role of lactobacilli in the control and maintenance of the vaginal bacterial microflora, *Rev. Infect. Dis.,* 12, 856, 1990.

17. **Handsfield, H.H.,** Recent developments in STDs: I. Bacterial diseases, *Hosp. Pract. (Office Edition),* 26, 47, 1991.

18. **Frecentese, D.F. and Schreiman, J.S.,** Congenital syphilis in Nebraska: a case report, *Nebr. Med. J.,* 76, 330, 1991.

19. **Kirchner, J.T.,** Syphilis — an STD on the increase, *Am. Fam. Physician,* 44, 843, 1991.

20. **Wooldridge, W.E.,** Syphilis. A new visit from an old enemy, *Postgrad. Med.,* 89, 193, 1991.

21. **Jordan, W.C.,** Chancroid: a review for the family practitioner, *J. Natl. Med. Assoc.,* 83, 724, 1991.

22. **Thomason, J.L., Gelbart, S.M., and Scaglione, N.J.,** Bacterial vaginosis: current review with indications for asymptomatic therapy, *Am. J. Obstet. Gynecol.,* 165, 1210, 1991.

23. **Spiegel, C.A.,** Bacterial vaginosis, *Clin. Microbiol. Rev.,* 4, 485, 1991.

24. **Rapp, F.,** Sexually transmitted viruses, *Yale J. Biol. Med.,* 62, 173, 1989.

25. **Schulhafer, E.P. and Verma, R.S.,** Acquired immunodeficiency syndrome: molecular biology and its therapeutic intervention (review), *In Vivo,* 3, 61, 1989.

26. **Fathalla, M.F.,** Reproductive health: a global overview, *Early Hum. Dev.,* 29, 35, 1992.

27. **Weber, T., Hunsmann, G., Stevens, W., and Fleming, A.F.,** Human retroviruses, *Baillieres Clin. Haematol.,* 5, 273, 1992.

28. **McCarthy, K.H., Studd, J.W., and Johnson, M.A.,** Heterosexual transmission of human immunodeficiency virus, *Br. J. Hosp. Med.,* 48, 404, 1992.

29. **Haseltine, W.A.,** Molecular biology of the human immunodeficiency virus type 1, *FASEB J.,* 5, 2349, 1991.

30. **Horwitz, M.S., Boyce-Jacino, M.T., and Faras, A.J.,** Novel human endogenous sequences related to human immunodeficiency virus type 1, *J. Virol.,* 66, 2170, 1992.

31. **Miles, S.A.,** Pathogenesis of human immunodeficiency virus-related Kaposi's sarcoma, *Curr. Opinion Oncol.,* 4, 875, 1992.

32. **Buchbinder, A. and Friedman-Kien, A.E.,** Clinical aspects of epidemic Kaposi's sarcoma, *Cancer Surv.,* 10, 39, 1991.

33. **Thin, R.N.,** Management of genital herpes simplex infection, *Int. J. STD & AIDS,* 2, 313, 1991.

34. **Arvin, A.M.,** Relationships between maternal immunity to herpes simplex virus and the risk of neonatal herpesvirus infection, *Rev. Infect. Dis.,* 13(Suppl.11), S953, 1991.

35. **Sparks, J.M.,** Vaginitis, *J. Reprod. Med.,* 36, 745, 1991.

36. **Ngeow, Y.F. and Soo-Hoo, T.S.,** Incidence and distribution of vaginal yeasts in Malaysian women, *Mycoses,* 32, 563, 1989.

37. **McCormack, W.M., Starko, K.M., and Zinner, S.H.,** Symptoms associated with vaginal colonization with yeast, *Am. J. Obstet. Gynecol.,* 158, 31, 1988.
38. **Wilson, J.D., Jones, B.M., and Kinghorn, G.R.,** Bread-making as a source of vaginal infection with *Saccharomyces cerevisiae.* Report of a case in a woman and apparent transmission to her partner, *Sex. Trans. Dis.,* 15, 35, 1988.
39. **Cunha, B.A.,** Treatment of pelvic inflammatory disease [see comments], *Clin. Pharm.,* 9, 275, 1990.
40. **Boyd, M.E.,** Cesarean section, *Can. J. Surg.,* 31, 10, 1988.
41. **Barrasso, R.,** HPV-related genital lesions in men, *IARC Sci. Publ.,* 119, 85, 1992.

INDEX